OXFORD CLINICAL NEPHROLOGY SERIES

Infections of the Kidney and Urinary Tract

Oxford Clinical Nephrology Series

Prevention of progressive chronic renal failure
Edited by A. Meguid El Nahas, Netar P. Mallick, and Sharon Anderson

Analgesic and NSAID-induced kidney disease
Edited by J. H. Stewart

Dialysis amyloid
Edited by Charles van Ypersele and Tilman B. Drüeke

Infections of the kidney and urinary tract
Edited by W. R. Cattell

Polycystic kidney disease
Edited by Michael L. Watson and Vicente E. Torres

To subscribe to this series, see subscription information and order form at the back of this book.

Infections of the Kidney and Urinary Tract

Edited by

W. R. CATTELL
Consultant Physician and Nephrologist

Oxford New York Tokyo
OXFORD UNIVERSITY PRESS
1996

Oxford University Press, Walton Street, Oxford OX2 6DR

Oxford New York
Athens Auckland Bangkok Bombay
Calcutta Cape Town Dar es Salaam Delhi
Florence Hong Kong Istanbul Karachi
Kuala Lumpur Madras Madrid Melbourne
Mexico City Nairobi Paris Singapore
Taipei Tokyo Toronto
and associated companies
Berlin Ibadan

Oxford is a trade mark of Oxford University Press

Published in the United States
by Oxford University Press Inc., New York

A catalogue record for this book is available from the British Library.

Library of Congress Cataloging in Publication Data
Infections of the kidney and urinary tract / edited by W. R. Cattell.
p. cm. — (Oxford clinical nephrology series)
Includes index.
ISBN 0–19–262441–5 (Hbk)
1. Urinary tract infections. I. Cattell, W. R. II. Series.
[DNLM: 1. Urianry Tract Infections. 2. Kidney Diseases. WJ 151 I43 1966]
RC901.8.I49 1996
616.1—dc20
DNLM/DLC *95–40050*
For Library of Congress *CIP*

ISBN 0 19 262441 5

Typeset by EXPO Holdings, Malaysia

Printed in Great Britain by
Bookcraft (Bath) Ltd, Midsomer Norton, Avon

PREFACE

The purpose of this book is to update and refresh all those concerned in the care of patients with urinary tract infection (UTI). It is deliberately multi-disciplinary and brings together the expertise and authority of those actively involved in the field. In planning the book it was clearly recognized that publicaiton of any new medical text must be justified by a genuine need. In the case of urinary tract infection the need is overwhelming, as many senior clinicians believe that UTI and its treatment is becoming a forgotten subject with serious consequences for patient care. The flood of research papers, symposia, and medical texts which followed the seminal work of Kass in the 1950s has, with some sterling exceptions, largely dried up in the last ten years, despite the fact that many important advances have been made by those few still actively engaged in research. Major textbooks on renal medicine or urology do contain excellent chapters on the subject but space restricts detailed review. More importantly, those texts are large and expensive and rarely reach the bookshelves of family physicians, microbiologists, consultants in infectious diseases, or clinical pharmacologists all of whom play their part in this multi-disciplinary subject. In consequence new knowledge and practice appear not to reach the non-specialist.

The first six chapters of the book provide 'core' information on diagnostic criteria, pathogenesis, laboratory and radiological investigations, natural history, and treatment. Subsequent chapters deal with specific patient groups where the usual pattern of UTI may be modified, such as children, diabetics, men, elderly people, and pregnant women. Chapters are also included on tuberculosis and fungal diseases. Each chapter reviews current knowledge and practice and, where possible, gives clear conclusions and guidelines. While primarily designed to be a practical update on our understanding and management of UTI, it is hoped that this book will also serve as a stimulus for both basic scientists and clinicians to elucidate further the many problems still remaining in the prevention and treatment of this common condition. The preparation of any multi-author book takes time while information on the subject moves on. Every effort has been made to keep as up to date as possible but inevitably some information will have come to light between the proofing and publication.

In preparing this book I have been immensely fortunate in recruiting a team of enthusiastic and committed experts to contribute chapters. I have also had the continuing support and critical advice of the Series Editor — Professor David Kerr. Without them there would be no book.

London W.R.C.
February 1996

CONTENTS

CONTRIBUTORS

G. D. Abbott Department of Paediatrics, Christchurch School of Medicine, Christchurch, New Zealand

Ross R. Bailey Department of Nephrology, Christchurch Hospital, Christchurch, New Zealand

M. J. Bendall Consultant Physician, Department of Health Care of the Elderly, Queen's Medical Centre, Nottingham, UK

W. R. Cattell Consultant Physician and Nephrologist, Harley Street, London, UK

Susan A. Dilly Consultant Histopathologist, St. George's Hospital, London, UK

Paul L. Drury Medical Director, Auckland Diabetes Centre, Auckland, New Zealand

John B. Eastwood Consultant Physician/Senior Lecturer in Medicine, St. George's Hospital, London, UK

Kenneth F. Fairley Epworth Hospital, Richmond, Victoria, Australia.

John M. Grange National Heart and Lung Institute, London, UK

David Greenwood Department of Microbiology, Queens Medical Centre, Nottingham, UK

R. J. Hay St John's Institute of Dermatology, Guys Hospital, London, UK

Priscilla Kincaid-Smith Department of Pathology, The University of Melbourne, Parkville, Victoria, Australia

Alasdair D. R. Mackie Senior Registrar, Department of Endocrinology, Addenbrooke's Hospital, Cambridge, UK

A. B. MacLean Department of Obstetrics and Gynaecology, The Royal Free Hospital, London, UK

L. E. Nicolle Departments of Internal Medicine and Medical Microbiology, University of Manitoba, Winnipeg, Canada

David J. Riden Chief Resident, Department of Urology, Northwestern University Medical School, Chicago, Illinois, USA

Anthony J. Schaeffer Herman L. Kretschmer Professor and Chairman, Northwestern University Medical School, Chicago, Illinois, USA

Richard Slack Department of Microbiology, Queens Medical Centre, Nottingham UK

Judith A. W. Webb Department of Diagnostic Radiology, St Bartholomew's Hospital, London, UK

Hugh Whitfield Consultant Urologist, Harley Street, London, UK

Martin J. Wiselka Department of Infectious Diseases, Groby Road Hospital, Leicester, UK

Dose-schedules are being continually revised and new side-effects recognized. Oxford University Press makes no representation, expressed or implied, that the drug dosages in this book are correct. For these reasons the reader is strongly urged to consult the drug company's printed instructions before administering any of the drugs recommended in this book.

1
Urinary tract infection: definitions and classifications

W. R. Cattell

Introduction

Infection of the urinary tract is one of the most common and most extensively studied infections encountered in clinical practice. The need for a separate chapter on definitions and classifications may thus seem unnecessary. It is, however, an area where in the past and even to date significant confusion has existed in agreeing the criteria for diagnosis, the natural history of the disease, and the criteria for 'cure' of infection. In part, this is due to changing criteria and concepts which may yet continue to change. For these reasons it is felt desirable at the outset to re-examine current definitions and classifications and to seek a common terminology for application throughout this monograph.

Urinary tract infection describes a condition in which there are microorganisms established and multiplying within the urinary tract whether within the bladder, prostate, collecting systems, or kidney. It is most often due to bacteria but may also involve fungal infection and, more rarely, viral infection (the last is not dealt with in this monograph). Schistosomiasis may also affect the urinary tract but again is not included.

In general, urinary tract infection (UTI) is characterized by the presence of bacteria in bladder urine. Exceptions include chronic bacterial prostatitis, infected renal cysts, or perinephric abscess.

Bacteriuria literally means the 'demonstration of bacteria in a voided urine sample'. It may be the result of contamination of the sample during voiding or be due to true bladder bacteriuria where microorganisms are established within the bladder. Prior to the introduction of quantitative urine culture by Kass (Kass and Finland 1956), the significance of bacteriuria was confused and ill understood.

Significant bacteriuria The introduction by Kass of quantitative culture of clean-catch midstream samples of urine (MSSU) to define the concentration of bacteria in urine (colony-forming units; CFU per ml) must be considered a major milestone in the road to understanding UTI. His demonstration that 100 000 (10^5) or more of the same organism per ml of urine indicated bladder bacteriuria in asymptomatic women led to this bacterial count being accepted as evidence of 'significant bacteriuria': the gold standard for defining UTI.

Time and further study have, however, clearly shown that a blanket application of this criterion for the diagnosis of UTI in all patients is flawed. This applies especially to symptomatic young women and men and has confused understanding of the natural history of UTI especially in former group. Thus, almost 30 years ago careful community studies showed that less than 50 per cent of symptomatic young women had 'significant bacteriuria' on the basis of a colony count of $\geqslant 10^5$ per ml and were labelled as having the acute urethral syndrome (Gallagher *et al.* 1965; Mond *et al.* 1965). This was despite the fact that these women closely resembled those with significant bacteriuria in terms of age, clinical presentation, marital status, and response to treatment. Careful follow-up showed that over 50 per cent of these women subsequently developed significant bacteriuria (O'Grady *et al.* 1970). A suspicion therefore arose that a cut-off point of $\geqslant 10^5$ CFU per ml was too high in symptomatic young women. Support for this comes from the work of Stamm and colleagues who found that at least one-third of women with acute coliform infections of the urinary tract had less than 10^5 bacteria per ml in MSSU (Stamm *et al.* 1980, 1981). They subsequently reported that a colony count of $\geqslant 10^2$ coliform organisms per ml of urine in symptomatic young women had a sensitivity of 95 per cent and specificity of 85 per cent for bladder bacteriuria (Stamm *et al.* 1982). They also suggested that the presence of pyuria ($\geqslant 8$ white blood cells per cubic mm of urine) in conjunction with a bacterial count of $\geqslant 10^2$ coliform organisms per ml increases the probability of true bladder bacteriuria (Stamm *et al.* 1980, 1982). Whether the same criteria can be applied where there is infection with other bacteria remains to be confirmed.

There are relatively few studies of what constitutes significant bacteriuria in men. Those of Lipsky and colleagues do, however, support the use of $\geqslant 10^3$ CFU per ml of urine as evidence of bladder bacteriuria (Lipsky 1989).

The acid test of bladder bacteriuria is culture of a urine sample obtained by suprapubic aspiration (SPA). Bladder urine is normally sterile. Thus, the presence of any bacteria (except skin contaminants) in such a sample indicates bladder bacteriuria. Culture of urine obtained by SPA is particularly valuable in symptomatic patients with equivocal results on culture of MSSU.

The criteria for diagnosing significant bacteriuria must therefore vary with the clinical situation. Those now proposed are set out in Table 1.1.

Pyuria The importance attached to the demonstration of pus cells in the urine has waxed and waned over the past 40 years. General acceptance of significant bacteriuria as defined by Kass as the gold standard for the diagnosis of UTI and recognition that pyuria was not regularly observed in the presence of bacteriuria, especially in asymptomatic individuals, led to the belief that microscopy of urine was not essential for the diagnosis of UTI. This is now recognized to be too sweeping a generalization. The work of Stamm and his colleagues has clearly shown the importance of detecting pyuria in symptomatic young women with low bacterial counts (Stamm *et al.* 1980). It may be reasonable to omit urine microscopy in screening programmes, such as are used for pregnant women, but it must remain an essential part of the examination of the urine in symptomatic

Table 1.1 Criteria for diagnosis of significant bacteriuria

Symptomatic women
$\geq 10^2$ coliform organisms/ml urine plus pyuria;
or
$\geq 10^5$ of any pathogenic organism/ml urine;
or
any growth of a pathogenic organism from urine obtained by suprapubic aspiration (SPA).
Symptomatic men
$\geq 10^3$ pathogenic organisms/ml urine.
Asymptomatic patients
$\geq 10^5$ pathogenic organisms/ml urine in two consecutive samples.

patients. Whether its place can be taken over by the use of chemical methods, such as the leucocyte esterase test, remains controversial.

Aside from its role in the diagnosis of UTI, the presence of pyuria is also an important indicator of other diseases of the urinary tract.

Definition of pyuria Critical to the diagnostic value of pyuria is general acceptance of criteria for its definition. Traditional methods of expressing white blood cell counts in urine as numbers per high power field is now generally accepted as being inaccurate (Stamm 1983). White blood cell or pus cell counts should be expressed per cubic mm of uncentrifuged urine. This is facilitated by the introduction of automated laboratory methods. A white blood cell count of $\geqslant 8$ per cubic mm is now widely accepted as indicative of pyuria (Stamm *et al.* 1980).

White cell excretion rates, although in theory more accurate, are cumbersome to perform and not without error. They are now rarely if ever used. Staining of white blood cells in the urine is also rarely required, except possibly in children when the presence of tubular cells may confuse counting (Chapter 7, p. 165).

Clinical terminology

Several attempts have been made to rationalize the clinical terminology in respect to UTI (Kaye 1972; MRC 1979; Kunin 1987). Most have been only partly successful. Traditional terminology is deep rooted and difficult to change.

Cystitis Although literally meaning 'inflammation of the bladder', this term is almost universally used to describe a clinical syndrome characterized by frequency and dysuria. Recommendations that the term 'cystitis' be replaced by 'the frequency and dysuria syndrome' has had very limited success. This probably does not matter very much, provided that it is clearly understood that the clinical syndrome may or may not be due to inflammation of the bladder.

There is, however, much to commend qualification of the term to 'bacterial cystitis' or 'abacterial cystitis' to distinguish clearly those with bacteriuria from those without. This can only be done retrospectively when the results of urine cultures and microscopy are available including, where appropriate, culture of urine samples obtained by SPA. The distinction is especially important in repeatedly or persistently symptomatic patients when, in the absence of bacteriuria, an alternative cause for symptoms must be sought (Stamm *et al.* 1980).

Urethral syndrome Included under the heading 'abacterial cystitis' are those patients often labelled as having the urethral syndrome. This singularly inappropriate diagnosis still enjoys widespread use. There is little evidence that a urethral disorder is present. Most are women who are intermittently bacteriuric sometimes with 'low count bacteriuria' (O'Grady *et al.* 1970; Stamm *et al.* 1980). This diagnosis should be abandoned.

Acute pyelonephritis Although localization studies have shown that distinguishing between upper and lower tract infection on clinical grounds can be inaccurate it is generally accepted that a clinical syndrome characterized by fever, loin pain, and tenderness; accompanied by significant bacteriuria indicates bacterial infection of the kidney and thus the need for therapy that achieves high tissue concentrations of antibacterial drugs. It now seems probable that definitive evidence of acute bacterial infection of the kidney is best provided by computed tomography (CT) scanning and the demonstration of 'lobar nephronia' (Lee *et al.* 1980) now to be called 'acute pyelonephritis' (Chapter 4, p. 82). CT Scanning is, however, rarely indicated except possibly in very ill high-risk patients such as diabetics.

The use of the term 'acute pyelitis', suggesting infection confined to the renal pelvis, has now been abandoned.

Chronic pyelonephritis; reflux nephropathy It is now generally accepted that this is a radiological diagnosis where there is evidence of focal scarring of the kidneys with associated calyceal abnormality indicating renal damage due to a combination of vesicoureteric reflux (VUR) and infection usually in infancy or early childhood (Chapter 7).

Asymptomatic or covert bacteriuria This refers to patients found to have significant bacteriuria following routine urine culture. It implies infection (or colonization) of the urinary tract in the absence of any declared symptoms by the patient. Careful history-taking may, however, reveal that in some, often elderly women, minor symptoms, such as nocturia or urgency have been accepted as 'normal', yet can be eliminated by eradication of bacteriuria. The relevance of asymptomatic bacteriuria as a cause of potential morbidity in various population groups remains controversial, but is more clearly defined in pregnant women (Chapter 9).

Upper versus lower tract infections These terms may be used as alternatives to the more commonly used 'cystitis' or 'pyelonephritis'. A clear distinction on clinical grounds is, however, inaccurate and the use of localization studies has become unfashionable. Interest in distinguishing upper from lower UTI stemmed mainly from the belief that infection involving the kidneys was more difficult to eradicate and could also indicate some complicating factor (see below). Treatment duration for clinical pyelonephritis has, however, been shortened and indeed a pragmatic approach for distinguishing lower from upper tract infection is the response to single-dose or short-course therapy (Chapter 6). With a caveat in respect to patients with 'complicated UTI' the need to distinguish accurately upper from lower tract infection has become less acute.

Response to treatment: cure, treatment failure, relapse and re-infection There has, in the past, been considerable confusion in the use of terminology relating to the response to antibacterial treatment in patients with UTI. This was particularly indiscriminate in the reporting of the results of new drug treatments and new antibacterial drug regimens. Confusion was largely due to the potential for recurrence of infection in a small population of women.

There are four possible outcomes to antibacterial therapy in patients shown to be bacteriuric: 'cure', treatment failure, relapse, or re-infection.

'Cure' and treatment failure Most often, and especially in the isolated 'one-off' episode of infection, treatment with an appropriate antibacterial agent leads to permanent resolution of symptoms and eradication of bacteriuria—the patient is '*cured*'. Occasionally, symptoms do not improve and bacteriuria is not eradicated. Treatment of that episode of infection has failed, most often due to the prescription of an antibacterial agent to which the organism is resistant. This may be called *primary treatment failure*.

Confusion in terminology develops when symptoms and bacteriuria are eliminated by treatment, and then for both to recur within days or weeks. There are then two possible reasons: relapse or re-infection.

Relapse This describes a situation in which symptoms and bacteriuria are eliminated by treatment but infection has not been eradicated from the urinary tract. Symptoms and bacteriuria usually recur within 10 to 14 days. Urine culture yields the same organism as was originally present, most accurately identified as the same bacterium on the basis of serotyping (for *Escherichia coli*). Less accurate but clinically convenient identification is usually based on comparison of its sensitivity to antibiotics. Relapse also indicates treatment failure. It most often occurs where there are complicating factors present such as stones, scarred or cystic kidneys, or bacterial prostatitis. All are conditions where penetration of the antibacterial drugs to the site of bacteria is reduced. *Re-infection* of the urinary tract with the same organisms within 10 to 14 days is theoretically possible (see below), but the presence of one of the factors mentioned above strongly supports relapse.

The importance of distinguishing relapse from re-infection is the need in the former to seek complicating factors making eradication of infection difficult. All patients require renal imaging if not previously carried out.

Re-infection is the most common cause for recurrence of UTI. Appropriate treatment eradicates the initial infection but UTI recurs within weeks or months with a different or occasionally the same organism. This is *not* failure in treatment of the initial infection but reflects the potential in this individual for re-invasion of the urinary tract whether due to impaired bladder defence mechanisms, persisting colonization of the periurethral area, or colonization by new bacteria following a change in flora during treatment.

In reporting the results of new drug treatments or new treatment regimens it is essential that the trial protocol is designed to identify primary treatment failure versus relapse or re-infection.

Complicated versus uncomplicated UTI For many years a distinction has been made between UTI in patients with anatomically and functionally normal urinary tracts and in whom there are no other associated conditions, such as diabetes, sickle-cell disease, or immunosuppression, compared to infection in those with such complicating factors (Fig. 1.1). The reasons for this were the belief that patients with uncomplicated UTI were easily treated and were unlikely to sustain permanent kidney damage or to develop a severe life-threatening situation due to septicaemia. Clinicians commonly reassure patients on these points on the basis of the clinical setting and renal imaging. This concept has been challenged in recent years with the demonstration that patients with acute pyelonephritis may in fact develop renal scarring (Meyrier *et al.* 1989; Soulen *et al.* 1989). Indeed, one of the authors contributing to this monograph deems it appropriate to include pyelonephritis in the chapter on complicated UTI (Chapter 8). Just how common and serious a problem this is remains to be clarified by careful documentation and follow-up of patients with pyelonephritis using more sophisticated renal imaging such as ultrasound, CT, or DMSA (dimercaptosuccinicacid) scanning. The initial

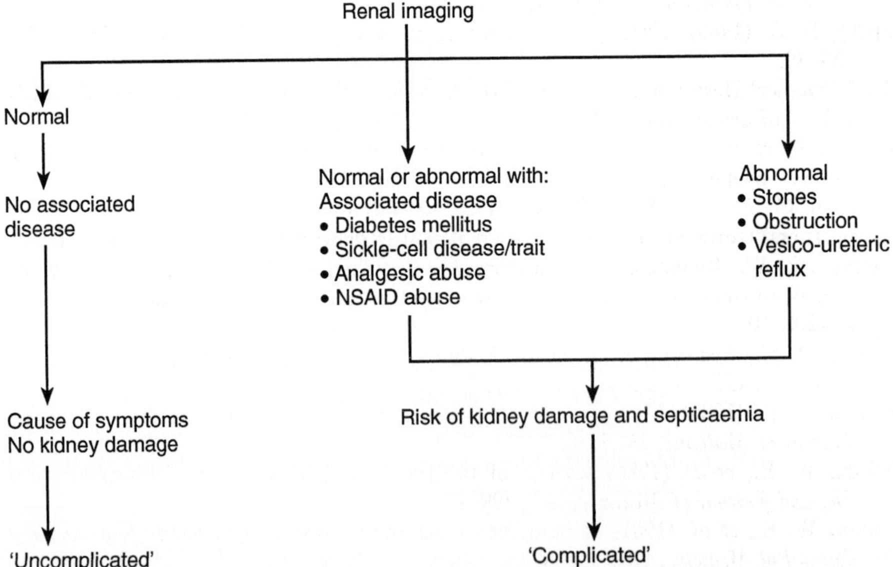

Fig. 1.1 Classification of uncomplicated and complicated urinary tract infection (UTI).

impression is that it may be more likely to develop in patients with diabetes or with VUR—both conditions already meriting a diagnosis of 'complicated UTI'. Suffice it to say that clinicians may feel it wise to be less confident that 'uncomplicated' acute pyelonephritis in adult life does not produce permanent renal scarring although the functional significance of this would seem to be small (Chapter 8).

Conclusion

A clear internationally agreed terminology in respect of the diagnosis, natural history and response to treatment of UTI is now possible. The use of this terminology is essential for a common understanding of current and future developments in this field.

References

Gallagher, D. I. A., Montgomerie, J. Z., and North, J. D. K. (1965). Acute infection of the urinary tract and the urethral syndrome in general practice *British Medical Journal*, **1**, 622–6.

Kaye, D. (1972). Important definitions and classifications of urinary tract infection. In *Urinary tract infection and its management*, (ed. D. Kaye), p. 1. Mosby, St. Louis.

Kass, E. H. and Finland, M. (1956). Asymptomatic infections of the urinary tract. *Transactions of the Association of American Physicians*, **69**, 56–64.

Kunin, C. M. (1987). An overview of urinary tract infections terminology. In D*etection, prevention and management of urinary tract infection*, (4th edn), p. 1 Lea & Febiger, Philadelphia.

Lee, J. K. T., McClennan, B. L., Melson, G. L., and Stanley, R. J. (1980). Acute focal bacterial nephritis: emphasis on gray scale sonography and computed tomography. *American Journal of Roentgenology*, **135**, 87–92.

Lipsky, B. A. (1989). Urinary tract infection in men. *Annals of Internal Medicine*, **110**, 135–50.

MRC (Medical Research Council) (1979). Bacteriuria Committee. Recommended terminology of urinary tract infection. *British Medical Journal*, **2**, 717–19.

Meyrier, A. *et al.* (1989). Frequency of development of early cortical scarring in acute primary pyelonephritis. *Kidney International*, **35**, 696–703.

Mond, N. C., Percival, A., Williams, J. D., and Brumfitt, W. (1965). Presentation, diagnosis and treatment of urinary tract infection in general practice. *Lancet*, **1**, 514–16.

O'Grady, F. W., Richards, B., McSherry, M. A., O'Farrell, S. M., and Cattell, W. R. (1970). Introital enterobacteria, urinary infection and the urethral syndrome. *Lancet*, **1**, 1208–10.

Soulen, M. C., Fishman, E. K., and Goldman, S. M. (1989). Sequelae of acute renal infections; CT evaluation. *Radiology*, **13**, 423–6.

Stamm, W. E. (1983). Measurement of pyuria and its relation to bacteriuria. *American Journal of Medicine*, **75**, 53–8.

Stamm, W. E., *et al.* (1980). Causes of the acute urethral syndrome in women. *New England Journal of Medicine*, **303**, 409–15.

Stamm, W. E., *et al.* (1981). Treatment of the acute urethral syndrome. *New England Journal of Medicine*, **304**, 956–8.

Stamm, W. E., *et al.* (1982). Diagnosis of coliform infections in acutely dysuric women. *New England Journal of Medicine*, **305**, 463–8.

2

Bacterial and host factors in the pathogenesis of urinary tract infections

Martin J. Wiselka

Introduction

Urinary tract infection (UTI) is an important cause of morbidity and mortality. Most infections are caused by enteric bacteria that colonize the lower urethra and ascend the urinary tract. The development of infection depends on the virulence of the infecting organism and the integrity of the host defence mechanisms. This chapter will discuss the nature of these bacterial and host factors and their role in the pathogenesis of disease.

Bacteriology of urinary tract infections

There are important differences in the spectrum of bacteria infecting previously healthy individuals compared to those with urinary tract abnormalities or other underlying disease (Table 2.1). *Escherichia coli* is responsible for approximately 85 per cent of community-acquired infections, with Proteus and Klebsiella spp. occurring infrequently (Bryan and Reynolds 1984). *Staphylococcus saprophyticus* is associated with over 20 per cent of episodes of bacteriuria in young women, but rarely causes severe symptoms (Wallmark *et al.* 1978). A far wider range of organisms are associated with UTI in patients who have structural abnormalities of the urinary tract or are immunosuppressed.

Routes of infection

The majority of bacteria responsible for UTI are bowel commensals that ascend the urinary tract (Cox *et al.* 1968; Grunberg 1969). Evidence for the importance of the ascending route of infection include long-term follow-up studies of women suffering from recurrent infections. These studies showed that colonization of the lower urethra with faecal organisms occurred shortly before the development of symptomatic UTI (Stamey *et al.* 1971). Healthy women have an increased risk of developing UTI compared to men, as they have a shorter urethra which may become contaminated more easily (Hinman 1966; Bran *et al.* 1972). Ascending infection is also associated with the presence of indwelling urinary catheters, vesicoureteric reflux, and urinary stasis resulting from prostatic hypertrophy, hydronephrosis, or stones.

Table 2.1 Microbiology of uncomplicated and complicated urinary tract infection

Organism	Community-acquired in previously healthy host	Hospital-acquired and/or impaired host defences
Gram-negative bacteria	*Escherichia coli* Klebsiella Proteus	*Escherichia coli* Klebsiella Proteus Pseudomonas Enterobacter Serratia Citrobacter Salmonella
Gram-positive bacteria	*Staphylococcus saprophyticus*	*Staphylococcus epidermidis* Enterococci Lactobacilli Group B streptococci
Mycobacteria		*Mycobacterium tuberculosis* Atypical mycobacteria
Mycoplasmas		Ureaplasma
Fungi		Candida Aspergillus Cryptococcus
Viruses		Cytomegalovirus Adenovirus

Haematogenous spread of infection is relatively less important in the urinary tract, but occasionally follows episodes of generalized septicaemia. A wide range of organisms are associated with blood-borne infection, including Salmonella spp., Enterococci, *Staph. aureus, Mycobacterium tuberculosis*, and Candida spp. These infections are most commonly seen in severely ill or immunocompromised patients. There is little evidence for the spread of organisms into the urinary tract via the lymphatic system.

Animal models of infection

Animal studies have played an important role in the investigation of bacterial virulence and the pathogenesis of urinary tract infection. Early difficulties were encountered in establishing a good animal model of ascending infection. This led to the realization that the species of animal was of crucial importance, as many bacterial virulence factors have a narrow species-specificity.

A mouse model of ascending infection was developed by Hagberg *et al.* (1983*a*). Bacteria are introduced into the bladder using a plastic catheter and virulent organisms ascend the ureters to cause renal infection. Pathological changes in the kidney correlate closely with bacterial localization of infection and histological features allow a distinction to be made between bacterial colonization, pyelitis, and pyelonephritis (Johnson *et al.* 1992). Although the mouse is a good model of ascending infection, the findings in animal experiments must be interpreted with caution as host factors are of great importance and results obtained from animal experiments may not be applicable to human disease.

A haematogenous model of infection has also been described in the mouse (Ivanyi *et al.* 1983). Bacteria injected intravenously are rapidly cleared by the reticuloendothelial system in healthy animals and infection will only become established in the kidneys if they have previously been damaged by trauma or ureteric ligation.

Pigs and primates have also been experimentally infected with uropathogenic organisms (Roberts *et al.* 1984). However, these models have only a limited role in the investigation of UTI and are likely to be used mainly for testing candidate drugs or vaccines prior to human trials.

Bacterial virulence factors

Virulence may be defined as the capacity of an organism to cause disease. Bacteria which cause life-threatening infections in previously healthy people are clearly more virulent than those which only infect patients with urinary tract abnormalities or those who are immunocompromised. Bacterial virulence has been most extensively investigated in *E. coli* and known and putative *E. coli* virulence factors are shown in Fig. 2.1.

Bacterial adhesins

Bacteria which successfully invade the urinary tract must have the ability to withstand the process of urinary flow. Bacterial adherence to urinary epithelial cells is therefore one of the most important factors in the pathogenesis of infection. Further potential advantages of close adherence include the transfer of nutrients from the host cell to the bacterium and effective targeting of toxins to adjacent tissues to facilitate bacterial colonization.

The importance of adhesion is demonstrated by the observation that the adherence of bacterial isolates to uroepithelial cells *in vitro* corresponds closely with their ability to cause clinical disease (Fig. 2.2.) *Escherichia coli* obtained from patients with symptomatic UTIs adhere more strongly than faecal isolates (Varian and Cooke 1980), or isolates from patients with asymptomatic bacteriuria (Svanborg-Edén *et al.* 1976). These findings are supported by animal studies of experimental pyelonephritis in the mouse and primate which have shown that ascending infection may be prevented by anti-adhesin antibodies or the administration of epithelial cell-surface analogues which inhibit the adhesin-receptor interaction (Hagberg *et al.* 1983; Robert *et al.* 1984; Svanborg-Edén *et al.* 1982)

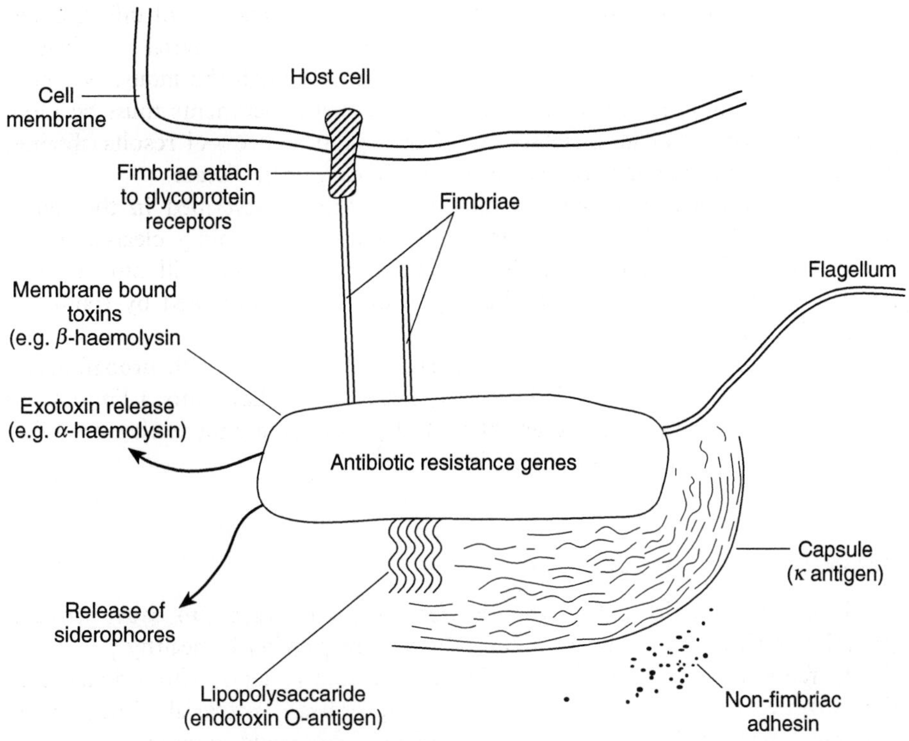

Fig. 2.1 Important virulence factors in uropathogenic *E. coli.*

Adherence of *E. coli* to uroepithelial cells correlates with the ability to agglutinate erythrocytes. Duguid *et al.* (1955) first demonstrated that bacterial haemagglutination was associated with the presence of filamentous projections on electron microscopy. These were termed fimbriae or pili and are approximately 10 nm in diameter. (Fig. 2.3) Fimbriae appear to be the most important mechanism mediating bacterial attachment to uroepithelial cells, as adherence is markedly reduced if cells are incubated with purified fimbriae or adhesin-specific antibody (Svanborg-Edén and de Man 1987).

Many distinct fimbrial adhesins have been identified in uropathogenic *E. coli.* Finer appendages known as fibrillae have also been described and some bacteria are surrounded by a diffuse layer of adhesin molecules, termed non-fimbrial or afimbrial adhesin. Adhesins bind to specific receptor ligands on the surface of uroepithelial cells and are classified into two major groups, type 1 or mannose-sensitive fimbriae, and mannose-resistant adhesins. Mannose-resistant adhesins are further classified on the basis of receptor specificity into those which adhere to P blood group antigens (P-fimbriae) and a diverse group of X-adhesins.

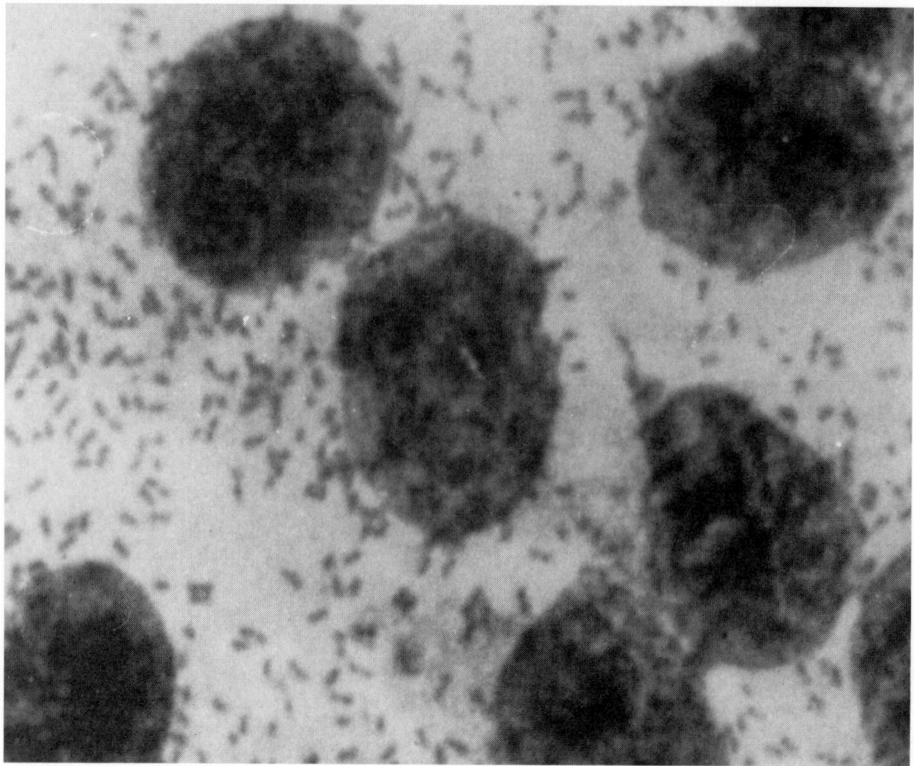

Fig. 2.2 Adherence of *E. coli* to cultured epithelial cells.

Type 1 fimbriae

Approximately 70 per cent of faecal and urinary isolates of *E. coli* possess type 1 fimbriae which bind to a mannose containing receptor (Abraham *et al.* 1988). Receptors incorporating D-mannose residues are widely expressed by mucosal cells in the lower urinary tract (Ofek *et al.* 1977; Fujita *et al.* 1989) and type 1 fimbriae are believed to play an important role in the colonization of the urethra and bladder (Schaeffer *et al.* 1987). Type 1 fimbriae may also protect bacteria against *in vitro* macrophage killing (Keith *et al.* 1990).

The molecular biology of type 1 fimbriae has been extensively investigated. Cloning of the type 1 fimbria revealed a cluster of genes (the *fim* cluster) responsible for fimbrial expression (Klemm *et al.* 1985). The *fim* cluster consists of eight genes (*fim* A–H) which code for the major and minor subunit proteins, transport functions, and regulation of adhesin expression. The bulk of the fimbria consists of repeated molecules of the major subunit protein (FimA), whereas the adhesin is located on a minor subunit (FimH). Electron microscopy using gold-conjugated anti-adhesin antibodies identified receptor binding sites at the tip and at long intervals on the lateral shaft of the fimbriae (Krogfelt *et al.* 1990). Regulation of gene expression and phase variation are important factors in the pathogenesis of infection and are controlled at the transcriptional level by the inversion of a 314 base pair segment of DNA (Eisenstein 1988).

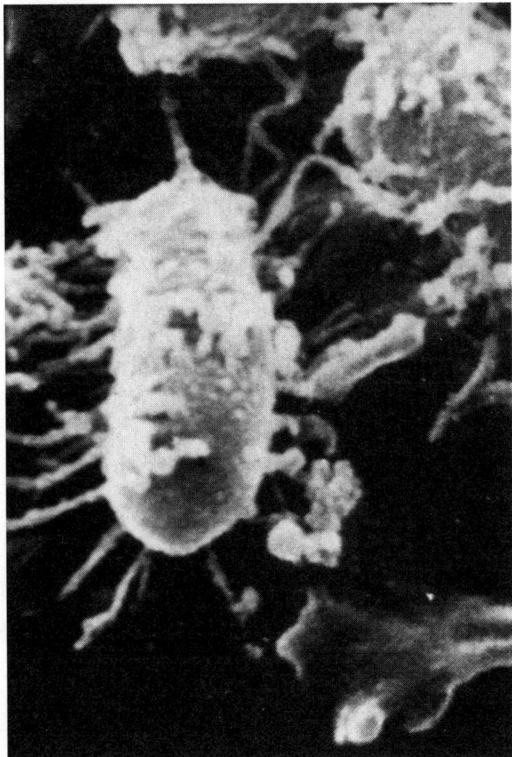

Fig. 2.3 Scanning electron microscopy of fimbriated *E. coli*.

P-fimbriae

These fimbriae bind to P blood group antigens that are widely expressed on erythrocytes and epithelial cells. The adhesin binds to a specific family of the glycosphingolipid, known as the globoseries glycolipid, and the actual receptor ligand has been identified as a digalactose complex Galα (1–4) Galβ (Kallenius *et al. 1981)*.

P-fimbriae are believed to be an important factor in the development of invasive infection, as bacteria expressing P-fimbriae are associated with pyelonephritis (Vaisanen *et al.* 1981), and a Gal-Gal pilus vaccine prevented renal infection in a mouse model of ascending pyelonephritis (O'Hanley *et al.* 1985*a*).

The P-fimbria has a complex heteropolymer structure consisting of a rigid helical stalk, approximately 10 nm in diameter, with a fine flexible fibrillum of 3 nm diameter extending from the distal tip. The *pap* gene cluster codes for P-fimbrial expression and has been extensively investigated in a series of elegant studies (Lindberg *et al.* 1987 Hultgren *et al.* 1991; Kuehn *et al.* 1992). The nucleotide sequence has been determined for the entire *pap* operon which comprises 11 separate genes. The functions of the individual genes were investigated by constructing a series of isogenic mutants and comparing the phenotypes associated with each mutant.

The *pap* genes code for separate structural, transport, and regulatory proteins. Fimbrial subunit components are transported by 'chaperone' proteins and assembled in a strictly regulated sequence. Six separate structural proteins are present in each P-fimbria. The bulk of the rigid fimbrial shaft consists of approximately 1000 repeated major subunit proteins (PapA) and is anchored to the bacteria by PapH protein. The distal fibrillar structure is composed mainly of repeated PapE subunits, but also contains the minor subunits papE and PapK. The actual adhesin which mediates Gal-Gal binding is a minor subunit known as papG which is located at the terminus of the fibrillin.

The molecular epidemiology of P-fimbriae has been investigated by colony hybridization of pathogenic *E. coli* isolates, using gene probes derived from fragments of the *pap* operon (Arthur *et al.* 1989*a*, Plos *et al.* 1990). These studies have shown that the majority of clinical isolates possess more than one copy of pap-related sequences. Fimbriae with related gene sequences include the F-adhesin, which is encoded by the *prs* (pap-related sequence) operon and binds to a Forssman antigen expressed by cells in the renal pelvis. Co-expression of pap-related adhesins was found to occur more frequently in pyelonephritic isolates than isolates from cystitis or faeces. The *pap* polymorphism is presumably caused by genetic recombination events. This process allows independent variability of major and minor subunit components and gives bacteria the potential for a high degree of antigenic variability and adhesin–receptor specificity.

X-adhesins

Other *E. coli* adhesins mediating mannose-resistant haemagglutination are termed X- adhesins. These include S-, F1c-, and G-fimbriae, and the non-fimbrial adhesins.

S (Moch *et al.* 1987) and F1C (Pere *et al.* 1987) fimbriae are closely related and bind to sialyl-galactoside residues which are expressed by cells in the kidney and upper urinary tract. S-fimbriae are strongly associated with *E. coli* strains causing neonatal bacteraemia and meningitis, but are also produced by some pyelonephritic isolates. G-fimbriae bind to *N*-acetylglucosamine residues. Their importance in UTI is unclear (Vaisanen-Rhen *et al.* 1983; Rhen *et al.* 1986).

Non-fimbrial adhesins

A variety of non-fimbrial adhesins have been described. These surround the bacteria like an adhesive protein capsule (Kroncke *et al.* 1990) and include the M-adhesin, adhesins which belong to the Dr-adhesin family, and a series of non-fimbrial adhesins (NFAs).

The M-adhesin appears to be unrelated to other adhesins described in *E. coli* and binds to the terminal amino acid sequence of the M blood group antigen located on glycophorin A (Rhen *et al.* 1986). The Dr family of adhesins bind to components of the Dr blood group antigen and include the Dr- or 075X-adhesin, the afimbrial adhesins AFAI and AFAIII, and the fimbrial adhesin F1845 (Nowicki *et al.* 1989, 1991). The pathological significance of Dr-adhesins is unclear, but they may have a role in colonization of the lower urinary tract as there is a high concentration of Dr-receptors in the bladder and Dr-adhesins were expressed by approximately 50 per cent of *E. coli* isolates from patients with cystitis, but fewer than 20 per cent of those with pyelonephritis (Johnson 1991).

A further series of non-fimbrial adhesins, denoted NFA1–4, have been described in uropathogenic isolates of *E. coli* (Goldhar *et al.* 1987; Grunberg *et al.* 1988; Hales *et al.* 1988; Hoschutzky *et al.* 1989). These adhesins are composed of single protein subunits which form high molecular weight aggregates. Immunoelectron microscopy of encapsulated bacteria expressing NFA4 revealed a composite structure surrounding the bacterium, with the capsule located proximally and the adhesin forming an outer coating over the capsular polysaccharide (Kroncke *et al.* 1990). It has been suggested that non-fimbrial adhesins might reduce bacterial antigenicity, but this has not been clearly demonstrated.

NFA1 and NFA2 share limited serological cross-reactivity and cross-inhibition of binding suggesting a common receptor component, although the nature of the receptor is not known. NFA-3 recognizes the N blood group antigen, NFA4 recognizes a blood group M-specific receptor, but is unrelated to the previously described M-adhesin. Isolates expressing NFA1–4 were all obtained from patients with UTI. The epidemiology and clinical significance of non-fimbrial adhesins have not been defined.

Bacterial lipopolysaccharide

Lipopolysaccharide in Gram-negative bacteria consists of three components; lipid A, a core region, and an outer polysaccharide. Lipid A anchors the cell wall to the bacterial outer membrane. The outer polysaccharide is of variable antigenicity and is known as the O antigen.

Lipopolysaccharide is believed to be an important virulence factor as uropathogenic strains of *E. coli* belong to a very restricted group of serotypes. Colonization of the urinary tract with a new O serotype is often associated with symptomatic infection and antibodies to lipid A can be detected after invasive bacterial infection.

Bacterial lipopolysaccharide may enhance virulence through a number of different mechanisms. Lipopolysaccharide is also known as endotoxin and has many effects on host cells. Endotoxin induces the host inflammatory response and is responsible for the clinical features of Gram-negative shock (Wolff 1991). In addition, lipopolysaccharide inhibits ureteric peristalsis (Teague and Boyarski 1968) and the O serotypes commonly associated with UTI are resistant to complement-mediated lysis (Johnson 1991).

Capsular polysaccharide

This polysaccharide is composed of linear repeated carbohydrate subunits which form a protective coat around the bacteria. Uropathogenic strains of *E. coli* express type II capsular polysaccharide which is acidic, highly charged, and relatively thin and patchy. The polysaccharide capsule determines the K antigen specificity of *E. coli*. Although over 80 capsular serotypes have been identified, only a small minority are associated with urinary infections (Kaijser *et al.* 1977). K1 polysaccharide is a sialic acid polymer which is poorly immunogenic and has an identical structure to the *Neisseria meningitis* group B capsule. K1 capsular polysaccharide is of particular clinical importance as K1 strains of *E. coli* are responsible for over 80 per cent of cases of neonatal meningitis (Robbins *et al.* 1974) and approximately 25 per cent of blood culture isolates (Pitt 1978).

Capsular polysaccharide is an important virulence factor as it inhibits the detection of O antigen, protects bacteria against neutrophil phagocytosis (Svanborg-Edén and de Man 1987), and inhibits complement-mediated killing (Leying *et al.* 1990).

The genes coding for the production of several capsular polysaccharides have recently been cloned (Echarti *et al.* 1983; Roberts *et al.* 1986). Approximately 17 kilobases (kB) of DNA is required for polysaccharide expression and the capsular gene cluster can be divided into three separate regions which encode polysaccharide biosynthesis and polymerization (region 1), translocation of polysaccharide to the cell surface (region 2), and post-polymerization modification (region 3) (Boulnois *et al.* 1987). Specific capsular serotypes are encoded by distinct structural genes located in region 2, however genes in region 1 and 3 are widely conserved among group II encapsulated strains of *E. coli*. This arrangement of the gene operon had been likened to a cassette, and allows separate structural genes to be inserted into conserved regions that code for their assembly and regulation.

Aerobactin

Iron metabolism is an important factor determining bacterial growth and division. One of the mechanisms mediating iron uptake in *E. coli* is the production of the siderophore aerobactin. This is a relatively small molecule of molecular weight 616 daltons that is secreted into the extracellular fluid. Aerobactin chelates Fe^{3+} and the aerobactin–iron complex is taken up by the bacterium through an outer membrane receptor protein. Aerobactin scavenges for iron in body tissues and fluids where it competes with similar host molecules including transferrin and lactoferrin. Aerobactin expression is associated with enhanced bacterial virulence in a murine model of UTI (Montgomerie *et al.* 1984). It appears to be an important factor in invasive UTI and is produced by over 75 per cent of *E. coli* isolates from blood cultures or pyelonephritis, but fewer than 50 per cent of isolates from other sites (Johnson *et al.* 1988).

The aerobactin operon consists of five genes (Johnson *et al.* 1991). Four genes code for aerobactin synthesis and the remaining gene codes for the outer membrane receptor protein. Aerobactin genes may be located on the bacterial chromosome or on plasmids, where they are frequently found in association with antibacterial resistance genes (e.g. pColV-K30). Other siderophores produced by

E. coli include enterochelin, which has a higher affinity for iron than aerobactin at neutral pH, but is probably of minor importance *in vivo*.

Haemolysin

Haemolysins are secreted polypeptide toxins which lyse erythrocytes. Two types of haemolysin are produced by *E. coli;* alpha-haemolysin is a 110 kDa protein, which may be chromosomal or plasmid coded and is secreted extracellularly, whereas beta-haemolysin is usually coded on the chromosome and is cell-associated (Hacker and Hughes 1985).

Haemolysin is believed to be an important factor in the pathogenesis of UTI as it is associated with extra-intestinal *E. coli* infection and approximately 75 per cent of pyelonephritic strains are haemolytic (O'Hanley *et al.* 1985*b*). Transfer of cloned haemolysin genes to non-haemolytic strains of *E. coli* leads to enhanced bacterial virulence (Hacker and Hughes 1985).

Haemolysin has *in vitro* toxic effects on many cells including polymorphonuclear leucocytes and renal tubular epithelium (Cavalieri *et al.* 1984). The *in vitro* cytolytic effects of haemolysin are potentiated by the presence of P-fimbriae (O'Hanley *et al.* 1991), possibly as a result of more effective toxin delivery in bacteria that are closely adherent to host cells. Haemolysin may be an important factor in pyelonephritis as it causes membrane damage in the kidney and inhibits host defences. In addition, the increased iron availability resulting from haemolysis may enhance bacterial growth and multiplication.

Other virulence factors

Uropathogenic *E. coli* produce a number of other significant virulence factors including cytotoxins, proteases, and factors which appear to inhibit smooth muscle and reduce ureteric peristalsis (Teague and Boyarski 1968). The plasmid ColV is frequently associated with uropathogenic *E. coli* and encodes several possible virulence determinants. These include production of colicin and other antibiotic resistance genes, factors which enhance fimbrial and haemolysin production, and products that inhibit host phagocytosis and complement-mediated killing.

Co-ordinated expression of virulence determinants

A range of factors are believed to contribute to bacterial virulence. These products include particular lipopolysaccharide and capsular antigens, adhesins, and haemolysin. Molecular studies have shown that the genes coding for many of these virulence determinants are linked together in a block of genetic information (Low *et al.* 1984; Svanborg-Edén and de Man 1987; High *et al.* 1988).

Comparison of the genotype and phenotype of organisms isolated from different sites in the urinary tract show that the expression of virulence factors is controlled and co-ordinated during the pathogenesis of ascending infection. A single isolate of *E. coli* may possess several distinct adhesins with gene expression regulated by environmental conditions. Bacteria are therefore able to vary their phenotype depending on the location of infection. This property is known as phase variation. Strains that possess both type 1 and P-fimbrial genes predominantly express type 1 fimbriae in the bladder and P-fimbriae in the kidney (Kiselius *et al.* 1989). The ability to undergo phase variation may be clinically significant, as type 1 fimbriae adhere strongly to the bladder epithelium but appear to enhance bacterial phagocytosis in the kidney (Svanborg-Edén *et al.* 1984), whereas P-fimbriae receptors are concentrated on renal tubular cells.

Other uropathogens

The role of *E. coli* has received particular attention due to its overwhelming importance in UTI but many of the other Gram-negative organisms have similar virulence factors. Type 1 mannose-sensitive fimbriae are expressed by a wide range of Gram-negative organisms (Abraham *et al.* 1988). In addition, *Proteus mirabilis*, *Klebsiella pneumoniae*, *Providencia stuartii*, and *Pseudomonas aeruginosa* have all been shown to express fimbrial adhesins which mediate mannose-resistant haemagglutination (Mobley *et al.* 1988; Koga *et al.* 1993; Bahrani *et al.* 1993). A range of Gram-positive organisms also have the ability to adhere to uroepithelial cells, including *Staph. epidermidis*, *Staph. saprophyticus* (Schmidt *et al.* 1988), and *Enterococcus faecalis* (Guzman *et al.* 1989). *Staphylococcus epidermidis* and certain Enterobacteriacae attach strongly to foreign body material and form a surrounding biofilm. This process is believed to be an important factor in the pathogenesis of catheter-associated infections.

Tarkkanen *et al.* (1992) investigated virulence factors in 39 urinary Klebsiella isolates. All pathogenic strains were found to be encapsulated. A total of 27 distinct antigens were identified in this series of isolates and infection was not associated with any particular capsular serotype. All strains agglutinated human erythrocytes and reacted with a type 3 fimbria-specific probe. The iron scavenger, enterochelin, was expressed by all isolates but aerobactin was not identified.

Production of urease is thought to be the most important virulence factor in Proteus spp. isolated from urinary infections. Urease splits urea into carbon dioxide and ammonia which is toxic to renal cells, alkalinizes the urine, and forms magnesium ammonium phosphate. Proteus infection is one of the factors associated with the production of renal stones. Evidence for the contribution of urease to pathogenicity includes the observation that acetohydroxamic acid, a potent urease inhibitor, reduced renal damage caused by Proteus in the rat (Musher *et al.* 1975), and more recent studies showing attenuated virulence of urease-negative Proteus mutants in a mouse model of ascending infection (Jones *et al.* 1990). A number of other bacteria produce urease including *Ureaplasma urealyticum*, *Staph. saprophyticus*, and certain strains of *Klebsiella pneumoniae* and *Pseudomonas aeruginosa*.

Host defence factors

Host defence factors include the anatomy of the urinary tract, flow and composition of urine, local and systemic immunity and the commensal flora of the distal urethra. Bacterial virulence and host defence factors are summarised in Table 2.2.

Table 2.2 Bacterial and host factors in the pathogenesis of urinary tract infection

Bacterial virulence factors	Host defence factors
Adhesins	*Urinary flow*
Type 1 fimbriae	
P-fimbriae	*Urinary composition*
X-adhesins	pH and solute concentration
	Free oligosaccharide residues
Lipopolysaccharide	Uromucoid
	Sloughed epithelial cells
Capsular polysaccharide	*Ureteric peristalsis*
Siderophores	*Commensal flora around lower urethra*
Aerobactin	
Enterochelin	*Host immunity*
	Local secretory immunoglobulin
Haemolysin	Polymorphonuclear phagocytosis
	Complement-mediated killing
Urease	Cell-mediated immunity
Antibiotic resistance genes	

Structure of the urinary tract

The urethra

The majority of uncomplicated UTIs occur in women. Females have a greater susceptibility to ascending infection as the female urethra is relatively short and the vaginal introitus may become contaminated with faecal organisms (Bran *et al.* 1972). Urinary flow characteristics are important in the initiation of bladder infection. Backflow of urine in the female urethra has been observed during micturition (Hinman 1966). This process will facilitate the spread of colonizing bacteria into the bladder.

Host defence mechanisms operating in the lower urethra include the flow of urine and the resident bacterial flora colonizing the vaginal introitus. This flora normally includes Lactobacilli, Bacteroides, Streptococci, Corynebacteria, and *Staphylococcus epidermidis* (Marrie *et al.* 1980). The presence of Lactobacilli appears to inhibit colonization of the lower urethra with *E. coli* as vaginal flushes with Lactobacilli eradicated *E. coli* from the lower urinary tract in cynomolgus monkeys (Herthelius *et al.* 1989), and prevented recurrent UTI in susceptible women (Bruce and Reid 1988).

The bladder

The most important defence mechanisms operating in the bladder are bladder emptying and the antimicrobial properties of the bladder mucosa (Cox and Hinman 1961). Conditions in the bladder correspond to a static chamber and the frequency of voiding and residual volume are crucial factors in the development of bladder infection (O'Grady and Cattell 1966*a)*. Bladder emptying effectively removes the majority of infecting bacteria and women with bacteriuria showed a dramatic reduction in bacterial count after fluid loading and hourly micturition (Cattell *et al.* 1970). A residual volume of more than 1 ml is associated with bacteriuria and a poor response to treatment (Shand *et al.* 1970).

The bladder mucosa also plays a significant role in the removal of infecting bacteria (Cox and Hinman 1961; Norden *et al.* 1968). Defence mechanisms operating at the mucosal surface include secretory immunoglobulin and the presence of a covering layer of mucin containing glycosaminoglycan polysaccharide. The importance of the mucin layer was demonstrated by Parsons *et al.* (1978) who destroyed the coating mucopolysaccharide with dilute hydrochloride acid and showed that this resulted in a great increase in observed bacterial adherence.

The ureter

Ureteric defence mechanisms include urinary flow and the vesicoureteric valves which prevent reflux of urine during bladder emptying. Ureteric or intra-renal obstruction and vesicoureteric reflux are associated with a high risk of renal infection (Siegel *et al.* 1980). The peristaltic action of the ureter causes turbulent flow of urine which contributes to the elimination of ascending bacteria (O'Grady and Cattell 1966*b*). Diminished ureteric peristalsis during pregnancy may contribute to the increased incidence of pyelonephritis (Patterson and Andriole 1987).

The kidney

Bacterial colonization of the renal medulla occurs readily under favourable conditions. However, the cortex is considerably more resistant to infection (Freedman and Beeson 1958). Possible reasons for the increased susceptibility of the renal medulla include the presence of a high concentration of bacterial adhesin receptors and local physical conditions, with a high concentration of solutes and low oxygen concentration favouring bacterial growth.

Antibacterial properties of urine

The composition of urine has an important influence on bacterial infection and the integrity of local host defence mechanisms. Cox and Hinman (1961) showed that urine was generally a good bacterial culture medium. However, some components of urine may inhibit bacterial growth (Kaye 1968). The antibacterial activity of urine does not appear to result from a lack of nutrients but is associated with increasing urea, solute and ammonia concentrations, and low pH. In a large community study, Waters *et al.* (1967) found that the median value for urine pH was less in males than females and urine osmolality was greater in men. These findings would be consistent with a greater inhibitory role in men. The overall importance of urine composition in the pathogenesis of ascending infection remains unclear as urine production and concentration vary significantly at different times of day and the composition of urine has significant effects on phagocytic function and complement activation (Chernew and Braude 1962).

One of the most important defence mechanisms in the urinary tract is the production of uromucoid or Tamm–Horsfall protein which traps bacteria and prevents colonization. Attachment of *E. coli* to uromucoid is mediated by type 1 fimbriae (Orskov *et al.* 1980). Bacterial adhesins will also bind to free oligosaccharide residues in the urine, resulting in the aggregation and elimination of infecting organisms (Jarvinen and Sandholm 1980).

A further host defence mechanism is the rapid shedding of viable cells from the urinary epithelium following bacterial infection. Bacteria bound to these sloughed cells will be eliminated in the urine (Aronson *et al.* 1988).

Host immunity in the urinary tract

Host immune mechanisms operating in the urinary tract include local and systemic antibody production, complement-mediated killing, neutrophil phagocytosis, and cell mediated immunity.

Secretory IgA and IgG are normally found in urine. Secretory IgA and IgG inhibit bacterial adhesion and the interaction between antigen and antibody activates complement (Svanborg-Edén and Svennerholm 1978; Rene *et al.* 1982). A range of antibodies are detected in the serum following pyelonephritis. These antibodies are directed against various bacterial components including fimbriae, O antigens, and capsular polysaccharide. Lower urinary tract infections are not usually associated with a significant serum antibody response, and humoral immunity is therefore thought to play a relatively minor role in the elimination of bacteria from the bladder.

The classical complement pathway is activated by the presence of specific antibody and the alternative pathway may be activated by bacterial surface antigens. The result of complement activation is bacterial killing. However, some serotypes are relatively resistant to complement lysis and these organisms appear to predominate in cases of pyelonephritis (Lomberg *et al.* 1984).

Phagocytosis of bacteria by neutrophils and macrophages occurs if organisms invade the bladder or kidney (Cobbs and Kaye 1967), but is probably of little importance in most lower urinary tract infections as the composition of urine inhibits phagocyte function.

The importance of cell-mediated immunity is also uncertain. T cell infiltration of the bladder and kidneys is associated with ascending infection in animal models of infection (Hjelm 1984). However, cell-mediated immunity is unlikely to play a major role in human urinary tract infections as patients with profound defects in T cell-mediated immunity do not have a greatly increased susceptibility to bacterial urinary tract infection.

Predisposing factors for the development of urinary tract infection

Genetic predisposition

Bacterial adherence to vaginal epithelial cells is increased in women who suffer from recurrent UTI (Schaeffer *et al.* 1981). The development of UTI is strongly influenced by host phenotype and the level of expression of adhesin receptors on host cells. Blood group determinants are of particular importance as they are recognized by many bacterial adhesins (Kinane *et al.* 1982). Approximately 75 per cent of the population are of blood group P1 and express P, P1, and P^k antigens on erythrocytes. Individuals of blood group P2 express low levels of P1 and P^k and have a reduced risk of developing recurrent pyelonephritis. Secretor status is also an important host factor and non-secretors have a threefold risk of developing recurrent urinary tract infections compared to secretors (Lomberg *et al.* 1986; Sheinfeld *et al.* 1989).

Females and sexual intercourse

The incidence of UTI in women shows a striking rise in early adult life and there is strong evidence for an association with sexual intercourse (Remis *et al.* 1987). In a study of pre-menopausal women with recurrent UTI the majority of infections occurred within 24 hours of sexual intercourse (Nicolle *et al.* 1982). Bran *et al.* (1972) showed that urethral milking led to ascending infection in healthy human volunteers. Infection following sexual intercourse is thought to occur by a similar mechanical effect leading to bacterial contamination of the lower urethra and bladder. A case-controlled study showed that diaphragm—spermicide use was also associated with an increased risk of developing UTI (Stamm *et al.* 1989).

Pregnancy

Prevalence studies have shown that 2–11 per cent of women have bacteriuria at some stage in pregnancy (Stenquist *et al.* 1989). The onset of bacterial colonization usually occurs between the 9th and 17th week of pregnancy. Several factors contribute to the increased susceptibility to upper urinary tract infection in pregnant women, including dilation of the collecting system and ureters, reduced ureteric peristalsis, and partial ureteric obstruction resulting from the enlarging uterus (Patterson and Andriole 1987). Hormonal changes during pregnancy are probably responsible for many of these physiological effects and oestrogen treatment in rats leads to hydronephrosis and associated infection (Andriole and Cohn 1964). Orlander *et al.* (1992) found that post-menopausal women on hormone replacement therapy (HRT) had an increased risk of developing urinary tract infections compared to those not receiving HRT, but there was no information on the relative frequency of sexual intercourse in the two groups.

Children

Young children have a relatively high incidence of UTI compared to older children or adolescents. Infections of the urinary tract occurring in the neonatal period are usually the result of bacteraemic spread rather than ascending infection and are associated with a severe systemic illness and poor prognosis. Breast-feeding gives some protection against UTI in the first six months of life (Pisacane *et al.* 1992)

Seventy-five per cent of UTIs occur in boys in the first three to six months of life, but only 10 per cent of infections occur in later childhood (Ginsburg and McCracken 1982; Spencer and Schaeffer 1986). The initial preponderance of infections in boys is thought to be related to the presence of the foreskin as uncircumcised boys have a 20-fold greater incidence of UTI (Herzog 1989). The gut is colonized with enteric organisms in the first weeks of life and *E. coli* is the cause of over 80 per cent of childhood urinary tract infections. *Klebsiella pneumoniae*, group D Streptococci, and other organisms cause occasional infections.

Congenital abnormalities of the renal tract, which predispose to the development of childhood urinary infections, include phimosis, posterior urethral valves, ureterocoele, and vesicoureteric reflux (Spencer and Schaeffer 1986). Radiographic abnormalities of the urinary tract are found in approximately 40 per cent of infected girls, but only 10 per cent of infected boys (Ginsburg and McCracken 1982; Snodgrass 1991). Vesicoureteric reflux can be demonstrated in nearly 50 per cent of infants with upper UTI (Siegel *et al.* 1980). Reflux is particularly important in the first two years of life but usually resolves in later childhood.

The elderly

The incidence of bacteriuria increases with age until 70 and then remains stable. The age-related rise in incidence is particularly marked in men and the overall incidence of infection in men and women is approximately equal after the age of 65 (Baldessarre and Kaye 1991). Bacteriuria in the elderly is often asymptomatic (Bakke and Vollset 1993).

Bacteriuria in the elderly often reflects general disability and is associated with the presence of underlying medical disease, institutionalization, and need for catheterization or instrumentation. Factors which contribute to the increased risk of infection in the elderly include urinary stasis resulting from prostatic hypertrophy in elderly men, decreasing attention to personal care and hygiene, presence of neuropathy causing inability to empty the bladder completely, declining immunity, and reduced secretion of uromucoid.

Diabetes mellitus

The incidence of bacteriuria and symptomatic urinary tract infections is increased in patients with diabetes. Complications of infection are also more common and include renal papillary necrosis, perinephric abscess, and fungal infection of the kidney. Diabetics appear to be particularly prone to Klebsiella infection (Lye *et al.* 1992).

Several factors are responsible for the increased risk of infection in diabetes. Glycosuria enhances growth and spread of many organisms including *E. coli* (Levison and Pitsakis 1984) and *Candida albicans* (Raffel *et al.* 1981). In addition, the presence of glycosuria inhibits phagocytosis and the host immune response (Chernew and Braude 1962). Diabetic neuropathy is associated with bladder paralysis and incomplete voiding resulting in urinary retention. Neurogenic incompetence of the vesicoureteric orifice causes ureteric reflux and kidneys damaged by diabetic nephropathy are more susceptible to ascending or haematogenous infection (Ellenberg 1976).

Obstructive uropathy

Urinary obstruction and stasis are associated with the development of bacterial infection in any part of the urinary tract. Hydronephrosis is a significant factor in the development of ascending and haematogenous renal infection (Rocha *et al.* 1958; Thorley *et al.* 1974). The most common reason for obstruction is benign prostatic hypertrophy in men. Other important causes of obstruction include congenital abnormalities and urinary calculi.

Urinary tract calculi

Approximately 10–15 per cent of calculi in the urinary tract are secondary to bacterial infection (Lerner *et al.* 1989). Infective stones are usually caused by Proteus and other urease-producing bacteria, although they may also occur in association with *E. coli* infection (Ohkawa *et al.* 1992). Stones resulting from bacterial infection are composed of magnesium ammonium phosphate (struvite). The presence of urinary calculi predisposes to urinary tract infection as they cause urinary obstruction and epithelial damage. Calculi may also harbour bacteria, which are difficult to eradicate, and act as a source of recurrent infection.

Catheterization

This is associated with a very high incidence of UTI. The risk of infection is considerably reduced using a closed rather than open catheter system, but bacteriuria will develop in 10–27 per cent of catheterized patients within five days (*Lancet* 1991). The frequency of catheter-associated infection is increased in elderly and vulnerable patients. The reasons for the greatly increased risk of infection include introduction of bacteria into the bladder during catheter insertion, and infection by organisms ascending the lumen or outer surface of the catheter.

Bacteria isolated from catheterized patients have been shown to adhere strongly to the catheter material (Roberts *et al.* 1993). Infection is associated with the formation of a biofilm on the surface of the foreign body, which consists of a collection of microorganisms and extracellular products. Bacteria within the biofilm are resistant to antibiotics and the presence of a foreign body is associated with a complex defect in polymorphonuclear function (Zimmerli *et al.* 1984). Catheter-associated infections therefore respond poorly to antibiotics and are difficult to eradicate.

Immunosuppression

Immunosuppression due to drug treatment or malignant disease is associated with an increased incidence and severity of UTI which may involve a wide spectrum of pathogens. Reasons for the increased susceptibility of these individuals include compromised host immunity, epithelial damage resulting from cytotoxic drugs, changes in commensal bacterial flora following the use of antibiotics, and the increased risks of hospitalization and catheterization. Renal transplantation is a specific situation when anatomical changes in the urinary tract are combined with underlying medical disease, catheterization, and immunosuppressive therapy to give a high risk of infection. Neutropenia is associated with an increased risk of haematogenous renal infection (Sobel 1987), particularly if the absolute neutrophil count is below 500×10^9 cells/litre.

The incidence of UTI appears to be slightly increased in patients infected with the human immunodeficiency virus (HIV), but urinary tract infections are not a major cause of morbidity or mortality. Kaplan *et al.* (1987) reviewed the notes of 60 AIDS patients seen over a five-year period and found that 52 per cent had at least one period of documented pyuria and 20 per cent had a symptomatic UTI. Welch *et al.* (1989) documented bacteriuria in 8 per cent of 125 urine specimens obtained from HIV-infected homosexuals and none of 36 samples from HIV negative homosexuals. However, bacteriuria was usually asymptomatic and clinically apparent urinary infections were rare. Approximately 20 per cent of bacterial infections in HIV positive children originate in the urinary tract (Bernstein *et al.* 1985; Kransinski *et al.* 1988). A wide range of organisms have been isolated from the UTI in HIV-positive patients including *Escherichia coli, Klebsiella pneumoniae, Pseudomonas aeruginosa*, Salmonella spp., *Cryptococcus neoformans, Mycobacterium tuberculosis*, atypical mycobacterial infection, adenovirus, and cytomegalovirus.

Conclusion

The development of urinary tract infection involves a complex interaction between pathogen and host. Predisposing factors for infection are well recognized, but the importance of urine composition and local immunity is still relatively poorly understood. Recent advances in molecular biology have led to an enormous increase in our understanding of bacterial virulence and pathogenesis of disease. The possible benefits of this research include the development of novel strategies for the prevention or treatment of UTI. Experimental studies have investigated a variety of possibilities including vaccination with purified adhesin or conjugated capsular polysaccharide, use of soluble receptor analogues to prevent adhesion, and vaginal flushing with Lactobacilli to inhibit growth of enteric organisms (O'Hanley *et al.* 1985*a*; (Kaijser *et al.* 1983; Bruce and Reid 1988; Cox and Taylor 1990). These approaches may find future clinical applications. However, uropathogenic bacteria possess a great diversity of virulence factors and no single strategy is likely to prevent the majority of urinary infections.

References

Abraham, S. N., Sun, D., Dale, J. B., and Beachey, E. H. (1988). Conservation of the D-mannose-adhesion protein among type 1 fimbriated members of the family enterobacteriaceae. *Nature*, **336**, 682–4.

Andriole, V. T. and Cohn, G. L. (1964). The effect of diethylstilboestrol on the susceptibility of rats of hematogenous pyelonephritis. *Journal of Clinical Investigation*, **43**, 1136–45.

Arthur, M., *et al.* (1989*a*). Structure and copy number of gene clusters related to the *pap* P-adhesin operon of uropathogenic *Escherichia coli. Infection and Immunity*, **57**, 314–21.

Arthur, M., *et al.* (1989*b*). Molecular epidemiology of adhesin and haemolysin virulence factors among uropathogenic *Escherichia coli. Infection and Immunity*, **57**, 303–13.

Aronson, M., Medalia, O., Amichay, D., and Nativ, O. (1988). Endotoxin-induced shedding of viable uroepithelial cells is an anti-microbial defence mechanism. *Infection and Immunity*, **56**, 1615–7.

Bahrani, F. K., Cook, S., Hull, R. A., Massad, G., and Mobley, H. L. T. (1993). *Proteus mirabilis* fimbriae: *N*-terminal amino acid sequence of a major fimbrial subunit and nucleotide sequences of the genes from two strains. *Infection and Immunity*, **61**, 884–91.

Bakke, A. and Vollset, S. E. (1993). Risk factors for bacteruria and clinical urinary tract infection in patients treated with clean intermittent catheterisation. *Journal of Urology*, **149**, 527–31.

Baldessarre, J. S. and Kaye, D. (1991). Special problems in urinary tract infection in the elderly. In *The medical clinics of North America*, (ed. D., Kaye), pp. 357–900, Saunders, Philadelphia.

Bernstein, L. J., Krieger, B. Z. Novick, B., Sicklick, M. J., and Rubinstein, A. (1985). Bacterial infection in the acquired immune deficiency syndrome of children. *Paediatric Infectious Diseases*, **4**, 472–5.

Boulnois, G. J., Roberts, I. S., Hodge, R., Hardy, K. R., Jann, K. B. and Timmis, K. N. (1987). Analysis of the K1 capsule biosynthesis genes of *Escherichia coli*: Definition of three functional regions for capsule production. *Molecular and General Genetics*, **208**, 242–6.

Bran, J. L., Levison, M. E., and Kaye, D. (1972). Entrance of bacteria into the female urinary bladder. *New England Journal of Medicine*, **286**, 626–9.

Bruce, A. W. And Reid, G. (1988). Intravaginal instillation of lactobacilli for prevention of recurrent urinary tract infections. *Canadian Journal of Microbiology*, **34**, 339–43.

Bryan, C. S. and Reynolds, K. L. (1984). Community-acquired bacteraemic urinary tract infection: Epidemiology and outcome. *Journal of Urology*, **132**, 490–3.

Cattell, W. R. *et al.* (1970). Effect of diuresis and frequent micturition on the bacterial content of infected urine; a measure of competence of intrinsic hydrostatic clearance mechanisms. *British Journal of Urology*, **42**, 290–5.

Cavalieri, S. J., Bohach, G. A., and Snyder. I. S. (1984). *Escherichia coli* alpha haemolysin: Characteristics and probable role in pathogenicity. *Microbiology Reviews*, **48**, 326–43.

Chernew, I. and Braude, A. L. (1962). Depression of phagocytosis by solutes in concentration found in the kidney and urine. *Journal of Clinical Investigation*, **41**, 1945–53.

Cobbs, C. G. and Kaye. D. (1967). Antibacterial mechanisms in the urinary bladder. *Yale Journal of Biology and Medicine*, **40**, 93–108.

Cox, C. and Hinman, F. (1961). Experiments with induced bacteruria, vesical emptying and bacterial growth on the mechanism of bladder defense to infection. *Journal of Urology*, **86**, 739–48.

Cox, F. and Taylor, T. (1990). Prevention of *Escherichia coli* K1 bacteraemia in newborn mice by using topical vaginal carbohydrates. *Journal of Infections Diseases*, **162**, 978–81.

Cox, C. E., Lucy, S. S., and Hinman, F. (1968). The urethra and its relationship to urinary tract infection. II. The urethral flora of the female with recurrent urinary tract infections. *Journal of Urology*, **99**, 632–8.

Duguid, J. P., Smith, I. W., Dempster, G., and Edmunds, P. N. (1955). Nonflagellar filamentous appendages ('fimbriae') and haemagglutination activity in *Bacterium coli*. *Journal of Pathology and Bacteriology*, **70**, 335–48.

Escharti, C., Hirschel, B., Boulnois G, J., Varley, J. M., Waldvogel, F., and Timmis, K. N. (1983). Cloning and analysis of the K1 capsule biosynthesis genes of *Escherichia coli*: Lack of homology with *Neisseria meningitidis* group B DNA sequences. *Infection and Immunity*, **41**, 54–60.

Eisenstein, B. I. (1988). Type 1 fimbriae of *Escherichia coli*: Genetic regulation, morphogenesis and role in pathogenesis. *Reviews in Infectious Diseases*, **10**, S341–4.

Ellenberg, M. (1976). Diabetic neuropathy. Clinical aspects. *Metabolism*, **25**, 1627–55.

Freedman, L. R. and Beeson, P. B. (1958). Experimental pyelonephritis. IV. Observations on infections resulting from direct inoculation of bacteria in different zones of the kidney. *Yale Journal of Biology and Medicine*, **30**, 406–14.

Fujita, K., Yamamoto, T., Yokota, T., and Kitagawa, R. (1989). In vitro adherence of type 1 fimbriated uropathogenic *Escherichia coli* to human ureteral mucosa. *Infection and Immunity*, **57**, 2574–9.

Ginsberg, C. M. and McCracken, G. H. (1982). Urinary tract infections in young infants. *Pediatrics*, **69**, 409–12.

Goldhar, J., Perry, R., Golecki, J. R., Hoschutzky, H., Jann, B., and Jann, K. (1987). Non-fimbrial mannose-resistant adhesins from uropathogenic *Escherichia coli* 083:K1:H4 and 014:k^2:H11. *Infection and Immunity*, **55**, 1837–42.

Grunberg, J., Perry, R. Hoschutsky, H., Jann, B., Jann, K., and Goldhar, J. (1988). Nonfimbrial blood group N-specific adhesin (NFA-3) from *Escherichia coli* 020: KX104:H-, causing systemic infection. *FEMS Microbiology Letters*, **56**, 241–6.

Grunberg, R. N. (1969). Relationship of infecting urinary organisms to the faecal flora in patients with symptomatic urinary infection. *Lancet*, **ii**, 766–8.

Guzman, C. A., Pruzzo, C., Lipera, G., and Calegari, L. (1989). Role of adherence in pathogenesis of *Enterococcus faecalis* urinary tract infection and endocarditis. *Infection and Immunity*, **57**, 1834–8.

Hacker, J. and Hughes. (1985). Genetics of *Escherichia coli* haemolysin. *Current Topics in Microbiology and Immunology*, **118**, 139–62.

Hagberg, L., Engberg, I., Freter, R., Lam, J., Olling, S., and Svanborg-Eden, C. (1983*a*). Ascending unobstructed urinary tract infection in mice caused by pyelonephritogenic *Escherichia coli* of human origin. *Infection and Immunity*, **40**, 273–83.

Hagberg, L., Hull, R., Hull, S., Falkow, R., Freter, R., and Svanborg-Eden, C. (1983*b*). Contribution of adhesion to bacterial persistence in the mouse urinary tract. *Infection and Immunity*, **40**, 265–72.

Hales, B. A., *et al.* (1988). Molecular cloning and characterisation of the genes for a non-fimbrial adhesin from *Escherichia coli. Microbial Pathogenesis*, **5**, 9–17.

Herthelius, M., Gorbach, S. L., Mollby, R., Nord, C. E., Petterson, L., and Winberg, J. (1989). Elimination of vaginal colonisation with *Escherichia coli* by administration of indigenous flora. *Infection and Immunity*, **57**, 2447–51.

Herzog, L. W. (1989). Urinary tract infections and circumcision. *American Journal of Diseases of Childhood*, **143**, 348–50.

High, N. J., Hales, B. A., Jann, K., and Boulnois, G. J. (1988). A block of urovirulence genes encoding multiple fimbriae and haemolysin in *Escherichia coli* 04:K12:H-*Infection and Immunity*, **56**, 513–17.

Hinman, F. (1966). Mechanism for the entry of bacteria and the establishment of urinary infection in female children. *Journal of Urology*, **96**, 546–50.

Hjelm, E. M. (1984). Local cellular immune response in ascending urinary tract infection: Occurrence of T-cells, immunoglobulin-producing cells, and Ia-expressing cells in rat urinary tract tissue. *Infection and Immunity*, **44**, 627–32.

Hoschutzky, H. Nimmich, W., Lottspeich, F., and Jann, K. (1989). Isolation and charaterization of the non-fimbrial adhesin NFA 4 from uropathogenic *Escherichia coli* 07:K98:H6. *Microbial Pathogenesis*, **6**, 351–9.

Hultgren, S. J., Abraham, S. N., and Normark, S. A. (1991). Chaperone-assisted assembly and molecular architecture of adhesive pili. *Annual Reviews in Microbiology*, **45**, 383–415.

Ivanyi, B., Ormos, J., and Lantos, J. (1983). Tubulointerstitial inflammation, cast formation and renal parenchymal damage in experimental pyelonephritis. *American Journal of Pathology*, **113**, 300–8.

Jarvinen, A. and Sandholm M. (1980). Urinary oligosaccharides inhibit adhesion of *E. Coli* onto canine urinary tract epithelium. *Investigative Urology*, **17**, 443–5.

Johnson, J. R. (1991). Virulence factors in *Escherichia coli* urinary tract infection. *Clinical Microbiology Review*, **4** 80–128.

Johnson, J. R., Mosely, S. L., Roberts, P. L., and Stamm, W. E. (1988). Aerobactin and other virulence factor genes among strains of *Escherichia coli* causing urosepsis. Association with patient characteristics. *Infection and Immunity*, **56**, 405–12.

Johnson, J. R., Berggren, T., and Manivel, J. C. (1992). Histopathologic–microbiologic correlates of invasiveness in a mouse model of ascending unobstructed urinary tract infection. *Journal of Infectious Diseases*, **165**, 299–305.

Jones, B. D., Lockatell, C. V., Johnson, D. E., Warren, J. W., and Mobley, H. O. (1990). Construction of a urease negative mutant of *Proteus mirabilis*: Analysis of virulence in a mouse model of ascending urinary tract infection. *Infection and Immunity*, **58**, 1120–3.

Kaijser, B., Hanson, L. A., Jodal, U., Lidin-Janson, G., and Robbins, J. B. (1977). Frequency of *Escherichia coli* K antigens in urinary tract infections in children. *Lancet*, **i**, 663–4.

Kaijser, B., Larsson, P., Olling, S., and Schneerson, R. (1983). Protection against acute ascending pyelonephritis caused by *Escherichia coli* in rats, using isolated capsular antigen conjugated to bovine serum albumin. *Infection and Immunity*, **39**, 142–6.

Kallenius, G., Svenson, S. B., Mollby, R., Cedergen, B., Hultberg, H., and Winberg, J. (1981). Structure of carbohydrate part of receptor on human epithelial cells for pyelonephritogenic *Escherichia coli*. *Lancet*, **ii**, 604–6.

Kaplan, M. S., Wechsler, M., and Benson, M. K. (1987). Urologic manifestations of AIDS. *Urology*, **30** 441–6.

Kaye, D. (1968). Antibacterial activity of human urine. *Journal of Clinical Investigation*, **47**, 2374–90.

Keith, B. R., Harris, S. L., Russell, P. W., and Orndorff, P. E. (1990). Effect of type 1 piliation on in-vitro killing of *Escherichia coli* by mouse peritoneal macrophages. *Infection and Immunity*, **58**, 3448–54.

Kinane, D. F., Blackwell, C. C., Brettle, R. P., Wier, D. M., and Winstanley. (1982). ABO, blood group, secretory state and susceptibility to recurrent urinary tract infection in women. *British Medical Journal*, **285**, 7–9.

Kiselius, P. V., Schwan, W. R., Amundsen, S. K., Duncan, J. L., and Schaeffer, A. J. (1989). In vivo expression and variation of *Escherichia coli* type 1 and P pili in the urine of adults with acute urinary tract infections. *Infection and Immunity*, **57**, 1656–62.

Klemm, P., Jorgenson, B. T., Van Die, I, de Ree, H., and Bergmans, H. (1985). The *fim* genes responsible for synthesis of type 1 fimbriae in *Escherichia coli*. *Molecular and General Genetics*, **199**, 410–4.

Koga, T., Ishimoto, K., and Lory, S. (1993). Genetic and functional characterisation of the gene cluster specifying expression of *Pseudomonas aeruginosa* pili. *Infection and Immunity*, **61**, 1371–7.

Krasinski, K., Borkowsky, W., Bonk, S., Lawrence, R., and Chandwani, S. (1988). Bacterial infection in human immunodeficiency virus-infected children. *Pediatric Infectious Diseases*, **7**, 323–8.

Krogfelt, K. A., Bergmans, H., and Klemm, P. (1990). Direct evidence that the *fim* H protein is the mannose-specific adhesin of *Escherichia coli* type 1 fimbriae. *Infection and Immunity*, **58**, 1995–8.

Kroncke, K. D., Orskov, I., Orskov, F., Jann, B., and Jann, K. (1990). Electron microscopic study of co-expression of adhesive protein capsules and polysaccharide capsules in *Escherichia coli* 04: K12:H-. *Infection and Immunity*, **58**, 2710–4.

Kuehn, M. J., Heuser, J., Normark., and Hultgren, S. (1992). P-pili in uropathogenic *E. coli* are composite fibres with distinct fibrillar adhesive tips. *Nature*, **356**, 252–5.

Lancet (1991). Editorial. Catheter-acquired urinary tract infection. **338**, 857–8.

Lerner, S. P., Gleeson, M. J., and Griffith D. P. (1989). Infection Stones. *Journal of Urology*, **141** 753–8.

Levison, M. E. and Pitsakis, P. G. (1984). Effect of insulin therapy on the susceptibility of the diabetic rat to *Escherichia coli*-induced pyelonephritis. *Journal of Infectious Diseases*, **150**, 554–60.

Leying, H., Suerbaum, S., Kroll, H. P., Stahl, D., and Opferkuch, W. (1990). The capsular polysaccharide is a major determinant of serum resistance in K1-positive blood culture isolates of *Escherichia coli*. *Infection and Immunity*, **58**, 222–7.

Lindberg, F., Lund, B., Johansson, L., and Normark, S. (1987). Localisation of the receptor-binding protein adhesin at the tip of the bacterial pilus. *Nature*, **328**, 84–7.

Lomberg, H., Hellstrom, M., Jodal, U., Leffler, H., Lincoln, K., and Svanborg-Edén, C. (1984). Virulence-associated traits in *Escherichia coli* causing first and recurrent episodes of urinary tract infection in children with and without vesicoureteric reflux. *Journal of Infectious Diseases*, **150**, 561–9.

Lomberg, H., Cedergren, B., Leffler, H., Nilsson, B., Carlstrom, A. S., and Svanborg-Edén, C. (1986). Influence of blood groups on the availability of receptors for attachment of uropathogenic *Escherichia coli*. *Infection and Immunity*, **51**, 919–26.

Low, D., David, V., Lark, D, Schoolnik, G., and Falkow, S. (1984). Gene clusters governing the production of haemolysin and mannose-resistant haemagglutination are closely linked in *Escherichia coli* serotype 04 and 06 isolates from urinary tract infections. *Infection and Immunity*, **43**, 353–8.

Lye, W. C., Chan, R. K. T., Lee, E. J. C., and Kumarasinghe, G. (1992). Urinary tract infections in patients with diabetes mellitus. *Journal of Infection*, **24**, 169–74.

Marrie, T. J., Swantee, C. A., and Hartlen, M. (1980). Aerobic and anaerobic urethral flora in healthy females in various physiological age groups and females with urinary tract infection. *Journal of Clinical Microbiology*, **11**, 654–9.

Mobley, H. L. T., *et al.* (1988). MR/K haemagglutination of *Providencia stuartii* correlates with adherence to catheters and with persistence in catheter-associated bacteruria. *Journal of Infectious Diseases*, **157**, 264–71.

Moch, T. H. Hoschutsky, J., Hacker, J., Kroncke, K. D., and Jann, K. (1987). Isolation and characterization of the α-sialyl-β-2,3-galactosyl-specific adhesin from fimbriated *Escherichia coli*. *Proceedings of The National Academy of Sciences of the USA*, **84**, 3462–6.

Montgomerie, J. Z., Bindereif, A., Neilands, J. B., Kalmanson, G. M., and Guze, L. B. (1984). Association of hydroxamate siderophore (aerobactin) with *Escherichia coli* isolated from patients with bacteraemia. *Infection and Immunity*, **46** 835–8.

Musher, D. M., Griffith, D. P., and Yawn, D. (1975). Role of urease in pyelonephritis resulting from urinary tract infection with *Proteus*. *Journal of Infectious Diseases*, **131**, 177–8.

Nicolle, L. E., Harding, G. K. M., Preiksaitis, J., and Ronald, A. R. (1982). The association of urinary tract infection with sexual intercourse. *Journal of Infectious Diseases*, **146**, 579–83.

Norden, C. W., Green, G. M., and Kass, E. H. (1968). Antibacterial mechanisms of the urinary bladder. *Journal of Clinical Investigation*, **47**, 2689–7000.

Nowicki, B., Svanborg-Eden, C., Hull, R., and Hull, S. (1989). A haemagglutinin on uropathogenic *Escherichia coli* recognises the Dr blood antigen. *Infection and Immunity*, **57**, 446–51.

Nowicki, B., Labigne, A., Moseley, S., Hull, R., Hull, S., and Moulds, J. (1991). The Dr haemagglutinin, afimbrial adhesins AFA-1 and AFA-3, and the F1845 fimbriae of uropathogenic and diarrhoea-associated *Escherichia coli* belong to a family of haemagglutinins with Dr receptor recognition. *Infection and Immunity*, **58**, 279–81.

Ofek, I., Mirelman, G., and Sharon, N. (1977). Adherence of *Escherichia coli* to human mucosal cells mediated by mannose receptors. *Nature*, **265**, 623–5.

O'Grady, F. and Cattell, W. R. (1966*a*). Kinetics of urinary tract infection. II. The bladder. *British Journal of Urology*, **38**, 156–62.

O'Grady, F. and Cattell, W. R. (1966*b*). Kinetics of urinary tract infection. I. Upper urinary tract. *British Journal of Urology*, **38**, 149–55.

O'Hanley, P., Lark, D., Falkow, S., and Schoolnik, G. (1985*a*). Molecular basis of *Escherichia coli* colonization of the upper urinary tract in BALB/c mice: Gal-Gal pili immunization prevents *E.coli* pyelonephritis in the BALB/c model of human pyelonephritis. *Journal of Clinical Investigation*, **75**, 347–60.

O'Hanley, P. *et al.* (1985*b*). Gal-Gal binding and haemolysin phenotypes and genotypes associated with uropathogenic *Escherichia coli*. *New England Journal of Medicine*, **313**, 414–20.

O'Hanley, P. O., Lalonde, G., and Ji, G. (1991). Alpha-hemolysin contributes to the pathogenicity of piliated digalactoside-binding *Escherichia coli* in the kidney: Efficacy of an alpha-hemolysin vaccine in preventing renal injury in the BALB/c mouse model of pyelonephritis. *Infection and Immunity*, **59**, 1153–61.

Ohkawa, M., Tokunaga, S., Nakashima, T., Yamaguchi, K., Orito, M., Hisazumi, H. (1992). Composition of urinary calculi related to urinary tract infection. *Journal of Urology*, **148**, 995–7.

Orlander, J. D., Jick, S. S., Dean, A. D., and Jick, H. (1992). Urinary tract infections and estrogen use in older women. *Journal of the American Geriatric Society*, **40**, 817–20.

Orskov, I., Ferencz, A., and Orskov, F. (1980) Tamm–Horsfall protein or uromucoid is the normal urinary slime that traps type 1 fimbriated *Escherichia coli*. *Lancet*, **i**, 887.

Parsons, C. L., Shrom, S. H., Harmon, P., and Mulholland, S. G. (1978). Bladder surface mucin: Examination of possible mechanisms for its antibacterial effect. *Investigative Urology*, **16**, 196–200.

Patterson, T. F. and Andriole, V. T. (1987). Bacteruria in pregnancy. *Infectious Diseases Clinics of North America*, **1**, 807–22.

Pere, A., Nowicki, B., Saxen, H., Siitonen, A., and Korhonen, T. K. (1987). Expression of P, type 1 and type 1C fimbriae of *Escherichia coli* in the urine of patients with acute urinary tract infection. *Journal of Infectious Diseases*, **156**, 567–74.

Pisacane, A., Graziano, L., Mazzarella, G., Scarpellino, B., and Zona, G. (1992). Breast feeding and urinary tract infection. *Journal of Pediatrics*, **120**, 87–9.

Pitt, J. (1978). K1 antigen of *Escherichia coli*: Epidemiology and serum resistance of pathogenic strains. *Infection and Immunity*, **22**, 219–24.

Plos, K., Carter, T., Hull, S., Hull, R., and Svanborg-Eden, C. (1990). Frequency and organisation of pap homologous DNA in relation to clinical origin of uropathogenic *Escherichia coli*. *Journal of Infectious Diseases*, **161** 518–24.

Raffel, L., Pitasakis, P. G., Levison, S. P., and Levison, M. E. (1981). Experimental *Candida albicans*, *Staphylococcus aureus*, and *Streptococcus faecalis* pyelonephritis in diabetic rats. *Infection and Immunity*, **34**, 773–9.

Remis, R. S., Gurwith, M. J., Gurwith, D., Hargrett-Bean, N. T., and Layde, P. M. (1987). Risk factors for urinary tract infection. *American Journal of Epidemiology*, **126**, 685–94.

Rene, P., Dinolfo, M., and Silverblatt, F. J. (1982). Serum and urogenital antibody response to *Escherichia coli* in cystitis. *Infection and Immunity*, **38**, 542–7.

Rhen, M., Klemm, P., and Korhonen, T. K. (1986). Identification of two new hemagglutinins of *Escherichia coli*, *N*-acetyl-d-glucosamine-specific fimbriae and a blood group M-specific agglutinin, by cloning the corresponding genes in *Escherichia coli* K12, *Journal of Bacteriology*, **168** 1234–42.

Roberts, I., *et al.* (1986). Molecular cloning and analysis of genes for production of K5, K7, K12, and K92 capsular polysaccharides in *Escherichia coli*. *Journal of Bacteriology*, **168**, 1228–33.

Roberts, J. A., Hardaway, K., Kaack, B., Fussell, E. N., and Baskin, G. (1984). Prevention of pyelonephritis by immunisation with P-fimbriae. *Journal of Urology*, **131**, 602–7.

Roberts, J. A., Kaack, M. B., Fussell, E. N. (1993). Adherence to urethral catheters by bacteria causing nosocomial infections. *Urology*, **41**, 338–42.

Robbins, J. B., *et al.* (1974). *Escherichia coli* K1 capsular polysaccharide associated with neonatal meningitis. *New England Journal of Medicine*, **290**, 1216–21.

Rocha, H., Guze, L. B., Freedman, L. R., and Beeson, P. R. (1958). Experimental pyelonephritis.III. The influence of localised injury in different parts of the kidney on susceptibility to bacterial infection. *Yale Journal of Biology and Medicine*, **30**, 341- 54.

Schaeffer, A. J., Jones, J. M., and Dunn, J. K. (1981). Association of *in vitro Escherichia coli* adherence to vaginal and buccal epithelial cells with susceptibility of women to recurrent urinary tract infection. *New England Journal of Medicine*, **304**, 1062–6.

Schaeffer, A. J., Achwan, W. R., Hultgren, S. J., and Duncan, J. L. (1987). Relationship of type 1 pilus expression in *Escherichia coli* to ascending urinary tract infection in mice. *Infection and Immunity*, **55**, 373–80.

Schmidt, H., Naumann, G., and Putzke, H. P. (1988). Detection of different fimbria-like structures on the surface of *Staphylococcus saprophyticus*.. *Zentralblatt für Bakteriology*, **A268**, 228–37.

Shand, D. G., Nimmon, C. C., O'Grady, F., and Cattell, W. (1970). Relation between residual volume and response to treatment of urinary infection. *Lancet*, **i**, 1305–6.

Sheinfeld, J., Schaeffer, A. J., Cordon-Cardo, C., Rogatko, A., and Fair, W. R. (1989). Association of the Lewis blood group phenotype with recurrent urinary tract infection in women. *New England Journal of Medicine*, **320**, 773–7.

Siegel, S., Siegel, B., and Sokoloff, B. Z. (1980). Urinary infection in infants and pre-school children. *American Journal of Diseases of Childhood*, **134**, 369–72.

Snodgrass, W. (1991). Relationship of voiding dysfunction to urinary tract infection and vesicoureteral reflux in children. *Urology*, **38**, 341–4.

Sobel, J. D. (1987). Pathogenesis of urinary tract infections: Host defenses. *Infectious Diseases Clinics of North America*, **1**, 751–72.

Spencer, J. R. and Schaeffer, A. J. (1986). Pediatric urinary tract infections. *Urological Clinics of North America*, **13**, 661–72.

Stamey, T. A., Timothy, M., and Miller, M. (1971). Recurrent urinary tract infections in adult women. The role of introital enterobacteria. *California Medicine*, **115**, 1–19.

Stamm, W. E., *et al.* (1989). Urinary tract infections: From pathogenesis to treatment. *Journal of Infectious Diseases*, **159**, 400–6.

Stenquist, K., *et al.* (1989). Bacteruria in pregnancy. *American Journal of Epidemiology*, **129**, 372–9.

Svanborg-Edén, C. and de Man, P. (1987). Bacterial virulence in urinary tract infection. *Infectious Diseases Clinics of North America*, **1**, 731–50.

Svanborg-Edén, C., and Svennerholm, A. N. (1978). Secretory IgA and IgG antibodies prevent adhesion of *Escherichia coli* to human urinary tract epithelial cells. *Infection and Immunity*, **22**, 790–7.

Svanborg-Edén, C., Hanson, L. A., Jodal, U., Lindberg, U., and Sohl Akerlund, A. (1976). Variable adhesion to normal urinary tract epithelial cells of *Escherichia coli* strains associated with various forms of urinary tract infection. *Lancet*, **ii**, 490–2.

Svanborg-Edén, C., *et al.* (1982). Inhibition of experimental ascending urinary tract infection by epithelial cell-surface analogue. *Nature*, **298**, 560–2.

Svanborg-Edén, C., *et al.* (1984). Influence of adhesins on the interaction of *Escherichia coli* with human phagocytes. *Infection and Immunity*, **44**, 672–80.

Tarkkanen, A-M., *et al.* (1992). Fimbriation, capsulation and iron-scavenging systems of Klebsiella strains associated with human urinary tract infection. *Infection and Immunity*, **60**, 1187–92.

Teague, N. and Boyarsky, S. (1968). Further effects of coliform bacteria on ureteral peristalsis. *Journal of Urology*, **99**, 720–4.

Thorley, J., Jones, S. R., and Sanford, J. P. (1974). Perinephric abscess. *Medicine*, **53**, 441–51.

Vaisanen, V., *et al.* (1981). Mannose-resistant haemagglutination and P antigen recognition are characteristic of *Escherichia coli* causing primary pyelonephritis. *Lancet*, **ii**, 1366–9.

Vaisanen-Rhen, V., Korhonen, T. K., and Finne, J. (1983) Novel cell-binding activity specific for *N*-acetyl-d-glucosamine in an *Escherichia coli* strain. *Science*, **159**, 233–6.

Varian, S. and Cooke, E. (1980). Adhesive properties of *Escherichia coli* from urinary tract infections. *Journal of Medical Microbiology*, **13**, 111–19.

Wallmark, G., Arremark, I., and Telander, B. (1978). *Staphylococcus saprophyticus*: a frequent cause of urinary tract infection among female outpatients. *Journal of Infectious Diseases*, **138**, 791–7.

Waters, W. E., Sussman, M., and Asscher, A. W. (1967). A community study of urinary pH and osmolality. *British Journal of Preventative and Social Medicine*, **21**, 129–32.

Welch, J., Pilkington, H., and Bradbeer, C. (1989). Urinary tract infections in men. *British Medical Journal*, **299**, 184.

Wolff, S. M. (1991). Monoclonal antibodies and the treatment of gram-negative bacteraemia and shock. *New England Journal of Medicine*, **324**, 486–7.

Zimmerli, W., Lew, P. D., and Walkvogel, F. A. (1984). Pathogenesis of foreign body infection. Evidence for a local granulocyte defect. *Journal of Clinical Investigation*, **73**, 1191–200.

3

Laboratory investigations in urinary tract infection

Richard Slack and David Greenwood

Introduction

Clinicians know that urinary tract infections (UTI) may present in a diverse or atypical manner. They also know that the critical requirement for the diagnosis of infection is the demonstration of microbes in the urine. Careful microbiological examination of urine samples from patients suspected of having UTI is thus essential in establishing the diagnosis. However, to a laboratory worker urine samples appear plentiful, homogeneous, easy to handle, and amenable to standardized 'factory methods'. Sheer numbers of samples and a low yield of positive results can all too easily diminish the lab workers' perception of the value of laboratory investigation of urine. Harmonizing these potentially different attitudes to the examination of urine is essential for effective laboratory investigation and successful clinical practice.

The size and nature of the laboratory workload

Examination of urine constitutes a large part of the workload of diagnostic microbiology laboratories in the United Kingdom and elsewhere. Nottingham Public Health Laboratory, which serves two 1200 bed teaching hospitals, several smaller units, and a local population of about 650 000, tests on average 150 000 urine specimens annually of which about 15 per cent are infected.

The reasons for requesting culture of urine are not always clearly identified to the laboratory. Table 3.1 shows an analysis of common reasons given on request cards sent with urine specimens to the Nottingham Diagnostic Laboratory.

For other hospital patients, for example those febrile individuals in whom bacteraemia is likely, culture of the urine is an important investigation for the localization of infection. In our hospital, the urine is the source of infection in over 50 per cent of patients with Gram-negative bacteraemia (Ispahani *et al.* 1987).

The value of a negative result is less clear. False negatives are probably common in the examination of urines from patients with UTI. Many specimens are collected for convenience during the middle of the day when the patient attends the clinic. Often this is during maximum diuresis which can reduce the count significantly (Cattell *et al.* 1970). Laboratory methods are often inadequate for detecting low numbers of bacteria and laboratories rarely attempt to isolate

Table 3.1 Reasons indicated on requests for urine culture received at Nottingham Public Health Laboratory

Reason	Requests (%)
Frequency-dysuria, acute UTI	36
Recurrent UTI	6
Abdominal pain, retention	9
Incontinence, enuresis	2
Pyrexia	4
Total (%)	(57)
Catheterized	9
Pregnancy	9
Routine screen	2
Total (%)	(20)
Renal failure	1
Hypertension/other medical conditions	5
Haematuria, proteinuria	11
Total (%)	(17)
No information	6

UTI, urinary tract infection.

unusual organisms. A negative result as part of a screening campaign may be meaningless if these factors are not considered.

A negative result in symptomatic patients may alter the perception of the value of urinalysis by clinicians. A survey conducted in the United Kingdom by the Public Health Laboratory Service (PHLS 1978) showed that only 14 per cent of general practitioners would stop antibiotic therapy on receipt of a negative culture report whereas nearly 50 per cent of hospital staff would react to a negative result. Many patients will be treated before the result could be known and indeed, some will have received antimicrobial agents before the specimen is collected!

The workload imposed on the microbiology laboratory in examining urine samples is enormous and, in many cases, unjustified (Table 3.1). To develop an optimum role for the laboratory in the investigation of UTI re-examination of the indications for and extent of laboratory investigations is required.

Indications for and extent of laboratory investigations

Increasing awareness of the cost–benefit of all forms of investigations must focus attention on the indications for and extent of laboratory examination of urine samples (Fowlis *et al.* 1994). Clearly this must take account of the diagnostic problem and must involve a dialogue between clinicians and microbiologists.

In the context of urinary tract infection, the primary question is usually 'does this patient have infection or not?' There are however supplementary questions:

'does treatment depend on and await the result of the laboratory investigation?'; 'will the result alter treatment?', 'will the investigation identify urinary tract abnormalities complicating urinary tract infection?'; 'does a negative culture exclude UTI?' In respect to the first two it is common practice for clinicians to commence treatment in acutely symptomatic patients prior to obtaining the results of a pre-treatment urine culture. This calls into question the value of sending urine samples in the first place. In respect to the last two, microscopy may be of more value than culture.

Review of the indications for sending urine samples to the laboratory must also raise the question as to the role of the doctor, nurse, or clinic assistant in carrying out 'on the spot' urine testing. What is the place of dip-stick testing for blood, protein, nitrite, and leucocyte esterase as a screening procedure? Should the doctor carry out microscopic examination of the urine in the surgery or clinic? Can such procedures reduce the need for and cost of laboratory investigations?

There is no general agreement on most of these points and indeed the problem is addressed elsewhere in this book (Chapter 6). There can be no simple universal answer as the need for and value of investigations vary with particular clinical circumstances. A mixture of routine chemical urinalysis in the surgery/clinic and despatch of selected urines to the laboratory would seem most sensible. Thus, in screening for asymptomatic bacteriuria in, for example, pregnant women or diabetics, routine urinalysis and culture of urine samples should suffice. In acutely symptomatic young women a pre-treatment urine sample for microscopy and culture is desirable as is a post-treatment urine examination to ensure eradication of infection and the absence of persisting pyuria. However, in practice, this is not always possible and for those women it is probably unnecessary, provided sticks testing is carried out before and after the acute episode. Of special importance are those women, or men, with recurrent symptoms suggestive of UTI who require careful pre- and post-treatment urine microscopy and culture. These patients must also be identified in the request form to the laboratory. Routine culture of urine samples from patients with long-standing indwelling bladder catheters, who are otherwise well, is a waste of laboratory resources.

Criteria for diagnosis of UTI

Urine culture

By convention, the diagnosis of urinary tract infection has required demonstration that bacteria are established in the bladder ('bladder bacteriuria'). Exceptions include totally obstructed, infected upper urinary tracts, bacterial prostatitis and, occasionally, renal or peri-renal abscess. It has long been recognized that the presence of bacteria in a midstream specimen of urine (MSU), particularly in women, may be the result of contamination of the urine by organisms present in the distal urethra or vulval area. The classic studies by Kass (1956) of quantitative urine culture were designed to distinguish between true bladder bacteriuria and contamination. These studies showed that in asymptomatic women and women with pyelonephritis a cut-off point of 10^5 or more of the same organism per ml of a clean-catch MSU identified true bladder bacteriuria (i.e. 'significant bacteriuria'). The finding of 10^5 bacteria per ml on one occasion gives a 70 per cent chance of significance which is increased to 95 per cent for two urines infected with the same strain. The neat division between contamination and 'significant bacteriuria' is shown in Fig. 3.1 adapted from Kass's work. Although this concept was designed for screening populations for asymptomatic bacteriuria it has subsequently been used to define significant bacteriuria in all patients with UTI.

Time and further study have cast serious doubt on the general application of this criterion, especially in symptomatic young women and in men. Thus, early studies of symptomatic women in general practice (Gallagher *et al.* 1965) suggested that less than 50 per cent had UTI on this criterion. Sequential studies of recurrently symptomatic women indicated that on occasion they had urine samples yielding more than 10^5 of the same organism per ml but on other occasions did not (O'Grady *et al.* 1973). Consideration of the hydrokinetic clearance of bladder bacteriuria in response to fluid loading clearly indicated the potential for lower bacterial counts in urine obtained from patients with genuine infection (Cattell *et al.* 1970).

Stemming from these observations there developed the concept of 'low count bacteriuria', studied in detail by Stamm and his colleagues in Seattle. There is

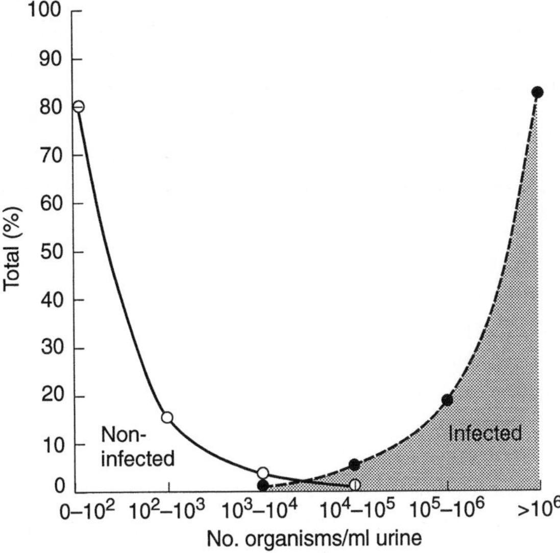

Fig. 3.1 Theoretical distribution of viable bacterial counts in early morning specimens of urine obtained from a large population of subjects with asymptomatic bacteriuria (●) and uninfected control (○). (From Asscher 1980.)

Table 3.2 Comparison of diagnostic tests of acute UTI in 187 patients

	Sensitivity	Specificity	Pred Value	
			Positive	Negative
Pyuria	0.91	0.50	0.67	0.83
MSU any coliform	1.00	0.71	0.79	1.00
$\geq 10^2$/ml	0.95	0.85	0.88	0.94
$\geq 10^5$/ml	0.51	0.99	0.98	0.65
Urethra + coliform	0.69	0.85	0.84	0.72
Vagina + coliform	0.81	0.73	0.77	0.77

MSU, midstream sample of urine.
(From Stamm *et al.* 1982.)

now considerable evidence for accepting lower bacterial counts as evidence of urinary infection in symptomatic women. Stamm *et al.* (1982) have proposed that a count of 10^2 or more of the same organism per ml of urine, if associated with pyuria (see below), can be taken as evidence of lower tract infection in symptomatic women with a sensitivity of 95 per cent and a specificity of 85 per cent (Table 3.2). Some have doubted the general application of this criterion (Kunin *et al.* 1993) but there has been no serious challenge to the concept that rigid adherence to a finding of 10^5 or more organisms per ml of urine is not necessary for the diagnosis of UTI in symptomatic women.

In men, the studies of Lipsky *et al.* (1987) have shown that a colony count of 10^3 or more of the same organism per ml of MSU urine has a sensitivity and specificity for true bacteriuria of 97 per cent.

The interpretation of urine culture results must, however, also take account of other factors.

Transient bacteriuria

It is highly probable that many symptomatic women may have transient bacteriuria, spontaneous clearance being achieved especially in association with a high fluid intake. Failure to obtain a urine culture early in the course of their illness may then miss bacteriuria (Cattell *et al.* 1975). Transient asymptomatic bacteriuria has also been demonstrated in relation to sexual intercourse and may represent transient 'colonization' of the bladder without tissue invasion (Buckley *et al.* 1978; Hooton *et al.* 1991).

Fluid intake

A high fluid intake with frequent voiding results in a dramatic fall in the urinary concentration of bacteria in infected women (Cattell *et al.* 1970). Samples obtained under such circumstances and especially when collected late in the day may yield only low bacterial counts. Ideally, samples should be obtained on first waking in the morning.

Strains of bacteria vary in their propensity to grow in urine and patients vary in their ability to clear organisms from the urinary tract. The hydrodynamic variables have been well studied using mathematical models and timed urine collections in patients at various stages of diuresis. Patients with anatomical abnormalities, for example a residual volume in the bladder over 20 ml, have difficulty in ridding the urinary tract of bacteria and counts rarely fall below 10^5 org/ml (Cattell *et al.* 1970).

Administration of antimicrobial drugs

The taking of such drugs prior to collection of an MSU will invalidate the results. This is especially likely to occur when patients self-treat with antibacterials 'left over' from a previous course of treatment. Surveys where urine has been tested for antimicrobial activity have shown the presence of antimicrobial agents in up to 16.5 per cent of urine samples, although the laboratory has often not been informed of any treatment (Pelling 1982).

Suprapubic aspiration of urine

The problem of interpreting 'low count bacteriuria' can be resolved by obtaining urine samples by suprapubic aspiration (SPA). Bladder urine is normally sterile. The recovery of any uropathogens in a sample obtained by SPA in symptomatic women indicates infection. This should always be carried out in symptomatic women in whom the results of culture of repeated MSU are equivocal. SPA is especially useful in the investigation of neonates and infants in whom 'clean-catch' urines are often unsatisfactory. SPA urine samples are collected at some inconvenience to the patient and clinician and should be treated with the same degree of care afforded to CSF samples. The specimen should be processed immediately or refrigerated if there is any delay. The urine should be inoculated on to a dried agar plate using a Pasteur dropping pipette or 0.1 ml spread over the surface. Such methods will detect 10^2 bacteria per ml with a degree of confidence.

Pyuria

Acceptance of quantitative urine culture as a gold standard for the diagnosis of UTI in the 1960s and the observation that not all patients with 'significant bacteriuria' had pyuria led to some workers dismissing the value of pyuria as an indicator of urinary infection. In part, this related to inaccurate methods for quantifying leucocytes in urine samples and, possibly, a failure to distinguish between asymptomatic often transient bacteriuria ('colonization') and symptomatic infection.

The presence of leucocytes in a clean-catch MSU may, as with bacteriuria, represent contamination of the sample by leucocytes from the urethra or introitus or may be due to an inflammatory reaction within the bladder as a consequence of bacterial invasion. The presence of large numbers of squamous epithelial cells on microscopy of urine samples is suggestive of contamination during collection. Many studies (reviewed by Stamm 1983) have shown a close correlation between 'significant bacteriuria' and the presence of 10 or more white blood cells per cubic mm in a fresh unspun urine sample. This cut-off point correlates with measurement of white cell excretion rates which is itself too cumbersome for routine use.

The need to identify pyuria has gained considerable relevance with the introduction of the concept of 'low count bacteriuria' in symptomatic women. Thus, the coexistence of pyuria and low bacterial counts of uropathogenic organisms in these women supports a diagnosis of infection rather than contamination.

In the majority of acutely symptomatic women white blood cell counts (WBC) of > 100 per mm^3 are commonly recorded. Lower counts ($\geqslant 10$ WBC per mm^2) are, however, significant. To identify confidently such low counts accurate methods are required to count leucocytes in urine samples. The widely used practice of expressing white blood cells per high-powered field in a centrifuged urine deposit has been shown to have a coefficient of variation of about 40 per cent, unless very carefully standardized (Stamm 1983). This method also correlates poorly with measurement of white cell excretion rates. In contrast, the counting of leucocytes in unspun urine samples in a haemocytometer correlates well with measured white cell excretion rates as does counting using an inverted microscope with a low-power objective and a microtitration tray or well slide (Mansell and Peacock 1973). The advent of automated systems may make this easier and less labour-intensive.

The finding of sterile pyuria (significant numbers of white cells with no significant bacterial growth) is itself important as an indicator of some urinary abnormality and must be confirmed with a repeat specimen unless an obvious cause is present such as concurrent administration of antibiotics.

Collection and transport of specimens

The reliability of the results of urine examination depend not only on laboratory expertise but on the care with which the specimen has been collected from the patient and maintained during transport to the laboratory. Examination of contaminated, old, or poorly preserved specimens is a waste of laboratory time. Urine should be collected before the administration of antimicrobial agents. If the patient is receiving any antimicrobial treatment this should be stated on the request form.

Specimen collection

Bladder urine is normally sterile but the anterior urethra is usually colonized with microorganisms. In the female, the periurethral area may be heavily colonized with bacteria including potential pathogens, and a substantial number of these organisms may enter the urine unless precautions are taken to prevent it. To minimize contamination in women, the external urethral orifice and the vulva

Table 3.3 Collection of mid-stream specimens of urine (MSSU)

Female

- The patient's bladder should be full (desperate to go).
- The patient removes underpants and stands over the toilet pan.
- The labia are separated using the left hand.
- The vulva is cleansed front to back with sterile swabs.
- The patient voids downward into the toilet and continues until 'half-done'.
- Without stopping the urine flow the sterile container is plunged into the stream of urine with the right hand. Only a small volume is required.
- The patient then completes voiding into the toilet.

Male

- The patient's bladder should be full.
- The foreskin, if present, is retracted.
- The glans penis is cleaned with a sterile swab.
- The patient voids into the toilet until 'half-done'.
- Without stopping the urine flow, the sterile container is plunged into the stream of urine.
- The patient then completes voiding into the toilet.

should be rinsed thoroughly with soap and water and dried. The use of disinfectants must be avoided. The labia should be held wide apart throughout voiding. The first portion of urine, which flushes the urethra, is discarded and, *without stopping*, a midstream sample should be obtained (Table 3.3). In males, the foreskin should be fully retracted and the glans penis may or may not be washed with soap and water. A midstream sample is again obtained. Urine samples should be collected in a sterile disposable container or directly into a sterile specimen bottle. Ideally, samples should be collected if possible early in the morning before the washout effect of drinking fluid.

In elderly or obese women, and those in ethnic groups who may have a poor understanding of English, nurse assistance may be required to obtain satisfactory samples. Diagrams illustrating correct methods for collecting a midstream sample may be of value.

A properly collected MSU is adequate for most diagnostic purposes. Catheterization carries a risk of introducing organisms into the bladder and should be avoided unless required for other reasons. In patients at the extremes of age, from whom it may be difficult to obtain a satisfactory midstream specimen, suprapubic needle aspiration of bladder urine after antiseptic cleansing of the skin is a safe and effective way of obtaining an uncontaminated sample. In some obese patients SPA may be guided by ultrasonography.

Transport of specimens

As a counsel of perfection, urine should be examined within one hour of collection. Delay may result in the proliferation of contaminant bacteria, the death of fastidious microorganisms, and the deterioration of cellular constituents. In practice, it is not usually possible to examine the urine immediately in which case it should be refrigerated as soon as possible. Most urinary pathogens will remain viable without significant multiplication if held at 4 °C although white cells, red cells, and casts may not be well preserved. With adequate refrigeration, urines can be reliably examined bacteriologically 24 hours after collection. Specimens more than 48 hours old should be regarded as unsatisfactory.

An alternative method of preserving urine for microbiological examination is by the use of chemical agents. Boric acid has a long history of use in this way and is satisfactory provided the concentration is strictly controlled at 1.8 per cent w/v (Porter and Brooke 1969). There are obvious difficulties in ensuring that this is achieved in practice. Prepared universal containers are manufactured to overcome some of these problems.

The simplest and most effective way of avoiding problems of bacterial overgrowth during transportation is by the use of dip-inoculum methods. In this technique, urine is passed over, or applied to, a suitable culture medium accommodated on sterile spoons (Mackey and Sandys 1965), slides (Guttman and Naylor 1967), or as slants (Greenwood and Slack 1982) in specimen bottles. The medium absorbs a finite amount of urine and bacteria, deposited on the agar surface, grow into colonies. Use of differential media facilitates identification and the recognition of mixed growths. Commercial versions of the test are widely available. Since the culture is made as soon as the specimen is passed, problems in delay of examination are effectively circumvented. However, optimal growth conditions are unlikely to be provided during transport and the samples still need to be incubated before examination in the laboratory. It is important to note that the laboratory does not receive the patient's urine if this method is used so that microscopy and chemical testing cannot be carried out. If microscopy or other tests are required, a separate request must be made and sent with the appropriate specimen.

The shelf life of these various dip-slides/spoons is limited. Before use they should be checked to ensure the medium has not deteriorated or separated.

Special procedures

Localization studies

During the 1960s and 1970s there was considerable interest in studies designed to localize the site of infection within the urinary tract. Most accurate was the relatively invasive method developed by Stamey and colleagues (Meares and Stamey 1968) which involved ureteric catheterization following cystoscopy and bladder washout. A more simple technique was introduced by Fairley *et al.* (1967) in which the catheterized bladder was rinsed with a 1 per cent solution of neomycin plus Elase (a proprietary mixture of fibrinolysin and deoxyribonuclease).

Various other methods have been proposed as indicators of kidney involvement. These include: the detection of serum antibody titres against the infecting organism (Percival *et al.* 1964); the antibody-coated bacteria test (Thomas *et al.* 1974); the excretion of β_2-microglobulin (Schardijn *et al.* 1979); and the demonstration of lactic acid dehydrogenase, or other low molecular weight proteins. The first two of these tests are potentially specific for bacterial infection while the remainder are merely non-specific indicators of renal damage. None of these tests is free from interpretive difficulties as an indicator of upper tract involvement in urinary infection, and none has proved sufficiently useful to warrant use as a routine procedure.

Prostatic infection

In the male, infection may involve or be confined to the prostate. Meares and Stamey (1968) devised a technique which seeks to differentiate urethral, prostatic, and bladder infection. The first portion of urine (ca 10 ml) is collected and designated 'voided bladder 1' (VB-1); a midstream specimen is then collected (VB-2). The patient then stops micturating and a sample of prostatic secretion is collected by prostatic massage (expressed prostatic secretion; EPS). Finally, the patient continues to empty the bladder and the first portion passed after prostatic massage is collected (VB-3). All four specimens are examined by microscopy and by quantitative culture. Interpretation of the results is discussed in Chapter 13.

Urethral and vaginal swabs/smears

Symptoms due to urethritis or vaginitis may mimic those of 'cystitis'. In one study, 10 of 16 sexually active young women with frequency/dysuria who had sterile pyuria were shown to be infected with *Chlamydia trachomatis* (Stamm *et al.* 1980). Collection of high vaginal or urethral swabs/smears is standard practice in departments of genitourinary medicine but rarely done by clinicians dealing with suspected UTI. There is much to commend taking such samples particularly in symptomatic young women with pyuria and sterile urine cultures.

The flora of the normal vagina does not normally include aerobic uropathogens. However, colonization of the vagina with *Escherichia coli* is recognized to precede and be associated with UTI. Persistent colonization may predispose to recurrent infections. This may be especially important in post-menopausal women with hormone deficiency vaginitis (Raz and Stamm 1993) and women using the diaphragm plus spermicidal jelly (Hooton *et al.* 1991). Identifying persistent vaginal carriers of *E. coli*, save for research purposes, is not part of normal practice. Why this is so is unclear and it would appear to be an area requiring more detailed evaluation.

Organisms causing urinary tract infection

Common pathogens

Urinary tract infection whether acquired in the community or in hospital is most commonly caused by *E. coli*. This reflects the predominance of *E. coli* in the aerobic flora of the gut, from whence organisms commonly causing urinary infection generally originate. Any of the numerous O (somatic), H (flagellar), and K (capsular) antigenic types of *E. coli* may be involved but those belonging to serogroups 02, 04, 06, 07, 08, 018, and 085 are more common than others (Grüneberg *et al.* 1968). Other properties including the possession of fimbriae (associated with the ability to adhere to the uroepithelium), haemolysins, and K antigens are also more commonly exhibited by strains of *E. coli* isolated from infected urine (Brooks *et al.* 1980) but no one factor nor combination of factors is strongly correlated with the ability to cause infection (O'Grady 1979). Microbial factors in the pathogenesis of UTI are dealt with in Chapter 2.

Other bacteria that are commonly involved in urinary tract infection in domiciliary practice are *Klebsiella aerogenes*, *Proteus mirabilis*, *Enterococcus (Streptococcus) faecalis*, and *Staphylococcus saprophyticus*. The latter organism is particularly prevalent in infection in young women. In patients in hospital a much more varied range of organisms may be found. Types encountered may include a wide variety of coliform organisms, *Pseudomonas* (notably *P. aeruginosa*), staphylococci, streptococci, and yeasts (notably *Candida albicans*). Mixed infections are uncommon except in patients with indwelling catheters, anatomical abnormalities of the urinary tract, or urinary calculi.

The spectrum of organisms isolated in Nottingham Public Health Laboratory during a three-month period from urine samples submitted from hospital patients, women attending an antenatal clinic, and patients presenting to general practitioners, is shown in Table 3.4. Differences in the incidence of various pathogens found in males and females of different age groups have been analysed by Maskell (1982) (Table 3.5).

Organisms that possess the ability to split urea, notably *Proteus* spp., *Klebsiella* spp. staphylococci, and certain corynebacteria (group D2), render the urine highly alkaline and create conditions favourable to the precipitation of magnesium ammonium phosphate (struvite). These organisms are therefore often implicated in struvite stone formation in the bladder, particularly in catheterized patients.

Fastidious organisms

As mentioned previously, using a criterion of 10^5 or more of the same organism per ml of urine as evidence of significant bacteriuria, some 50 per cent of symptomatic women do not have infection (Gallagher *et al.* 1965). Such women were labelled as having the 'urethral syndrome'. It is now clear that the majority of such women have bladder infection with 'low count bacteriuria' and pyuria (Stamm *et al.* 1980). However, if urine samples taken from such women are

Table 3.4 Resistance to selected antimicrobial agents among 4357 bacteria isolated between November 1987 and January 1988 in the Nottingham Public Health Laboratory

Agent	Break-point	Percentage of isolates resistant													
		E. coli		*Klebsiella* spp.		*Proteus* spp.		Other Gram-neg. bacilli		Enterococci		Staphylococci		Streptococci	
		Hosp	Comm	Hosp	Comm	Hosp	Comm	Hosp	Comm	Hosp	Comm	Hosp	Comm	Hosp	Comm
Ampicillin	10	48	42	92	87	28	10	95	95	1	0	87	83	3	0
Sulphonamides	128	36	25	21	17	11	4	15	10	100	82	30	6	44	31
Trimethoprim	5	18	15	17	11	22	12	12	18	6	2	29	8	6	6
Nitrofurantoin	50	4	5	26	13	99	100	18	19	0	0	0	0	3	0
Nalidixic acid	10	3	1	7	3	3	2	3	2	100	100	100	100	100	100
Cephalexin	16	14	13	29	33	31	16	45	80	97	100	15	0	49	36
Number		1347	1424	233	141	290	156	60	38	176	71	172	143	79	27
															4357

Hosp, hospital inpatients; Comm, community (general practice + antenatal clinic).

Table 3.5 Age and sex differences in the isolation of various organisms from UTI in domiciliary practice

	Number of isolates in each age and sex category*							
	0–15 years		16–35 years		36–55 years		>55 years	
Organism	M	F	M	F	M	F	M	F
Escherichia coli	15	108	10	192	26	114	42	102
Proteus spp.	17	9	2	15	3	12	7	15
Klebsiella spp.	0	2	0	3	0	5	5	7
Staphylococci	2	6	0	36	2	3	1	1
Other organisms	7	12	3	17	3	14	16	13
Total	41	137	15	263	34	148	71	138

*Organisms isolated over a three-month period, January–March 1976 in Portsmouth Public Health Laboratory. M, male; F, female. (From Maskell 1982.)

subjected to prolonged culture or if culture is carried out under microaerophilic or anaerobic conditions, significant counts of organisms with more demanding growth requirements can be recovered from a substantial number of specimens. Organisms that have been recognized in this way include lactobacilli, corynebacteria, microaerophilic streptococci, *Haemophilus* spp., *Gardnerella vaginalis*, *Ureaplasma ureolyticum*, and various anaerobes. Chlamydia and neisseria are not commonly isolated from urine even under appropriate conditions although these organisms may, of course, cause urethritis.

The significance of fastidious organisms isolated from urine has been the subject of much debate. The arguments for and against an aetiological role for these organisms have been rehearsed by Maskell (1986) and Hamilton-Miller and his colleagues (1986). In general, it seems safe to conclude that all of these fastidious bacteria are occasionally found as true aetiological agents although the role of lactobacilli as the putative cause of frequency and dysuria in the absence of conventional urinary pathogen (the so-called 'urethral syndrome') in young women remains doubtful.

Viruses

Viruria can be demonstrated in many viral diseases but is generally an incidental excretory manifestation of a viraemic phase of infection. Renal complications are associated with haemorrhagic fever caused by viruses of the Hantaan group and herpes simplex may invade the urethra and perhaps even the bladder. These circumstances apart, no convincing evidence has yet been presented for the involvement of viruses in urinary tract infection and virological examination of urine is rarely useful to diagnose UTI although it is of value for cytomegalovirus (CMV) infection in immunocompromised patients.

Laboratory methods

General

Examination of urine has fascinated physicians from the time of Hippocrates and has played a major part in the diagnosis of many medical conditions. Depiction of the physician 'water-gazing' abound in paintings, particularly those of the fifthteenth to seventeenth centuries (Wershub 1970) (Fig. 3.2). Early 'water doctors' had to rely on simple inspection of colour and clarity, smell, and taste of the urine. These characteristics may still be used at the bedside to assist clinicians. If on macroscopic inspection the urine appears crystal clear there is a 95 per cent predicted value for a negative result on urine culture. However, because of the frequent presence of crystals, a cloudy urine is not necessarily likely to yield significant bacteriuria. Acidification with 2 per cent acetic acid will remove much of this debris but to confirm UTI, microscopy and urine culture is required.

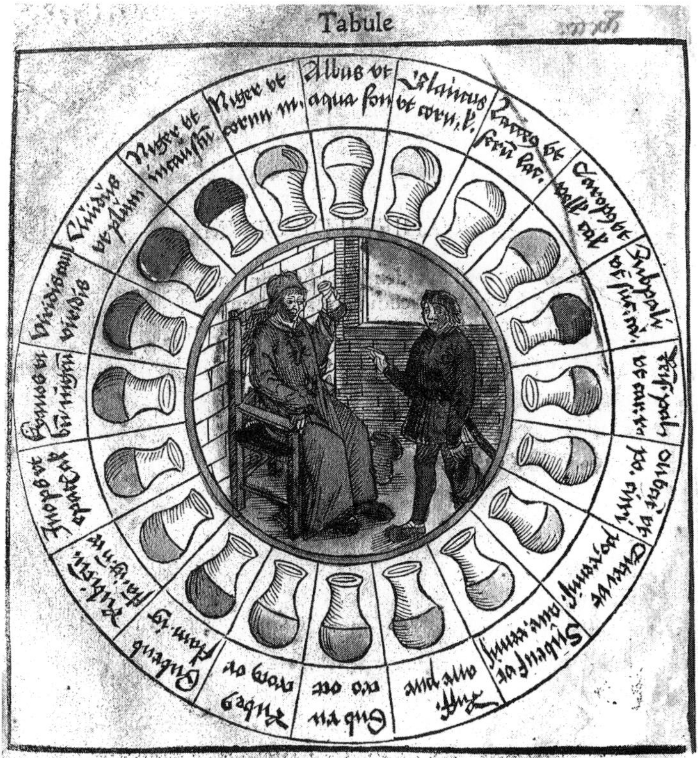

Fig. 3.2 Water gazing (Wellcome Institute, London)

Chemical testing

Testing for commonly found analytes is an important part of the examination of urine at the bedside and in the clinic. In the past, before the advent of filter-paper strips impregnated with reagents, this was a time-consuming process often left to junior nurses or medical students. Many potentially dangerous chemicals were mixed in side rooms or corners of clinics with potentially infectious clinical specimens. There is probably no case for this form of 'home chemistry' to return to clinical settings, as simple test kits suitable for use in the ward, clinic, or surgery (or even by the patients themselves) have been developed. Modern practitioners, who are being increasingly pressured by the manufacturers of these diagnostic reagents, should remember that safety standards and quality control are as important by the bedside as in the laboratory.

Protein

Urinary protein, usually albumin, which used to be determined by precipitation with sulphosalicylic acid, can be tested by sticks such as Albustix (Ames). These methods are sufficiently specific and sensitive to detect a glomerular leak of plasma proteins but will not measure bacterial protein. A patient may therefore have significant bacteriuria and remain negative for protein. Conversely, many non-infective medical conditions give rise to proteinuria.

Nitrites

Most Gram-negative bacteria reduce nitrate to nitrite. The Griess test is based on detecting nitrite either using freshly prepared reagents (sulphanilic acid and α-naphthylamine in acetic acid) or a commercial dipstick (Ames; Boehringer Mannheim). False positives are rare in freshly voided samples as nitrite is not found in sufficient concentration without bacteriuria. However, delay in testing contaminated non-refrigerated samples may yield false positive results. The principal disadvantage of the nitrite test is its relatively low sensitivity. Early morning or concentrated urines should be tested to detect nitrite as a significant period for incubation in the bladder is required. Some uropathogens such as enterococci and *Staph. saprophyticus* do not reduce nitrate. Some diets may lack sufficient nitrate although this is not usually a problem. Occasionally, other constituents in urine, such as ascorbic acid, may interfere with the test and give false negative results.

Leucocyte esterase

This enzyme, unique to neutrophils, can be detected chemically by a colour reaction. This has been incorporated into a dipstick test combined with nitrite determination (Chemstrip LN, Boehringer Mannheim). The sensitivity has been adjusted to correlate with careful microscopy—a change in colour indicates 10 or more leucocytes per mm^3. Positive reactions with both tests on fresh urine samples give a high predictive value of UTI but false negatives will sometimes occur, especially if the specimen is taken during a diuretic phase.

Practical use

Although each test by itself has a poor predictive value in diagnosing UTI, used in combination, they are much better at screening out negative urines. A urine clear to the naked eye and negative on both nitrite and leucocyte esterase testing is 99 per cent certain of being uninfected. New screening methods may potentially save laboratory resources and be cost-effective.

Direct microscopy

Microscopy of the urine may be performed directly without staining or centrifugation on a standard glass slide or a well-slide (Mansell and Peacock 1973). These simple methods are laborious and inaccurate but these disadvantages can be partly overcome by the use of an inverted microscope and a microtitration tray with a low-power objective. In this way a relatively large volume (100 μl) may be counted quickly. Leucocyte counts correlate with those obtained using a haemocytometer (Mansell and Peacock 1973).

The standard method used in many centres is to centrifuge a well-mixed urine sample at 3000 g for 5 minutes and count the number of cells per high power field (hpf). At least 5 fields should be counted. More than 5 white blood cells per hpf is taken to indicate pyuria. This method is, however, inaccurate and the results correlate poorly with white cell excretion rates. In contrast, leucocyte counts carried out on unspun fresh samples of urine using a haemocytometer do correlate well with timed white cell excretion rates.

Pyuria

Pyuria is abnormal and indicates inflammation within the urinary tract. Inflammation may or may not be due to infection also being associated with the presence of stones, interstitial nephritis (including analgesic nephropathy), the presence of foreign bodies, etc. Persisting pyuria following successful treatment of urinary infection must always raise the suspicion of some underlying abnormality in the urinary tract. 'Sterile pyuria' must still focus attention on the possibility of renal tuberculosis.

Microscopy may also identify other abnormalities such as microscopic haematuria or the presence of urinary casts. Whether microscopy to identify these, in suspected cases, is the role of the laboratory or should be done by the clinician is debatable.

Care must be taken in not confusing pyuria with the excretion of malignant cells or renal tubular cells in the urine.

Whether microscopic examination should be carried out on all urine samples sent to the laboratory is debatable. This is particularly so in samples sent specifically to exclude infection in asymptomatic patients in whom Stix testing has been negative. Microscopy cannot be carried out if only dip-slides/spoons are sent to the laboratory.

Stained deposits

Gram stain of a urine deposit provides a simple test for the diagnosis of UTI. The method is, however, labour-intensive and does not accurately correlate with bacteriuria assessed by culture techniques. Attempts have recently been made to automate the process and correlate it with bacterial culture. A machine to stain and read urines by Gram (Bac-T-Screen) and by using acridine dyes to distinguish human and bacterial DNA (Lipsky *et al.* 1985) is undergoing trials.

Direct culture

The demonstration of significant numbers of bacteria in clean-catch MSU is essential for the confident diagnosis of urinary tract infection. Culture of a causal organism also permits testing for sensitivity to antibacterial agents.

Media

Simple nutrient agar, particularly if enriched with sheep or horse blood, will allow the growth of most urinary pathogens but media selective for Enterobacteriaceae which will stop Proteus from swarming are preferable. MacConkey's bile salt agar (MacConkey 1908) meets these criteria and also allows the differentiation of lactose and non-lactose fermenting organisms. However, the frequent variations in selectivity between batches of MacConkey agar makes it far from ideal for performing viable counts to quantify coliforms in urine, to note contamination and to observe colonial morphology. Different approaches to this dilemma have been taken on each side of the Atlantic. In the United States various types of media are used for isolation and identification but sheep blood agar is usually retained for quantification. In the United Kingdom, CLED (cystine-lactose electrolyte-deficient medium) developed by Mackey and Sandys (1966) is widely used as the sole plate for urine bacteriology. CLED medium (Oxoid CM301) has all the advantages of MacConkey agar and is not so inhibitory. Full details have been described by Sandys (1978). CLED supports the growth of relatively fastidious organisms (Maskell 1982) if incubated in 7 per cent carbon dioxide. As with all media preparation, attention to detail in autoclaving and adjustment of pH is critical. *Proteus* spp. may begin to swarm on poorly prepared media and the growth of streptococci may be inadequate. CLED is a good medium for surface viable counting as colonial size of Enterobacteriaceae after overnight incubation is not as large as on blood agar yet sufficient to allow good differentiation between genera.

Inoculation

Whether or not one accepts rigidly Kass's criteria for significant bacteriuria it is still necessary to estimate bacterial numbers in urine. The standard method is to inoculate the surface of the agar plate with a fixed volume of urine which is adequately spread or diluted so that individual colony-forming units (CFUs) can be counted after incubation. The simplest and most common method is the use of a calibrated bacteriological loop. Loops can be calibrated by use of a dye-dilution method in which the colour produced by a loopful of dye (accurately measured photometrically) is compared with a known standard. Loops made in this way should be soldered to maintain their volume. Alternatively, disposable standard plastic loops can be purchased. An economical variant of this method involves use of a multipoint inoculator to inoculate plates which can then be read automatically by a digitalized camera scanner such as Mastascan (Mast Laboratories Ltd).

Most of the loop methods are at best semi-quantitative as a small volume of sample is taken without duplicates and the viscosity of the urine will affect the volume delivered. Most infected urines have counts of 10^6 CFU/ml or greater and the results by these techniques are satisfactory.

However, low counts (below 10^4 CFU/ml) cannot be detected as the volume inoculated is often as low as 0.001 ml. Accuracy may only be achieved by using a 'pour plate' in which a serial dilution of urine in saline is added to molten agar and well mixed. This method is expensive in time and reagants and is thus not suited to routine screening. If 'low count bacteriuria' is suspected and especially in patients with recurrent or persisting symptoms, the laboratory should be specifically asked to undertake 'pour plate' methods. Conversely, a urine sample should be obtained by suprapubic aspiration.

Atmospheric conditions

It is normal practice in clinical microbiology laboratories to incubate all plates aerobically at 35–37 °C overnight (18–20 hours). Culture for fastidious and unusual organisms involves use of a carbon dioxide incubator providing an atmosphere of 5–7 per cent CO_2, microaerophilic or anaerobic conditions and prolonged incubation for up to 7 days. The consensus view at present (Hamilton-Miller *et al.* 1986) does not appear to favour routine use of this approach except in patients with conditions, such as renal abscesses, which may well contain anaerobes or microaerophilic streptococci.

Sexually transmitted diseases, such as gonorrhoea and chlamydial urethritis, may be diagnosed by isolation of the pathogen from spun urine deposits on chocolate agar or cycloheximide treated McCoy cells. The best results however are obtained by culture of samples taken directly from the anterior urethra in males and the cervix in females. Both organisms commonly causing urethritis, *N. gonorrhoeae* and *C. trachomatis*, are delicate microbes that require careful specimen handling and transport. Swabs should be placed immediately into special media and processed as soon as possible. Gonococci survive for a few hours in bacteriological transport media (for example Stuart's) with added charcoal to inactivate toxic substances. Chlamydia need different conditions and specimens should be placed in a special transport medium which is similar to a viral medium without antibiotics. However, because *C. trachomatis* is heat-labile, refrigeration or freezing is essential if there is to be a delay before cell culture inoculation. Because of these constraints, non-cultural methods are increasingly used. Antigen detection by immunoassay (e.g. ELISA) of urine is becoming a popular non-invasive method for the diagnosis of chlamydial infection. Amplified gene probe methods (e.g. PCR and LCR) have undergone clinical studies and will become more widely available although the cost may constrain widespread use.

Identification

The methods used to identify significant bacterial isolates to genus or species level are identical to those used in any diagnostic microbiology laboratory and can be found in standard texts (Cowan 1974; Edwards and Ewing 1972; Collee *et al.* 1989; Murray *et al.* 1995). The difficult decision is how far should such an identification be taken given the constraints of time and cost. To the clinician dealing with an acutely symptomatic patient, the identity of the uropathogen is of less concern than its antimicrobial susceptibility. In contrast, in order to distinguish between relapse and re-infection it is necessary not only to identify the isolate to species level but to perform additional tests such as serotyping. As a compromise many laboratories identify all urinary pathogens to the genus level (e.g. *Proteus*, *Klebsiella*, etc.). The 'antibiograms'—the antimicrobial sensitivity profile—will also aid recognition. All typing methods are better at selecting differences between organisms rather than identifying that bacteria are identical. If two indistinguishable strains are found on separate occasions from the same individual a relapse of UTI is likely. This should point the clinician to investigate for some underlying pathology of the urinary tract (Murray *et al.* 1995). If similar organisms are found from a cluster of patients in hospital, cross-infection should be suspected.

Another advantage of bacterial identification is to aid in predicting antimicrobial susceptibilities. Thus, *Pseudomonas aeruginosa* has intrinsic resistance to many oral antimicrobial agents and nitrofurans are always ineffective against *Proteus* spp. because of urinary alkalinization. In addition, in cases of Gram-negative bacteraemia the identity of the blood culture isolate can be compared with that from the urine. Confirmation of similarity is evidence of the source of the bacteraemia.

Indirect methods

Blood culture

Blood cultures are regularly carried out in ill febrile patients and may give a clue to the presence of urinary infection. Thus, approximately half the episodes of Gram-negative bacteraemia in hospital practice are secondary to infection of the urinary tract (Ispahani *et al.* 1987).

Methods used vary between laboratories and automated techniques (e.g. BacTec) employing commercially available specimen bottles are becoming more common. Whichever method is available there are three important principles in taking blood for culture. First, a good aseptic technique including careful skin disinfection; secondly, taking an adequate volume of blood (10 ml); and thirdly, rapid transport to an incubator. Duplicate samples should be taken at a separate venepuncture.

Antibody test

Serum agglutinins to *Escherichia coli* antigens have been used to distinguish between upper and lower urinary tract infection (Percival *et al.* 1964). Unfortunately, the unreliable nature of serum responses to gut flora have made this a poor predictor. Urinary antibodies to infecting strains may be used to screen samples. If a common pool of coliform antigens is used the test can show past or present contact with uropathogens. Enzyme immunoassays (ELISA) are relatively cheap and easy to automate and have been used to screen for UTI (McGowan *et al.* 1991).

Infecting strains may become coated with host antibody. It was thought that the antibody-coated bacteria test would readily distinguish upper from lower urinary tract infection. If quantification is performed this may improve the correlation.

Calculi

Although only a minority of renal stones are infected the presence of an infected calculus may cause serious problems and is a major cause for relapsing bacteriuria. As bacteriuria is usually present it is rarely necessary to isolate bacteria from stones passed spontaneously or removed by the surgeon. It may, however, be valuable in determining whether prior therapy has sterilized the calculus. For bacteriological examination, stones removed at surgery are washed three times in phosphate-buffered saline and then crushed using a sterile pestle and mortar. Some of the chippings are then placed in liquid media (brain heart infusion and thioglycollate broths) and on agar plates to exclude laboratory contamination. Previous treatment with antimicrobials often reduces the bacterial numbers on the surface of the stone but viable organisms can be cultivated from the crushed calculus. *Proteus mirabilis*, the commonest cause of infective stones, may, like other enterobacteria, exist in a cell wall deficient form after treatment with a β-lactam antibiotic. These can be recovered from media of high osmolality (> 400 mOsm/kg). In addition to *P. mirabilis* other *Proteus* species, staphylococci, klebsiellae, and, occasionally, *Pseudomonas aeruginosa* and other Gram-negative bacteria may be isolated.

Automated methods

Apart from the automation of inoculation and reading of surface counts described above, there are a variety of new methods, usually employing expensive machines, which can take the tedium out of urine examination and, if used to full capacity, reduce staff requirements. Technical manipulation is minimal but so is technician satisfaction. These large expensive and impersonal machines are often rigidly programmed so that user-flexibility is lost. Most new methods depend on detection of organisms by one of the following:

(1) turbidimetry;
(2) bioluminescence;
(3) filtration and staining;
(4) particle counting.

Turbidimetry

Although many infected urines are turbid to the naked eye this simple test is not sufficiently accurate. A change in turbidity after incubation of urine diluted into a fluid growth medium correlates well with initial bacterial numbers although slow-growing organisms may be missed. This principle has been used in commercial instruments designed for antibiotic sensitivity testing: Autobac, AutoMicrobic (Vitek), Abbot, and Cobas systems. It is usually necessary to incubate the specimen for at least 5 hours to obtain a satisfactory result.

Bioluminescence

Minute quantities of ATP may be assayed by using the firefly luciferase system. Endogenous mammalian ATP is first removed before bacterial ATP can be measured. There are commercial systems developed using the principle of bioluminescence: Lumac, Monolight, and Amerlite. These methods are expensive in capital outlay and reagents and involve more technical time and expertise than automated turbidimetry.

Filtration and staining

This method is a sophisticated and automated method of direct microscopy. A fixed volume of urine is passed through a filter which is then stained either with safranin (Bac-T-Screen) or acridine orange (Autotrak) (Lipsky *et al.* 1985). The main practical problem is the interpretation of contamination (false positives). It will be possible in the future to use probes for bacterial DNA linked to a colorimetric system to hybridize with filtered urine. In this system, DNA specific for *E. coli* is covalently linked to a colour-generating system. Urine is filtered on to a nitrocellulose membrane and heated to split bacterial DNA adherent to the membrane. Labelled DNA is then added and 'hybridizes' to the split DNA on the filter. After washing, the concentration of *E. coli* DNA is measured on a colorimetric system. At present, this system is not sensitive enough to detect less than 10^5 org/ml (Carter *et al.* 1989). Although amplification systems will overcome this problem they will be too expensive for routine use.

Particle counting

The Coulter Channelyser is a particle counter which measures size, distribution, and numbers of particles passing through a narrow orifice by their altering the electrical current across it. This machine, designed for haematology, has been used to count microorganisms. Most bacteria are at the limit of detection with the standard 100 μm orifice and smaller holes tend to block easily. Improvements in handling the signals produced by these particle counters have led to the development of a commercial machine (Ramus) which counts both white cells and bacteria simultaneously using the 100 μm orifice (Alexander *et al.* 1981).

Fluorescent cell sorters (FACS) have the potential to count and size bacteria and white cells but have not been used commercially for this purpose because of expense and the amount of technical time necessary to process samples.

Limitations of automated methods

There are other physicochemical methods which can be used to detect bacteriuria such as electrical impedence, radiometry, and calorimetry. However, all the automated methods described have to satisfy a few simple criteria before they can be adopted by a clinical microbiology laboratory. Does the method save in cost? Are the savings in time of any value to the clinician and patient? Does the method distinguish between genuine bacteriuria and contamination? All that the methods can achieve at present is to screen out negative urines so that the 10–20 percent of potentially infected samples may be cultured by conventional means. For a large laboratory, there will often be a saving in time and cost provided staff can be redeployed and the work can be organized around the equipment—a real case of the machine running the person. These large capital developments beg the question; should we be examining all these urines anyway? Bedside screening using a dipstick method such as nitrite/leucocyte esterase is an attractive alternative. At least the result is available to the patient while in the clinic and may be of direct value in deciding management.

Antibiotic susceptibility testing

Testing of urinary isolates for sensitivity or resistance to antimicrobial drugs is part of every laboratory's stock in trade but it is doubtful whether it is necessary or helpful in many cases. Many urinary tract infections in domiciliary practice are treated successfully without seeking laboratory help. Treatment is normally offered at the time of the initial consultation so that when specimens are sent for laboratory investigation the patient is usually free of symptoms by the time culture and sensitivity results are available. In hospital, where there is more available access to the laboratory and patients more commonly suffer from intractable or difficult infections with resistant organisms, routine susceptibility testing is of more value. Testing does provide valuable data from both hospital and community settings on the prevalence of resistance—information which is useful in guiding primary therapy.

Antimicrobial susceptibility can be tested by any of the standard methods (Reeves *et al.* 1978; Lorian 1986). A restricted number of agents covering the commonly used oral compounds and reflecting local prescribing policies should be tested. Other agents need only be tested in selected cases.

The logistics of a busy service laboratory generally dictate that the method chosen should be rapid, simple, and economical. A convenient technique for laboratories handling large numbers of urinary isolates is the 'break-point' method in which cultures are spot-inoculated on to the surface of agar plates containing single concentrations of antimicrobial agents corresponding to the level at which organisms should be considered to be resistant (Waterworth 1981).

If the organism fails to grow at the chosen break-point it is reported as susceptible. If it grows it is considered resistant. Much controversy surrounds the choice of suitable break-points which are to some extent method-dependent. A working party of the British Society for Antimicrobial Chemotherapy (1991) has suggested break-points for most agents in common use but these refer principally to systemic infection. Higher values may be appropriate for infections that are confined to the urinary tract and for testing agents that are excreted in high concentration by the renal route.

Primary antibiotic sensitivity testing may be carried out on the initial urine culture. The break-point method has been used for such direct testing of infected urine but yields are very variable and sometimes there may be a mixed inoculum (Cheetham and Brown 1986). Alternatively, bacterial isolates are grown in broth until the culture is faintly turbid (10^7 CFU/ml) and 1 microlitre of this suspension is deposited on to the surface of each antibiotic-containing plate (inoculum 10^4 CFU per spot). The inoculum can be standardized more precisely by use of turbidity standards but this is not essential since inoculum effects are generally not pronounced when surface inoculation methods are used. The labour of inoculation can be considerably reduced by use of replicating devices, such as the Steers' replicator (Cheetham and Brown 1986), or an automatic multipoint inoculating device, such as the Denley inoculator (Denley Instruments Ltd, Billingshurst, Sussex, UK). Culture media should be free from inhibitors, notably thymidine, which interferes with the activity of trimethoprim and sulphonamides. Lysed horse blood contains thymidine phosphorylase, which eliminates this problem (Ferone *et al.* 1975). A semi-defined medium that is free from inhibitors and has been specifically designed for susceptibility testing is Iso-Sensitest agar (Oxoid CM 471). This has been widely used in the United Kingdom, where it has performed better than Mueller Hinton medium in quality control surveys (Snell *et al.* 1982; 1984). Since Iso-Sensitest agar is formulated to be free of inhibitors it is not necessary to supplement it with lysed blood but it is, nevertheless, advantageous to do this since the blood improves the nutritional properties and also enhances the background contrast which is helpful in reading the plates.

Spot-inoculated susceptibility test plates can be read with automatic plate scanning devices and labour can be further reduced by linking the output to computerized reporting systems.

Table 3.4 (p. 45) shows the break-points used for agents routinely tested in Nottingham Public Health Laboratory and shows results obtained with 4357 unselected urinary isolates tested over a three-month period.

Experimental models of UTI

Bladder models

The idea of constructing laboratory models of infection and its treatment has obvious attractions. The peculiar features of urinary tract infection, especially infection confined to the bladder, makes it a particularly suitable subject for *in vitro* modelling. In the infected urinary bladder, bacteria growing in the urine (which itself provides a highly variable substrate) are subjected to continuous dilution by the constant in-flow of ureteric urine. They are also periodically expelled when the patient micturates. The rate of production of urine is subject to diurnal variation and is affected by fluid intake. The frequency with which the patient micturates is also affected by diuresis and is commonly increased in cystitis. During treatment with antimicrobial agents, the bacterial population, which often exceeds the numbers used in conventional laboratory tests even when 'dense inocula' are used, is exposed to concentrations of drug that constantly change. Drug concentration depends on the renal handling of the agent, the integrity of renal function, the degree of diuresis, and the frequency of micturition. The behaviour of bacterial populations and their response to antibacterial agents in these dynamic conditions is hard to predict and much useful information has been obtained by the use of *in vitro* models that simulate the *in vivo* situation. Several models have been described that mimic, with varying degrees of sophistication, the conditions of exposure of bacteria to antibacterial agents in the treatment of urinary infection (Greenwood 1985*a*). Their use has been reviewed by Greenwood (Greenwood and O'Grady 1978; Greenwood 1985*b*) and Anderson (1985).

Clinical trials

The laboratory is often required to assist clinicians in the evaluation of new drugs. In order to comply with regulatory authorities, microscopy and simple chemistry of urine is performed before, during, and after the drug has been administered. Pharmacokinetic evaluation of new agents requires sequential collections of urine for assay. When antimicrobials are being evaluated, trials of efficacy in UTI are commonly performed. In these situations it behoves the organizer of the trial to inform and discuss the protocol with laboratory managers. Too many trials yield inadequate data because the information is collected retrospectively from laboratories without any prior consultation. Strains isolated from urine should be stored for further study and all records kept separately. The additional organization required is minimal and consists of proper labelling of urines from patients in a study.

Antimicrobial agents in urine

It is not usually necessary to measure the concentration of antimicrobial agents in bladder urine, except in pharmacokinetic studies, to judge compliance or for experimental purposes. Methods of assay appropriate to the study of urine are generally the same as those used for other body fluids (Edberg 1986). The method chosen will naturally vary with the agent under study and the degree of accuracy required. Methodological details can be found in standard texts. There are, however, many pitfalls for the unwary in the interpretation of results obtained in assays of antimicrobial agents in urine because of the variable nature of the fluid; because of the hydrokinetic features of the urinary tract and, sometimes, because of the metabolic form in which the drug is excreted.

Most antimicrobial agents are excreted to some extent by the renal route. For many, this is the principal mode of elimination and high concentrations are achieved in urine. A few compounds, notably hexamine (methenamine), nitrofurantoin, and the older quinolones, such as nalidixic acid, oxolinic acid, and cinoxacin, do not achieve therapeutically useful concentrations elsewhere and their use is virtually restricted to UTI. Other agents, although eliminated by the kidneys, are excreted chiefly as biologically inactive metabolites. For example, chloramphenicol is largely excreted as an inactive glucuronide conjugate. Some antibacterial agents including quinolones, sulphonamides, and isoniazid may be eliminated as varying proportions of several metabolic forms that may or may not retain antimicrobial activity.

Concentrations of drug achieved in bladder urine will depend not only on the excretion characteristics but also on the degree of diuresis, the residual volume remaining in the bladder after micturition, and the frequency of micturition. The contribution of these factors to the concentration of drug achieved and maintained in bladder urine has been calculated by Kawada *et al.* (1980). As might be expected, concentrations achieved are high but short-lived if a rapidly excreted agent is given to a patient with a normal (i.e. < 1 ml) residual bladder volume who is suffering from frequency of micturition. Conversely, a slowly excreted agent administered to a subject with an increased residual bladder volume who is micturating at intervals of two or more hours will achieve lower but more prolonged concentrations. During the night, when the flow of ureteric urine slows and micturition may be suspended entirely, the period for which drug concentrations are maintained will be further prolonged unless the compound is unstable or is inactivated for example by microbial enzymes.

The physicochemical constitution of urine may have a considerable influence on antibacterial activity (Edberg 1986). Thus, the activities of nitrofurantoin and fosfomycin are enhanced in acidic conditions, whereas aminoglycosides and quinolones (particularly the newer fluoroquinolones) exhibit depressed activity at low pH. Hexamine depends on acidic conditions for the generation of the active product of decomposition, formaldehyde, and is consequently inactive against urea-splitting organisms, such as *Proteus* spp, that render the urine alkaline. Variation in cation concentration may similarly affect the activity of aminoglycosides and to a lesser extent, quinolones.

The osmotic milieu, which can vary enormously depending on the degree of concentration of the urine, will affect the bacterial effect of β-lactam antibiotics against Gram-negative bacilli. High osmotic concentrations of urine reduce the cidal effect since bacterial death is dependent on cell rupture in dilute or normally concentrated urine. This may be particularly important with organisms, such as *Proteus mirabilis*, which exhibit a low intracellular osmolality (Greenwood and O'Grady 1972). Some samples of urine do not support bacterial growth apparently because of the presence of endogenous inhibitors (Kaye 1968) the precise nature of which is unclear.

Urine is a highly variable fluid formed as an efficient means of eliminating waste products, including drugs, from the body. Investigations of antibiotic concentrations in urine should therefore take into account the following factors:

1. The renal handling of the drug in health and disease and the integrity of renal function.
2. The form in which the agent is excreted; the degree of activity (if any) retained by any metabolites and the ability of the assay method chosen to discriminate between metabolic variants.
3. The effects of concomitant administration of drugs that may affect excretion (e.g. probenecid).
4. The hydrokinetic circumstances prevailing in the individual subject during the study: ureteric urine flow rate (degree of diuresis); residual bladder volume; frequency of micturition.
5. The composition of urine; pH; concentrations of cations or other potentially interfering substances; osmolality; presence of endogenous inhibitors of bacterial growth.

Bladder biopsies

Most specimens taken from the urinary tract at operation are examined only by conventional hispathological techniques. Light microscopy does not yield much to the diagnosis of conventional urinary infection although it may be crucial in identifying *Schistosoma haematobium* and tuberculosis. In patients with chronic bladder inflammation, biopsy will differentiate between specific infections and interstitial cystitis although often there may be only minor disruption of the urothelium with a subepithelial lymphocytic response. Electron microscopy, especially in the scanning mode (SEM), may aid in the evaluation of surface morphology of the bladder and the early detection of malignant changes. SEM can also show bacterial colonization of the urothelium. Culture of organisms from bladder biopsies may also be attempted. Using both these methods it is possible to show that many patients with chronic changes to the bladder carry microbes on a disrupted mucosa without having bacteriuria detected by conventional urine culture (Elliott *et al.* 1985). The precise relevance of this is the subject of debate.

Whither laboratory tests?

It is difficult to imagine the investigation of urinary tract infection without a confirmatory test for bacteriuria. Thus, the rapid methods that have been described are used to screen out presumptively negative urines, thereby greatly reducing the number requiring traditional 'culture and sensitivity'. This trend will continue, especially in health care systems where the cost of laboratory investigation is borne directly by the patient or requesting physician. Urine examination in the clinic offers not only the advantage of economy but also a rapid answer. In the future, the microbiology laboratory may well play a lesser confirmatory role in the diagnosis of UTI. The examination of urine by trained laboratory workers rather than by office or nursing staff will continue to be essential for isolation, identification, and sensitivity testing. Advances in DNA technology have made it possible to identify, quantify, and predict antimicrobial sensitivity of pathogens by direct application of DNA probes (Carter *et al.* 1989). Although non-radioactive probes are safer and can be used outside a laboratory, the stringent conditions and interpretation of results requires expertise. As market forces are driving diagnostic companies to produce these sophisticated tests for widespread use it is possible that dip-stick probes will be produced which could be used by a patient with recurrent urinary symptoms to confirm bacteriuria and suggest antimicrobials.

Urine examination is likely to be used far more frequently in the future as a diagnostic test for other infectious diseases. Pneumococcal antigen detection has been used for the diagnosis of pneumonia (Whitby *et al.* 1985) and this approach can be extended to other causes of pneumonia, such as Legionella, or to other diseases. Within the urogenital tract non-gonococcal urethritis may be confirmed without the necessity of urethral scraping. Improvements in the laboratory determination of localization of UTI are likely in the future.

These predictions imply a change in laboratory and clinical practice towards a more consumer led service. In clinical microbiology this will be most apparent in urine bacteriology which will cease to handle the largest number of specimens.

References

Alexander, M. K., Khan, M. S., and Dow, C. S. (1981). Rapid screening for bacteriuria using a particle counter, pulse-height analyser and computer. *J. Clin. Pathol.*, **34**, 194–8.

Anderson, J. D. (1985). Relevance of urinary bladder models to clinical problems and to antibiotic evaluation. *J. Antimicrob. Chemother.*, **15**, (Suppl. A), 111–15.

Asscher, A. W. (1980). *The challenge of urinary tract infections*. Academic Press, London. 1980.

British Society for Antimicrobial Chemotherapy Report (1991). A guide to sensitivity testing. *J. Antimicrob. Chemother.*, **27**, (Suppl. D): 1–50.

Barrow, G. I. and Feltham, R. K. A. (1993). *Cowan and Steel's manual for the identification of medical bacteria*, (3rd edn). Cambridge University Press.

Brooks, H. J. L., O'Grady, F., McSherry, M. A., and Cattell, W. R. (1980). Uropathogenic properties of *Escherichia coli* in recurrent urinary tract infection. *J. Med. Microbiol.*, **13**, 57–68.

Buckley, R. M., McGuckin, M., and MacGregor, R. R. (1978). Urine bacterial counts after sexual intercourse. *New Eng. J. Med.*, **278**, 321–4.

Carter, G. I., Towner, K. J., Pearson, N. J., and Slack, R. C. B. (1989). Use of a non-radioactive hybridisation assay for direct detection of gram-negative bacteria carrying TEM β-lactamase genes in infected urines. *J. Med. Microbiol.*, **28**, 113–17.

Cattell, W. R., Fry, I. K., Spiro, I. F., Sanderson, J. M., Sutcliffe, M. B., and O'Grady, F. W. (1970). Effect of diuresis and frequent micturition on the bacterial content of infected urine. *Brit. J. Urol.*, **42**, 290–5.

Cattell, W. R., Brooks, H. L., McSherry, M. A., Northeast, A., and O'Grady, F. (1975). Approach to the frequency dysuria syndrome. *Kidney Internat.*, **8**, 138–43.

Cheetham, P. and Brown, S. E. (1986). Technique for the culture and direct sensitivity testing of large numbers of urine specimens. *J. Clin. Pathol.*, **39**, 335–7.

Collee, J. D., Duguid, J. P., Fraser, A. G., and Marmion, B. P. (1989). *Mackie and McCartney practical medical microbiology*, (13th edn). Churchill Livingstone, Edinburgh.

Edberg, S. C. (1986). The measurement of antibiotics in human body fluids: techniques and significance In *Antibiotics in laboratory medicine*, (ed. V. Lorian), (2nd edn), 381–476. Williams & Wilkins, Baltimore.

Edwards, P. R. and Ewing, W. H. (1972). *Identification of enterobacteriaceae*, (3rd edn). Burgess, Minneapolis.

Elliott, T. S. J., Reed, L., Slack, R. C. B., and Bishop, M. C. (1985). Bacteriology and ultrastructure of the bladder in patients with urinary tract infections. *J. Infection.*, **11**, 191–9.

Fairley, K. F., Bond, A. G., Brown, R. B., and Habersberger, P. (1967). Simple test to determine the site of urinary tract infection. *Lancet*, **ii**, 427–8.

Ferone, R., Bushby, S. R. M., Burchall, J. J., Moore, W. D., and Smith, D. (1975). Identification of Harper–Cawston factor as thymidine phosphorylase and removal from media of substances interfering with susceptibility testing to sulphonamides and diaminopyrimidimes. *Antimicrob. Agents Chemother.*, **7**, 91–8.

Fowlis, G. A., Waters, J., and Williams, G. (1994). The cost effectiveness of combined rapid tests (Multistix) in screening for urinary tract infections. *J. Roy. Soc. Med.*, **87**, 681–2.

Gallagher, D. J. A., Montgomerie, J. Z., and North, J. D. R. (1965). Acute infection of the urinary tract and the urethral syndrome in general practice. *BMJ*, **1**, 622–66.

Greenwood, D. (1985*a*). An *in vitro* model simulating the hydrokinetic aspects of the treatment of bacterial cystitis. *J. Antimicrob. Chemother.*, **15**, (Suppl. A), 103–9.

Greenwood, D. (1985*b*). Models in the assessment of antimicrobial agents In *The scientific basis of antimicrobial chemotheraphy*, (ed. D. Greenwood and F. O'Grady), 323–9. Cambridge University Press.

Greenwood, D. and O'Grady, F. (1972). The effect of osmolality on the response of *Escherichia coli* and *Proteus mirabilis* to penicillins. *Br. J. Exp. Pathol.*, **53**, 457–64.

Greenwood, D. and O'Grady, F. (1978). An *in vitro* model of the urinary bladder. *J. Antimicrob. Chemother.*, **4**, 113–20.

Greenwood, D. and Slack, R. (1982). Urinary tract infection. *Br. J. Clin. Pharmacol.*, **13**, 619–30.

Gruneberg, R. N., Leigh, D. A., and Brumfitt, W. (1968). *Escherichia coli* serotypes in urinary tract infection: studies in domiciliary, ante-natal and hospital practice In *Urinary tract infection*, (ed. F. O'Grady and W. Brumfitt), pp. 68–79. Oxford University Press.

Guttman, D. E. and Naylor, G. R. E. (1967). Dip slide: an aid to quantitative urine culture in general practice. *BMJ*, **3**, 649–51.

Hamilton-Miller, H. M. T., Brumfitt, W., and Smith, G. W. (1986). Are fastidious organisms an important cause of dysuria and frequency?—The case against. In

Microbial disease in nephrology, (ed. A. W. Asscher and W. Brumfitt), 19–30. Wiley, Chichester.

Hooton, T. M., Hillier, S., Johnson, C. *et al.* (1991) *Escherichia coli* bacteriuria and contraceptive method. *JAMA*, **265**, 64–9.

Ispahani, P., Pearson, N. P., and Greenwood, D. (1987). An analysis of community and hospital acquired bacteraemia in a large teaching hospital in the United Kingdom. *Quart. J. Med.*, **63**, 427–40.

Kass, E. H. (1956). Asymptomatic infections of the urinary tract. *Trans. Assoc. Amer. Phys.*, **69**, 56–63.

Kawada, Y., Greenwood, D., and O'Grady, F. (1980). Factors affecting antibiotic concentrations in bladder urine. *Invest. Urol.*, **17**, 484–6.

Kaye, D. (1968). Antibacterial activity of human urine. *J. Clin. Invest.*, **47**, 2374–90.

Kunin, C. M., White, L. V., and Hua, T. H. (1993). A reassessment of the importance of 'low count' bacteriuria in young women with acute urinary symptoms. *Ann. Int. Med.*, **119**, 454–60.

Leigh, D. A. and Williams, J. D. (1964). Method for the detection of significant bacteriuria in large groups of patients. *J. Clin. Path.*, **17**, 498–503.

Lipsky, B. A., Plorde, J. J., Tenover, F. C., and Brancata, F. P. (1985). Comparison of the Automicrobic system, acridine organe-stained smears and Gram-stained smears in detecting bacteriuria. *J. Clin. Microbiol.*, **22**, 176–81.

Lipsky, B. A., Ireton, R. C., Fihn S. D., Hackett, R., and Berger, R. E. (1987). Diagnosis of bacteriuria in men: specimen collection and culture interpretation. *J. Infect. Dis.*, **155**, 847–53.

Lorian, V. (ed.) (1991). *Antibiotics in laboratory medicine*, (3rd edn). Williams & Wilkins, Baltimore.

MacConkey, A. T. (1908). Bile salt media and their advantages in some bacteriological examinations. *J. Hyg.* (*Camb.*), **8**, 322–4.

Mackey, J. P. and Sandys, G. H. (1965). Laboratory diagnosis of infections of the urinary tract in general practice by means of a dip-inoculum transport medium. *BMJ*, **2**, 1286–8.

Mackey, J. P. and Sandys, G. H. (1966). Diagnosis of urinary infections. *BMJ*, **1**, 1173.

McGowan, A. P., Marshall, R. J., Cowling, P., and Reeves, D. S. (1991). Measurement of urinary lipopolysaccharide antibodies by ELISA as a screen for urinary tract infection. *J. Clin. Path.*, **44**, 61–3.

Mansell, P. E. and Peacock, A. M. (1973). Direct microscopy of uncentrifuged urine. *J. Clin. Pathol.*, **26**, 724–5.

Maskell, R. (1982). *Urinary tract infection*, pp. 18–20. Edward Arnold, London.

Maskell, R. (1986). Are fastidious organisms an important cause of dysuria and frequency?—The case for. In *Microbial disease in nephrology*, (ed. A. W. Asscher and W. Brumfitt), pp. 1–18. Wiley, Chichester.

Meares, E. M. and Stamey, T. A. (1968). Bacteriologic localization patterns in bacterial prostatitis and urethritis. *Invest. Urol.* **5**, 492–518.

Murray, P. R., Baron, E. J., Pfuller, M. A., Tenover, F. C., and Yolken, R. H. (1995). *Manual of clinical microbiology*, (4th edn). American Society for Microbiology, Washington, DC.

Nicolaier, A. (1895). Über die therapeutische Verwendung des Urotropin (Hexamethylentetramin). *Dtsch. Med. Wochenschr.*, **21**, 541–3.

O'Grady, F. (1979). Urinary tract infection in women. *J. Roy. Coll. Phys.*, **13**, 70–3.

O'Grady, F. W., Charlton, C. A. C., Kelsey, Fry. I., McSherry, A., and Cattell, W. R. (1973). Natural history of intractable 'cystitis' in women referred to a special clinic In *Urinary tract infection*, (ed. W. Brumfitt and A. W. Asscher), pp. 81–91. Oxford University Press.

Pelling, W. (1982). Inhibitory substances in urine: an addition to the routine screen. *Med. Lab. Sci.*, **39**, 377–81.

Percival, A., Brumfitt, W., and De Louvois, J. (1964). Serum antibody levels as an indication of clinically unapparent pyelonephritis. *Lancet*, **ii**, 1027–33.

PHLS (Public Health Laboratory Service) (1978). *The bacteriological examination of urine: report of a workshop on needs and methods*. HMSO, London.

Porter, I. A. and Brooke, J. (1969). Boric acid preservation of urine samples. *BMJ*, **2**, 353–5.

Raz, R. and Stamm, W. E. (1993). A controlled trial of intravaginal estriol in post-menopausal women with recurrent urinary tract infection. *New Eng. J. Med.*, **329**, 753–6.

Reeves, D. S., Phillips, I., Williams, J. D., and Wise, R. (1978). *Laboratory methods in antimicrobial chemotherapy*, Churchill Livingstone, Edinburgh.

Sandys, G. H. (1978). Cystine-lactose electrolyte deficient medium. In *The bacteriological examination of urine. Report of a workshop on needs and methods*, 29–33 (PHLS monograph). HMSO, London.

Schardijn, G., Statius van Eps, L. W., Swaak, A. J. G., Kager, J. C. G. M., and Persijn, J. P. (1979). Urinary β_2 microglobulin in upper and lower urinary tract infections. *Lancet*, **i**, 805–7.

Snell, J. J. S., Brown, D. F. J., and Gardner, P. S. (1982). An antibiotic susceptibility testing trial organised as part of the United Kingdom national external micro-biological quality assessment scheme. *J. Clin. Pathol.*, **35**, 1169–76.

Snell, J. J. S., Brown, D. F. J., and Gardner, P. S. (1984). Comparison of results from two antibiotic susceptibility testing trials that formed part of the United Kingdom national external quality assessment scheme. *J. Clin. Pathol.*, **37**, 321–8.

Stamm, W. E. (1983). Measurement of pyuria and its relationship to bacteriuria. *Amer. J. Med.*, **75**, (Suppl. 1B), 53–85.

Stamm, W. E., Wagner, K. F., Amsel, R. *et al.* (1980). Causes of the acute urethral syndrome in women. *New Eng. J. Med.*, **303**, 409–15.

Stamm, W. E., Counts, G. W., Running, K. R., Fihn, S., Turck, M. and Holmes, K. K. (1982). Diagnosis of coliform infection in acutely dysuric women. *New Eng. J. Med.*, **307**, 463–8.

Thomas, V., Shelokov, A., and Forland, M. (1974). Antibody coated bacteria in the urine and the site of urinary tract infection. *New Eng. J. Med.*, **290**, 588–90.

Waterworth, P. M. (1981). Sensitivity testing by the break-point method. *J. Antimicrob. Chemother.*, **7**, 117–26.

Wershub, L. P. (1970). *Urology from antiquity to the 20th century*. Warren H. Green, St. Louis, MO.

Whitby, M., Kristinsson, K. G., and Brown, M. (1985). Assessment of rapid methods for the detection of pneumococcal antigen-detection in routine sputum bacteriology. *J. Clin. Path.*, **38**, 341–4.

4
Imaging in urinary tract infection

Judith A. W. Webb

Imaging techniques

Intravenous urography (IVU)

Intravenous urography is an important first-line imaging method that mainly provides structural diagnostic information on the urinary tract.

Plain films Preliminary plain films detect calcifications within the kidneys. A full-length film on inspiration and a coned renal area film on expiration are a good combination to decide whether calcifications overlying the kidneys are intra-renal. If doubt remains about the position of calcifications, these films may need to be supplemented by oblique renal views or plain renal tomography. Plain tomography is helpful in excluding renal calculi when the renal areas are overlain by bowel or when low-density calculi are suspected, for example, in Proteus urinary tract infection (Schwartz *et al.* 1984). Calcifications in the expected position of the ureters and bladder may also be detected on plain films but films following contrast medium excretion are necessary to know whether they lie within the urinary tract.

Contrast media The intravascular contrast media in current use are all derivatives of tri-iodinated benzoic acid. The older ionic agents have a high osmolality (approximately 1500 mOsm/kg) and consist of iodine-containing anions, such as iothalamate and diatriozoate, and cations, such as sodium and meglumine. The newer non-ionic agents, such as iohexol, iopamidol, and iopromide, have osmolalities approximately one-third of the ionic agents but cost significantly more—about 4 and 10 times the cost of the ionic agents in the United Kingdom and United States, respectively.

Side-effects of contrast media When given intravenously, contrast media often produce a sensation of warmth and tingling, and may induce a metallic taste. These effects are more common with ionic agents and should be considered normal: they do not constitute any 'allergy'. Approximately 5 per cent of subjects receiving ionic agents and 1 per cent receiving non-ionic agents have more serious side-effects (Shehadi 1975; Schrott *et al.* 1986; Palmer 1988). The majority of these reactions are moderate in severity and consist of bronchospasm, urticaria, vomiting, angioneurotic oedema, and hypotension. About 0.01 per cent receiving ionic agents will have serious side-effects, such as cardiac arrhythmias, cardiac arrest, convulsions, or loss of consciousness, and the incidence of these effects is believed to be 5 to 10 times less with non-ionic agents (Ansell 1970; Katayama *et al.* 1990; Palmer 1988). Death has been reported in 1 in 75 000 subjects receiving ionic agents (Hartman *et al.* 1982) and appears to occur 3 to 4 times less frequently with non-ionic agents (Katayama *et al.* 1990).

Contrast medium reactions are more likely if there is a history of previous reaction to contrast medium, of allergy, asthma, or heart disease (Ansell *et al.* 1980; Katayama *et al.* 1990). Their aetiology is poorly understood but appears to involve activation of the complement system (Lasser *et al.* 1980).

Because of the cost differential, ionic agents are still routinely used for urography in many hospitals. Non-ionic agents should be used in patients with increased risk of contrast medium reaction, in patients with impaired renal function or myeloma, and in the elderly and children.

Renal effects of contrast media In patients with normal renal function contrast media have no adverse effects on renal function. In approximately 10 per cent of patients with impaired renal function, intravenous contrast medium produces a rise in serum creatinine which is usually reversible (Berns 1989). The risk of inducing such further impairment of renal function is increased by dehydration, the use of large contrast medium doses, and diabetes mellitus (Byrd and Sherman 1979).

Value of urography

Urography gives a rapid overview of the kidneys, ureters, and bladder. It shows the detailed anatomy of the calyces, pelves, and ureters particularly well. It is the best method for detecting and localizing stones in the kidneys and ureters. Its disadvantages include the limited functional information it gives and the lack of information it provides concerning renal parenchymal structure and the nature of masses. It necessitates the use of contrast medium, which has a low but definite associated morbidity, and irradiation.

Ultrasonography (US)

Ultrasonography is a further first-line method for imaging the urinary tract which, like urography, provides mainly structural information.

Principles The technique uses high-frequency sound waves which are reflected from the surfaces of organs and from the structures within them. The reflected sound is used to generate a sectional image. Current equipment uses 'real-time' transducers which contain multiple sound generating elements that fire off in sequence, so that a moving image is produced. Individual image frames can be frozen and used to make hard copy.

In abdominal scanning, the flexibility of the technique, which allows images to be made in any sectional plane, is an advantage. US shows the consistency of tissues, whether they are fluid or solid, and so provides detailed images of parenchymal structure. Difficulties may be encountered with bone (e.g. ribs) or gas which reflect sound producing a bright echo with a black band (or acoustic shadow) behind it. The transducer can usually be angled around the ribs but gas in bowel precludes full examination of the retroperitoneum in most adult subjects. Fat transmits ultrasound poorly and reduces the resolution of the resultant images. Abdominal US scanning requires considerable skill to achieve its full potential—hence its reputation of operator-dependence.

Renal ultrasonography

Ultrasound is widely used for measuring renal length. Technique must be careful to ensure measurements are made in the true long axis and not from oblique scans. The lower limit of normal length for the adult kidney is considered to be 9.0 cm (Webb *et al.* 1984). US is a sensitive detector of pelvicalyceal system dilatation and of fluid collections within and around the kidney. It can differentiate cortex from medulla and can characterize masses as cystic or solid. It has the advantage over urography of not using either ionizing radiation or contrast medium.

Renal US provides less detailed anatomical information than urography. It does not show pelvicalyceal detail and does not visualize the normal ureter. It is less sensitive in detection of opaque renal stones than the combination of plain films and plain tomography (Middleton *et al.* 1988) and does not show the majority of ureteric stones. For this reason, if ultrasound is the only imaging method used, plain abdominal radiographs should also be obtained.

Bladder ultrasonography

Bladder calculi are detected as mobile echogenicities with associated acoustic shadows. Bladder wall thickness can be measured and bladder emptying can be assessed by measuring the bladder before and after voiding. The method is approximate and does not estimate small volumes accurately, but is quite adequate for the assessment of bladder outflow obstruction (Posten *et al.* 1983).

Transrectal ultrasound of the prostate (TRUS)

The technique of transrectal prostate ultrasound uses a high frequency (7.5 MHz) transducer in the rectum and provides high-resolution images of the prostate. Both longitudinal and transverse sections through the gland should be obtained using a biplanar transducer, a single transducer with a scanning plane which can be rotated from longitudinal to transverse, or two separate transducers. The peripheral zone, which occupies the posterior gland and extends into the apex, contains acinar tissue and may be involved both by prostatitis and adenocarcinoma. The transition zone which is affected by benign prostatic hypertrophy surrounds the upper urethra above verumontanum level. The periurethral glandular tissue is often also involved in prostatitis (Griffiths *et al.* 1990). Features suggestive of benign prostatic hypertrophy, carcinoma, prostatitis, and prostatic abscess can be detected. The technique can be used to guide the biopsy of focal abnormalities, either transrectally or transperineally, and the drainage of abscesses. Prophylactic antibiotics should be given before transrectal biopsy because the risk of sepsis is high (Thompson *et al.* 1982).

Doppler ultrasound

The Doppler principle is used to detect movement which is indicated by a change in frequency of the reflected US beam. With duplex Doppler, the US image is used to place the Doppler cursor in the vessel of interest to obtain flow spectra. A further development is that of colour Doppler in which blood flow in blocks of tissue is assessed and the direction of flow is colour-coded. This method makes it easier to detect small blood vessels (such as the arcuate arteries in the kidney) and place the Doppler cursor within them. Tissue vascularity can be assessed and the increased vascularity of neoplastic and inflammatory tissue can be detected.

Nuclear medicine

Renal imaging

Principles Nuclear medicine studies of the kidneys use radioactive tracers which are either excreted or taken up by the kidney. The most commonly used labelling agent is ^{99m}Tc (technetium). The gamma-ray photons which are emitted by the ^{99m}Tc are detected by a sodium iodide crystal which acts as a gamma-camera, emitting light when struck by the gamma-rays. The information obtained is mainly functional but structural information can also be obtained from the images, in particular an indication as to which areas of the parenchyma are functioning normally.

Static scanning Static renal scanning uses ^{99m}Tc-labelled dimercaptosuccinic acid (DMSA) which is taken up by the proximal tubular cells. Images are obtained three hours after an intravenous injection of the tracer. About 30 per cent of the injected dose is fixed by the proximal tubules and the uptake is proportional to the renal function.

The total uptake allows relative function between the kidneys to be assessed. The distribution of renal uptake is also important with diffuse or focal reduction in uptake occurring in acute pyelonephritis and reduced uptake with cortical defects when scars develop (Rushton and Majd 1992).

Dynamic scanning This uses agents that are excreted by the kidney either by glomerular filtration–^{99m}Tc-diethylamine triamine penta-acetic acid (DTPA)—or by glomerular filtration and tubular secretion–^{99m}Tc-mercaptoacetyl tryglycine (MAG 3).

Following an intravenous bolus of the tracer, serial computer frames are collected by using a gamma-camera at the patient's back. A rapid uptake phase occurs first during perfusion, glomerular filtration and/or secretion. Subsequently, counts over the kidney decrease as the tracer passes through the parenchyma, into the collecting system, and drains to the bladder. Quantitative assessments of perfusion, transit time, and relative renal function can be obtained.

Nuclear cystography

The appeal of nuclear medicine techniques for cystography compared to the radiographic micturating cystourethrography (MCU) relates to the reduced radiation dose, estimated to be between one-tenth and one-fiftieth of that given by the radiographic method (Willi and Treves 1983; Chapman *et al.* 1988). The reduced radiation dose is achieved with improved sensitivity because, unlike radiographic cystography, continuous monitoring is possible without increasing the radiation dose. The disadvantages of nuclear cystography relate to the lack of anatomical detail of the pelvicalyceal system, ureter, and urethra, and to the fact that it is only suitable in older children who are toilet trained.

Direct nuclear cystography (Willi and Treves 1983) In direct nuclear cystography the bladder is catheterized and filled by drip infusion with a dilute solution of ^{99m}Tc-DTPA. After removal of the catheter, the patient voids. Throughout bladder filling and voiding serial frames are recorded on the gamma-camera. The amount of tracer infused and voided is measured and any reflux can be quantified. The technique is sensitive for vesicoureteric reflux (VUR), despite the limited anatomical information it provides.

Indirect nuclear cystography (Merrick *et al.* 1977; Chapman *et al.* 1988) This technique has the advantage of avoiding bladder catheterization and is performed at the end of a ^{99m}Tc-DTPA dynamic renal study, using the tracer already present in the bladder. Serial frames from the gamma-camera are obtained during voiding. The method is at least as sensitive as the radiographic MCU for detecting significant reflux reaching the kidney.

Localization of infection

Radionuclide tracer techniques that localize infection may occasionally be required in the evaluation of UTI, for example to localize infection within a kidney in autosomal-dominant polycystic kidney disease if neither ultrasound nor computed tomography (CT) detect an atypical cyst. Possibilities are either the use of ^{67}Ga (gallium)-citrate or of leucocytes labelled either with ^{111}In (indium) or ^{99m}Tc. The leucocyte technique is only useful in approximately the first 10 days of infection and is more expensive and technically complex than the more widely used ^{67}Ga study, which is performed 48 hours after the injection of tracer. By this time, renal excretion of the tracer should be complete in subjects with normal renal function, and renal accumulation of tracer indicates an inflammatory process (Hampel *et al.* 1980).

Lower tract investigations

Micturating cystourethrography (MCU)

Principles In radiographic micturating cystourethrography the catheterized bladder is filled with contrast medium and the bladder and urethra are screened fluoroscopically during voiding. The technique provides excellent anatomical information but is unpleasant, especially for children, and necessitates the use of radiation.

An extension of the technique is the pressure–flow video-cystogram (or video-urodynamic study) which also provides functional information. Pressure lines attached to transducers are placed in the bladder and rectum to measure bladder and abdominal pressure respectively. The bladder is filled with contrast medium and bladder detrusor pressure is obtained by subtracting abdominal from bladder pressure. Bladder detrusor pressure is recorded together with urine flow rate at the same time that anatomical information is obtained by fluoroscopy.

Technique (Lebowitz *et al.* 1985) The procedure should be performed when the acute infective episode has been controlled by antibiotics. If the patient is not still taking antibiotics, an agent, such as nitrofurantoin, should be taken for 48 hours after the MCU. The patient empties the bladder which is then catheterized and slowly filled with dilute contrast medium. During bladder filling, intermittent fluoroscopy is performed to check for VUR. In young babies, the bladder catheter can be removed when they start to void. With older children and adults, the catheter is removed when the bladder feels full and they are then instructed to void. Fluoroscopy is carried out throughout voiding. If there is VUR, films that show the whole urinary tract should be obtained at the height of VUR, so that the grade of reflux can be assessed (p. 71). Detection of abnormalities of voiding is an important part of the assessment of children with VUR. An unstable bladder may be indicated by bladder trabeculation or by uninhibited contractions of the bladder during filling. When uninhibited contractions occur the bladder neck may open and bladder filling may stop or be reversed (Fotter *et al.* 1986; Seruca 1989). In males, urethral valves and their secondary obstructive effects should be sought on the voiding films.

A study in which repeated voidings around the urethral catheter were examined indicated that MCU is a reliable test for excluding VUR, but the use of more than one voiding cycle increases its reliability (S. Jequier and J. C. Jequier 1989). This study also showed that repeated voidings increased the accuracy of reflux grading. Clearly, the increased accuracy has to be weighed against the increased radiation dose.

Urethrography

This is used in adult males to define the anatomy of the anterior urethra, particularly to detect urethral strictures. It is usually combined with a voiding study to examine the posterior urethra and define the functional effect of any strictures.

Computed tomography (CT)

Computed tomography (CT) is a second-line urinary tract investigation that provides mainly anatomical information.

Very sensitive X-ray detectors provide multiple readings of X-ray absorption within each tissue 'slice'. The result is a cross-sectional image that shows great anatomical detail because the method is very sensitive to different tissue densities. For renal imaging, intravenous contrast medium is necessary for a full examination. Following an intravenous bolus of contrast medium, rapid sequence scans demonstrate the renal arteries and veins, and differential opacification of the cortex and medulla. Scans carried out later show homogeneous renal parenchymal enhancement and filling of the pelvicalyceal systems and ureters.

CT shows renal parenchymal abnormalities well and is a sensitive detector of collecting system dilatation and intrarenal fluid collections. Unlike US, it shows the retroperitoneum clearly and is a sensitive method of detecting renal and ureteric calculi. It provides a less detailed examination of pelvicalyceal anatomy than urography; and like urography, it provides little functional information, and necessitates the use of irradiation and contrast media.

Magnetic resonance imaging (MRI)

MRI techniques image the mobile protons that occur naturally in water. If a subject lies in a magnetic field, a proportion of the body's protons align with the field. They can be displaced by a radiofrequency pulse, and the radiofrequency signals that they emit as they return to equilibrium are used to generate sectional images in the axial, coronal, or sagittal planes. A variety of radiofrequency pulses may be used and the resultant images contain detailed information about the soft tissues in which the protons lie.

Experience in the use of MRI in patients with urinary tract infection is as yet anecdotal. The use of MRI has been limited by cost, limited machine availability, and slow scanning speed. Motion artefact and the inability of MRI to visualize calcium, which contains no mobile protons, have been particular problems in renal MRI. As scanning techniques improve and equipment becomes more readily available the use of MRI in the evaluation of complicated renal infection is likely to increase.

Reflux nephropathy

The term 'reflux nephropathy' was coined by Bailey in 1973 to encompass both the acute damage caused by reflux of infected urine and the long-term sequelae of this process. The great majority of imaging investigations in childhood UTI are directed towards diagnosing this condition in the hope that early identification will allow treatment to slow, arrest or prevent the development of renal scars.

Vesicoureteric reflux (VUR)

Because of the natural history of reflux nephropathy it is particularly important to detect vesicoureteric reflux (VUR) in infants and young children.

The radiographic micturating cystogram This remains the method of choice (Blickman *et al.* 1985). The intermittent and variable nature of VUR may make it difficult to detect. Reflux may occur during bladder filling or voiding, but is more likely to occur during voiding because of the higher intra-vesical pressure: in one series, 17 per cent of children only refluxed during voiding (Willi and Treves 1983).

Vesicoureteric reflux should be graded in severity using the categories recommended by the International Study Classification (Fig. 4.1) (Lebowitz *et al.* 1985):

Grade I: Reflux into the non-dilated ureter only.

Grade II: Reflux into the non-dilated ureter, pelvis, and calyces. The calyceal fornices remain sharp.

Grade III: Reflux with mild or moderate dilatation and/or tortuosity of the ureter, mild or moderate dilatation of the renal pelvis, no or slight blunting of the calyces/fornices.

Grade IV: Moderate dilatation and/or tortuosity of the ureter and moderate dilatation of the renal pelvis and calyces. The sharp forniceal angles of the calyces are lost but the majority of calyces still show papillary impressions.

Grade V: Gross dilatation and tortuosity of the ureter. Gross dilatation of the renal pelvis and calyces. Loss of the papillary impressions in the majority of calyces.

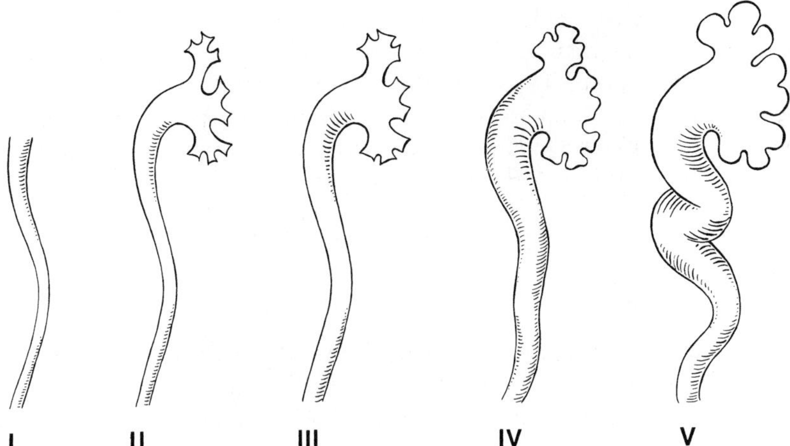

Fig. 4.1 Grades of vesicoureteric reflux: the International Study Classification. (After Lebowitz *et al.* 1985, by permission of the *Journal of Urology*.)

Accurate classification of the severity of reflux is important both for choosing appropriate management and for predicting the natural history of the condition. The more severe the reflux, the more severe the resultant scarring and associated renal damage (Smellie *et al.* 1975; Shah *et al.* 1978).

In some patients with severe VUR, intra-renal reflux is seen with contrast medium passing into the renal parenchyma in a lobar distribution (Fig. 4.2). This condition and its association with renal scarring were first recognized by Rolleston *et al.* (1974). It is estimated that intra-renal reflux occurs in between 3 and 28 per cent of patients with VUR (Cremin 1979; Thomsen 1985). Intra-renal reflux is a fleeting phenomenon which occurs at the height of severe VUR and high-quality images are necessary to show it.

Direct and indirect radionuclide cystography These methods appear to be as sensitive as micturating cystography in detecting significant VUR (Merrick *et al.* 1977; Willi and Treves 1983; Chapman *et al.* 1988). However, the anatomical detail obtained is generally considered insufficient for the initial assessment of VUR. It has been recommended that radionuclide cystography should be reserved for the follow-up of known VUR and after ureteric re-implantation, and for the evaluation of siblings of those with known VUR (Willi and Treves 1983; Lebowitz 1986).

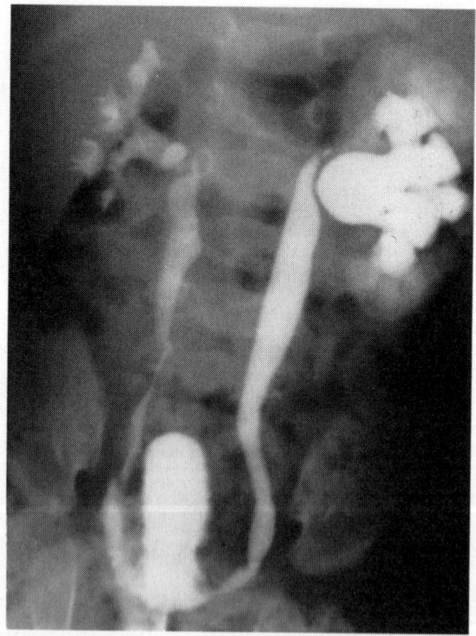

Fig. 4.2 Micturating cystogram in a 3-month-old child shows Grade II reflux on right, Grade V reflux, and intra-renal reflux on left. (Reproduced by permission of John Wiley & Sons.)

Intravenous urography This demonstrates the scars that may result from VUR and may also show a variety of indirect indicators of the reflux itself. Change in size and density of the pelvicalyceal systems and ureters, especially on the post-micturition film, and a large post-micturition bladder residue caused by the refluxed urine returning from the ureters to the bladder, are both indirect indicators of the presence of VUR (Fig. 4.3). With severe grades of VUR, striations caused by folds in the redundant collapsed pelvis and ureter may be seen (Friedland and Forsberg 1972) (Fig. 4.4).

Studies of the sensitivity of urography in detecting VUR suggest that it is reasonably sensitive in detecting more severe reflux. Thus Lanning *et al.* (1979) obtained a false negative rate of 6 per cent for detecting Grades II–V VUR with urography, compared to a false negative rate of 48–53 per cent for all grades of reflux. Cavanagh and Sherwood (1983) obtained similar results. Others, however, have noted that severe VUR can coexist with a normal IVU (Shah *et al.* 1978; Blickman *et al.* 1985).

Ultrasonography This is relatively insensitive for detecting collecting system dilatation caused by VUR, presumably because of the intermittent nature of

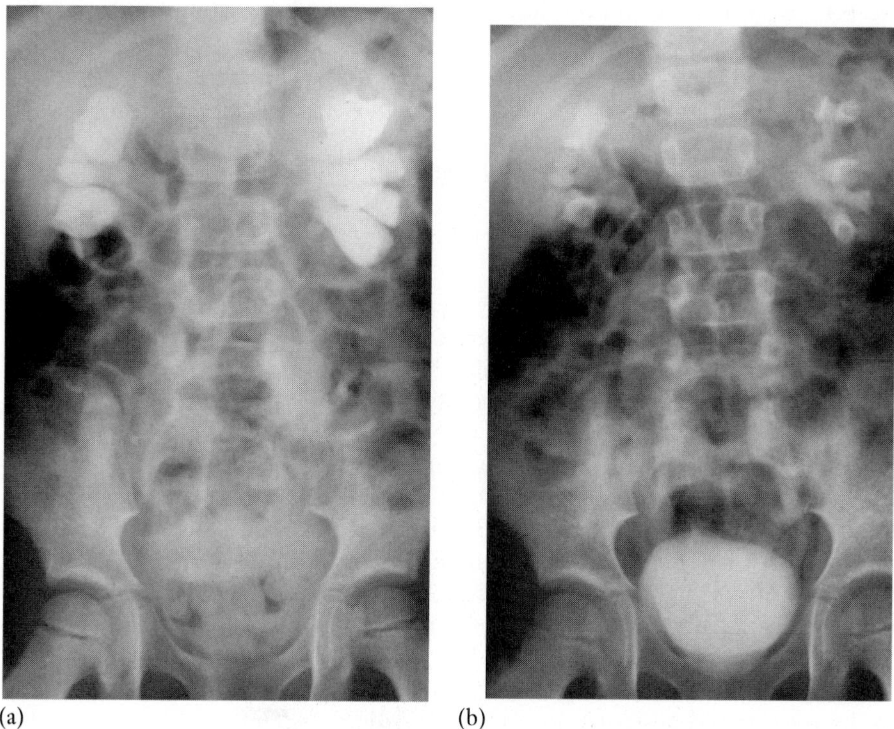

(a) (b)

Fig. 4.3 Bilateral vesicoureteric reflux with diffuse reflux nephropathy. Note markedly dilated calyces and diffuse parenchymal thinning on the 15-min film (a) with calyceal emptying and a large residual bladder volume on the post-micturition film (b). (Reproduced by permission of John Wiley & Sons.)

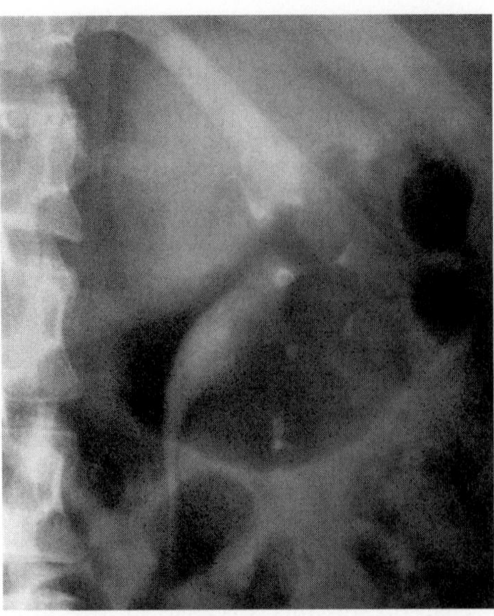

Fig. 4.4 Striations. Typical linear lucencies in an undistended renal pelvis. (Reproduced by permission of T. Sherwood and B. C. Decker.)

reflux. Indeed, it can miss even severe grades of VUR (Rickwood *et al.* 1992). Because there are many other causes of collecting system dilatation false positive scans occur frequently (Leonidas *et al.* 1985).

Renal scars

Urography has been used for many years to diagnose renal scars in reflux nephropathy and to follow their progress. Recently in many centres urography has been replaced by DMSA scanning, which is now widely regarded as the method of choice to detect scars, especially in young children.

DMSA scans The timing of these is important because during acute infection there may be patchy reduced uptake of isotope which does not persist subsequently. To detect true scars, DMSA scans at 2–3 months after the acute infective episode are necessary (Rushton and Majd 1992). However, since a high proportion of the abnormalities do persist, a case can be made for earlier DMSA scans to identify those at risk of renal damage and scarring (Verber and Meller 1989; Rushton and Majd 1992).

DMSA scans are sensitive detectors of scars (Fig. 4.5), including those lying on the anterior and posterior surfaces of the kidney. Several studies indicate that DMSA scanning is more sensitive than urography for detecting scars, and is especially sensitive in detecting early scars (Merrick *et al.* 1980; Monsour *et al.* 1987; Verber and Meller, 1989). Others have noted that DMSA scans can miss some scars, especially if they are polar (Smellie *et al.* 1988) or if the scarring is

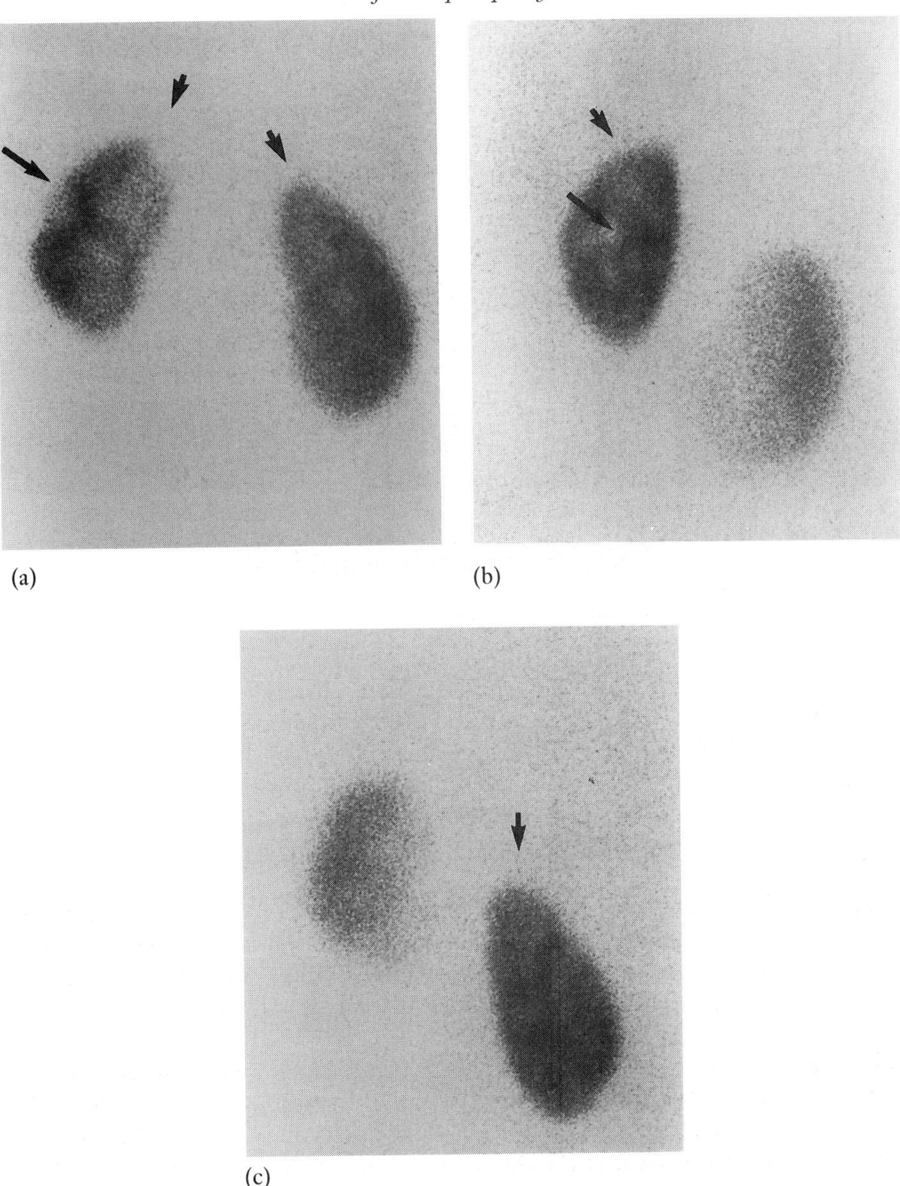

Fig. 4.5 Scars in reflux nephropathy. DMSA scan show focal scars (long arrows) and less obvious diffuse scars (short arrows) on posterior (a) and oblique (b,c) views. (Reproduced by permission of John Wiley & Sons.)

diffuse, particularly when the contralateral kidney is shrunken (Whitear *et. al.* 1990). Smellie *et al.* (1988) found that DMSA scanning underestimated the number of scars in approximately one-third of kidneys.

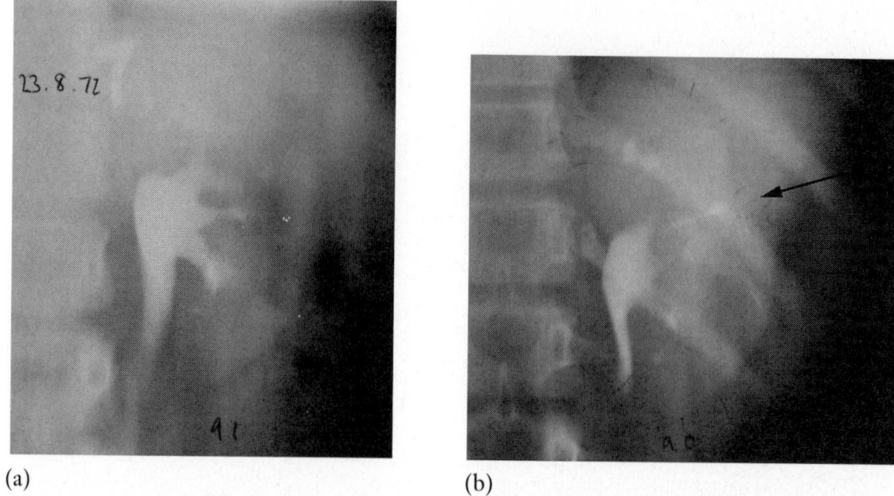

(a) (b)

Fig. 4.6 Reflux nephropathy: development of a scar in the upper lateral kidney (arrowed) (b), 4 months after a normal urogram (a). (By permission of H. M. Saxton.)

Urography Although it is less sensitive than DMSA scanning, urography remains a good method for detecting scars, for diagnosing the development of scars during follow-up (Fig. 4.6) and for following established scarring (Hodson and Wilson 1965; Smellie *et al.* 1988). It has the advantage of being more specific than DMSA since it also shows the typical associated calyceal clubbing of the full-blown scar of reflux nephropathy.

Ultrasonography This detects many scars (Fig. 4.7) but is insensitive compared to both urography and DMSA scanning, and can fail to detect large scars (Kangarloo *et al.* 1985; Rickwood *et al.* 1992; Tasker *et al.* 1993).

Renal growth

Reflux nephropathy causes impaired renal growth. Follow-up of renal growth has traditionally been by renal length measurement at *urography*. Although the method overestimates renal size because of urographic magnification, it is readily reproducible. In children, the parenchymal thickness is greater in relation to renal length than in adults (Hodson *et al.* 1975). Standard charts are available comparing renal length to height (Hodson 1979) and to vertebral height (Eklof and Ringertz 1976).

Ultrasonography In many centres this has replaced urography for follow-up of renal growth. Standard charts are available which compare ultrasonographic renal length and volume to patient size (Rosenbaum *et al.* 1984; Dinkel *et al.* 1985; Han and Babcock 1985). Ultrasonographic renal measurements are less readily repro-

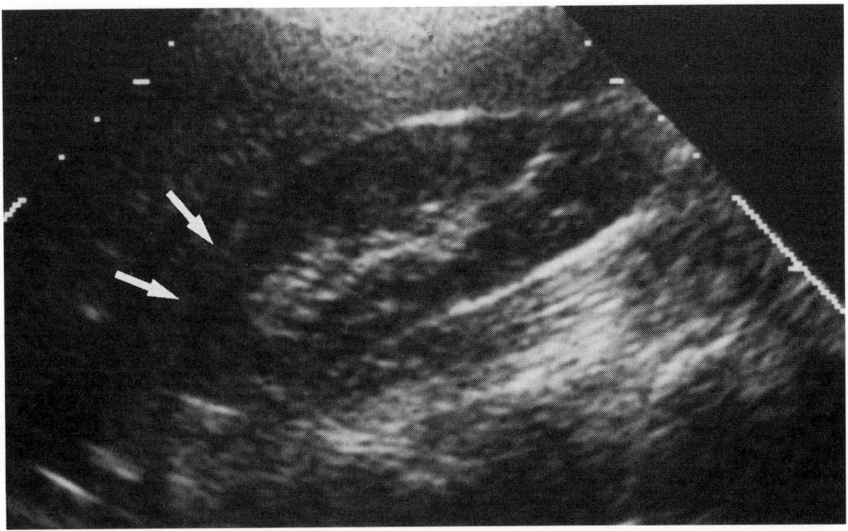

Fig. 4.7 Reflux nephropathy. Parenchymal thinning indicating a scar (arrowed) at the upper pole of the right kidney on longitudinal US scan.

ducible than radiographic measurements. Studies of inter- and intra-observer variation in renal length measurement in children have shown that observer error may lead to differences in measurement equal to between one and three years of normal renal growth (Schlesinger *et al.* 1991; Sargent and Wilson 1992).

Established reflux nephropathy: urographic features

The typical urographic finding in reflux nephropathy is a parenchymal scar with an underlying, blunted calyx (Hodson and Wilson 1965). Usually, the changes are focal and patchy both in site and severity (Hodson 1967) (Figs 4.8–4.11).

To detect parenchymal scarring the whole of the renal parenchyma must be assessed by measuring the distance from the apices of the papillae to the renal margin. The medial aspects of the renal poles must be assessed as well as the poles themselves and the lateral renal margin. At the poles there is lobar fusion during development with resultant compound calyces which are more susceptible to intra-renal reflux (Ransley and Risdon 1975*a*,*b*). For this reason, scarring is most commonly polar, with the upper poles more often affected than the lower, and the right kidney more often than the left (Hodson and Wilson 1965; Owen *et al.* 1985). Parenchymal thinning at the poles is typically associated with a smooth renal outline, but lateral scarring usually produces an irregular renal outline (Figs 4.9 and 4.11) Medial scarring at the poles causes the upper pole calyces to lie abnormally close to the spine and the lower pole calyces to lie unusually close to the ureter (Friedland *et al.* 1974).

The calyces underlying the scars are typically clubbed with smooth rounded outlines. Clubbed calyces with overlying scars also may occur when there has

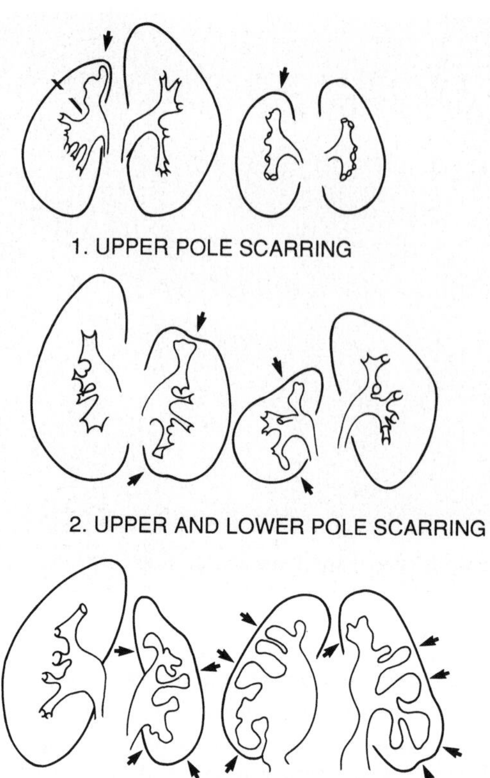

Fig. 4.8 Patterns of established reflux nephropathy. (After Hodson and Wilson 1965, by permission of the *British Medical Journal*.)

been focal obstruction, usually by a calculus in a calyceal infundibulum. Scarring due to infarction can be distinguished from that caused by reflux nephropathy because of the normal or minimally distorted underlying calyx. Calyceal clubbing in papillary necrosis is not associated with focal scarring, although in the late stages of the disease, following papillary sloughing, a 'wavy' renal outline may be seen. In tuberculosis, there is usually irregular destruction of the dilated calyces rather than the smooth clubbing which occurs in reflux nephropathy.

There is usually renal asymmetry, with one kidney reduced in size (Fig. 4.10), and reflux nephropathy may be unilateral. Compensatory hypertrophy of the parts of the kidney unaffected by scarring often occurs and the resultant bulge contributes to the irregular outline. If reflux nephropathy is unilateral there will usually be compensatory hypertrophy of the unaffected kidney (Fig. 4.10) (Hodson and Wilson 1965; Hodson 1967).

A number of variants of the typical reflux nephropathy pattern occur. There may be little or no calyceal deformity underlying the focal scars (Gedroyc *et al.* 1988). This pattern appears to be associated with smooth parenchymal thinning.

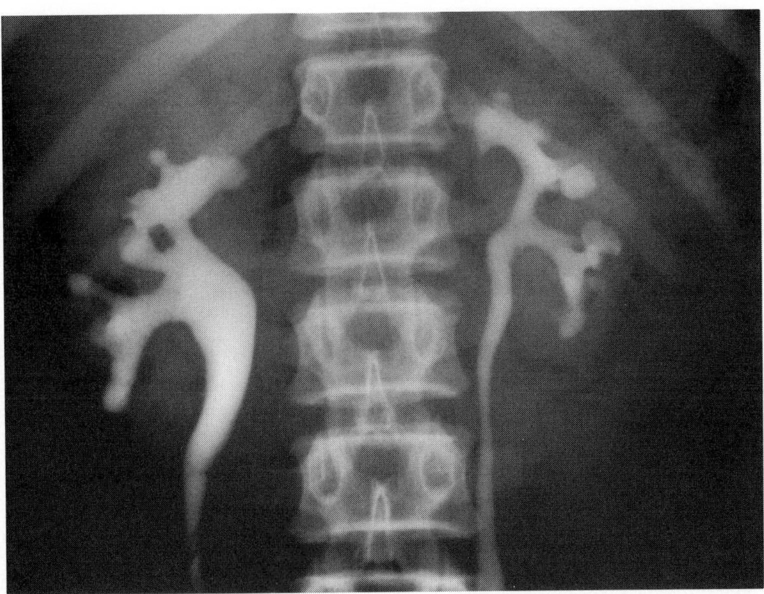

Fig. 4.9 Reflux nephropathy. Urogram shows multiple blunted calyces with irregular scarring in the right kidney, and more diffuse parenchymal loss in the left kidney. (Reproduced by permission of John Wiley & Sons.)

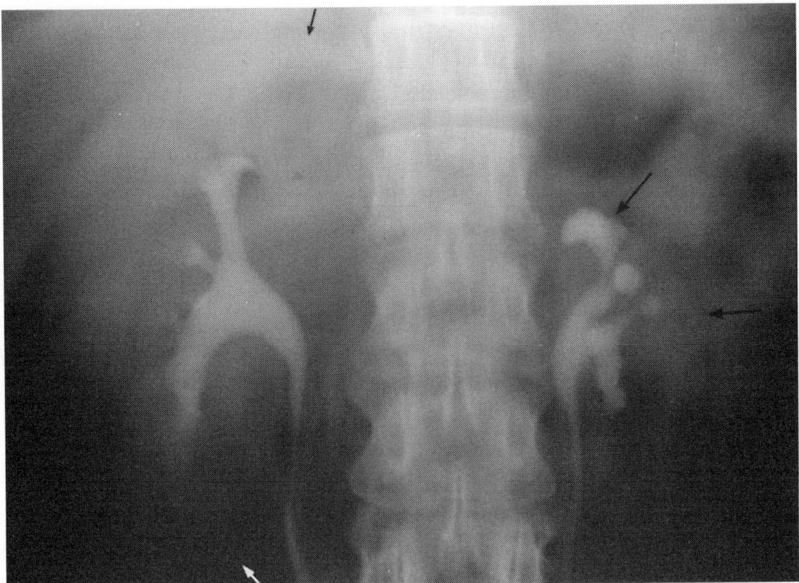

Fig. 4.10 Unilateral involvement in reflux nephropathy. Tomogram from IVU shows small irregular left kidney (outline indicated by long arrows) with blunted calyces and compensatory hypertrophy of right kidney (poles indicated by short arrows). (Reproduced by permission of B. C. Decker.)

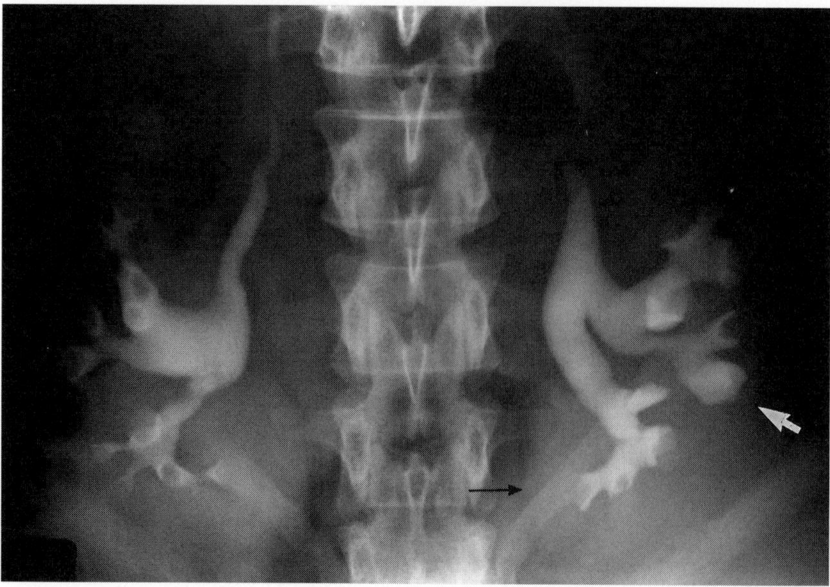

Fig. 4.11 Mild involvement in reflux nephropathy. Urogram shows blunted lateral calyx with overlying scar (white arrow) and parenchymal loss at medial upper pole (black arrow). (Reproduced by permission of B. C. Decker.)

In another variant, the process is diffuse involving the whole kidney with generalized parenchymal thinning and calyceal clubbing (Fig. 4.3) (Thomsen 1985). Diffuse reflux nephropathy is associated with severe high-pressure reflux and may be more difficult to detect early in its development. DMSA scans may fail to show the parenchymal thinning, especially if the contralateral kidney is abnormal (Whitear *et al.* 1990). The established condition appears identical to obstructive or post-obstructive atrophy and can only be distinguished by demonstrating that VUR is present.

In complete renal duplication the insertion of the lower pole moiety ureter into the bladder is usually at the normal level but commonly has an abnormally short intra-mural segment predisposing to reflux. Changes of reflux nephropathy may be seen in the lower pole moieties of such duplex kidneys (Fig. 4.24).

Adult urinary tract infection

The majority of adults with urinary tract infection (UTI) are not imaged during the acute infection. Imaging is usually necessary only if the diagnosis is in doubt, particularly if ureteric colic is suspected, or if there is severe loin pain or fever leading to the suspicion of either renal obstruction or sepsis. Most often, urography is used to differentiate patients with ureteric colic from those with pyelonephritis, and so a minority of patients with acute UTI have urography. US and/or CT are used to check for evidence of renal obstruction or sepsis.

With these methods, findings indicating interstitial nephritis progressing to suppuration may be detected. CT has emerged as a method that can show the evolution of the inflammatory process within the renal interstitium, and serial studies with CT have thrown new light on the long-term sequelae of acute renal infection in adults.

Acute urinary tract infection

Urography This is generally avoided in acute UTI because it only provides limited diagnostic information. In the minority of patients who have urography because of suspected ureteric colic, abnormality is detected in approximately 25 per cent (Little *et al.* 1965; Silver *et al.* 1976). The kidney may show swelling, either diffuse or focal, and there may be reduced nephrogram density and delayed poor pelvicalyceal filling with contrast medium of reduced density (Fig. 4.12).

In more severe acute pyelonephritis, there may be a dense, persistent nephrogram (Cattell *et al.* 1973) or a 'striated' nephrogram with alternating dense and lucent streaks (Fig. 4.13) (Davidson and Talner 1973). There may also be non-obstructive pelvicalyceal dilatation or no pelvicalyceal filling (Davidson and Talner 1973; Teplick *et al.* 1979).

Ultrasonography In moderate or severe acute pyelonephritis, ultrasonography may show renal swelling, either diffuse or focal (Fig. 4.14). Diffuse swelling may be associated with attenuation of the sinus echoes. Focal swelling may be isoechoic or hypoechoic compared to the normal parenchyma. The term 'acute lobar nephronia' was coined to describe focal hypoechoic solid masses in a lobar distribution occurring in acute pyelonephritis (Rosenfield *et al.* 1979; Lee *et al.* 1980). Occasionally, the focal masses may be hyperechoic because of haemorrhage within them (Rigsby *et al.* 1986).

Computed tomography CT scans are normal in patients with mild renal infection, but with more severe infection, a variety of changes occur. On the scans obtained without contrast medium, there may be renal swelling, diffuse or focal, and there may be patchy areas of low attenuation. Rarely, if the infection is haemorrhagic, high-density areas will be seen (Rigsby *et al.* 1986). After contrast medium enhancement the abnormalities appear much more dramatic. Band-like or wedge-shaped areas of reduced enhancement radiate from the renal papillae to the renal margin, with their bases at the renal margin. The borders of the abnormal areas are usually straight and well-defined, and the abnormalities enhance poorly, either homogeneously or patchily (Fig. 4.15) (Lee *et al.* 1980; Gold *et al.* 1983). Delayed scans may show dense staining of the previously poorly enhancing areas (Ishikawa *et al.* 1985). CT is more sensitive than US in detecting evidence of inflammatory involvement of the renal parenchyma (June *et al.* 1985; Soulen *et al.* 1989*a*).

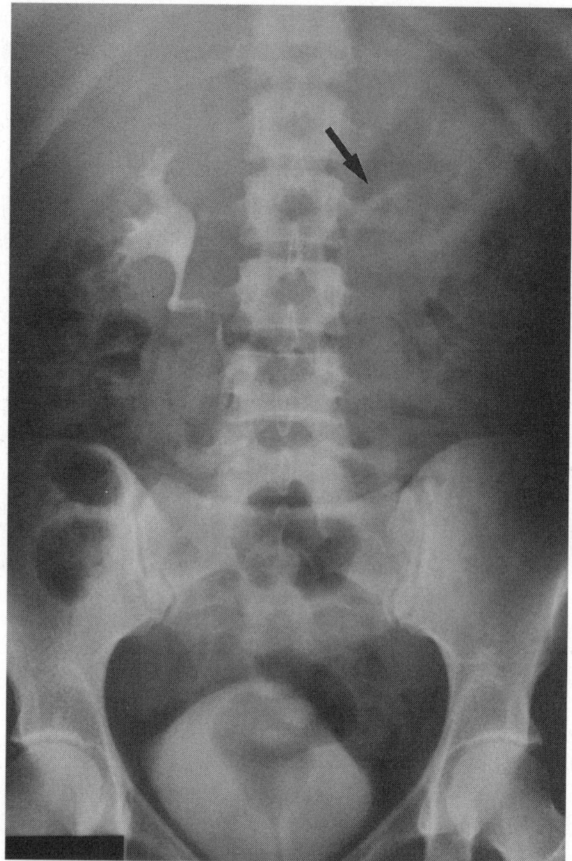

Fig. 4.12 Acute pyelonephritis. Urogram shows delayed faint pelvicalyceal opacification on left (arrowed).

As the changes of inflammatory involvement of the renal parenchyma have been recognized with US and CT, a large number of different terms have been coined—'acute lobar nephronia', 'acute bacterial nephritis', and 'lobar nephritis' being the most commonly used. This has led to confusion among clinicians and radiologists about what is being described and about the significance of the changes. The Society of Uroradiology has recently proposed a simplification of terminology for the CT and US appearances with all evidence of renal parenchymal inflammatory involvement being described as 'acute pyelonephritis'. This can then be further characterized by stating whether it is uni- or bilateral, focal or diffuse, and with or without swelling (Talner *et al.* 1994).

Follow-up studies of CT abnormalities These have provided interesting findings. Abnormalities of parenchymal contrast medium enhancement may persist for two months or more (Soulen *et al.* 1989*b*; Tsugayza *et al.* 1990). An unexpectedly

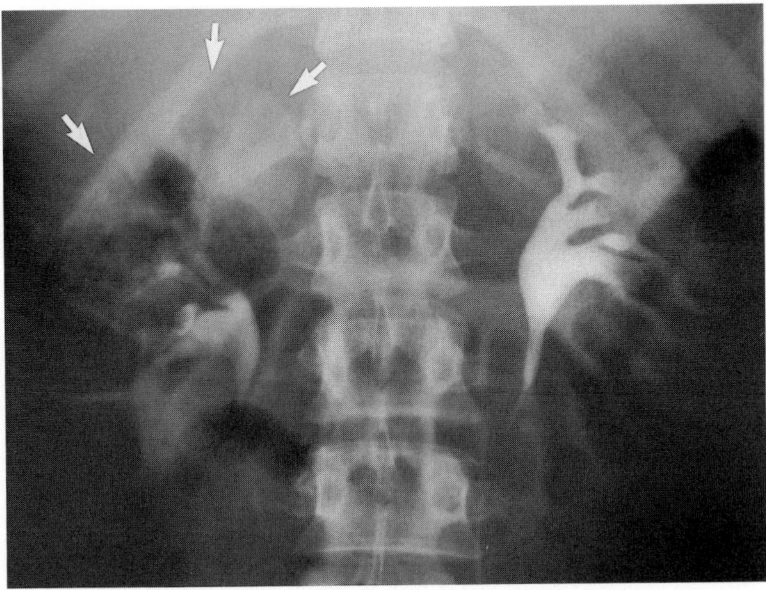

Fig. 4.13 Bilateral dense striated nephrograms seen at urography in acute pyelonephritis. Striations are best seen at the right upper pole (arrowed).

high incidence of scar formation has been found with up to 43 per cent of patients—admittedly those with severe renal infection—developing scars (Meyrier *et al.* 1989; Soulen *et al.* 1989*b*). To date, the best predictor of the likelihood of scar formation appears to be the extent of involvement shown by CT (Tsugaya *et al.* 1990).

DMSA scans There are limited data on the use of ^{99m}Tc-DMSA scintigraphy in adults with acute pyelonephritis. One study (Fraser *et al.* 1989), suggests that the method is more sensitive than CT in showing abnormalities in patients with acute pyelonephritis and normal urograms. The sensitivity of DMSA scans in detecting abnormalities in children with acute pyelonephritis is well recognized (Kass *et al.* 1992; Rushton and Majd 1992).

Emphysematous pyelonephritis

This is a rare and very severe form of renal infection in which gas-forming organisms produce air in the renal collecting system, renal parenchyma, and surrounding tissues. It is associated with diabetes, which was present in 87 per cent of a series of 50 (Michaeli *et al.* 1984), and also with obstruction.

Plain films demonstrate air in the renal parenchyma, the collecting system, and in the perinephric space. If urography is performed no contrast medium excretion occurs into the pelvicalyceal system (Fig. 4.16). US may show air in the renal parenchyma as echogenicities with associated shadows but may be unable to identify the kidney if a large amount of air is present. CT clearly

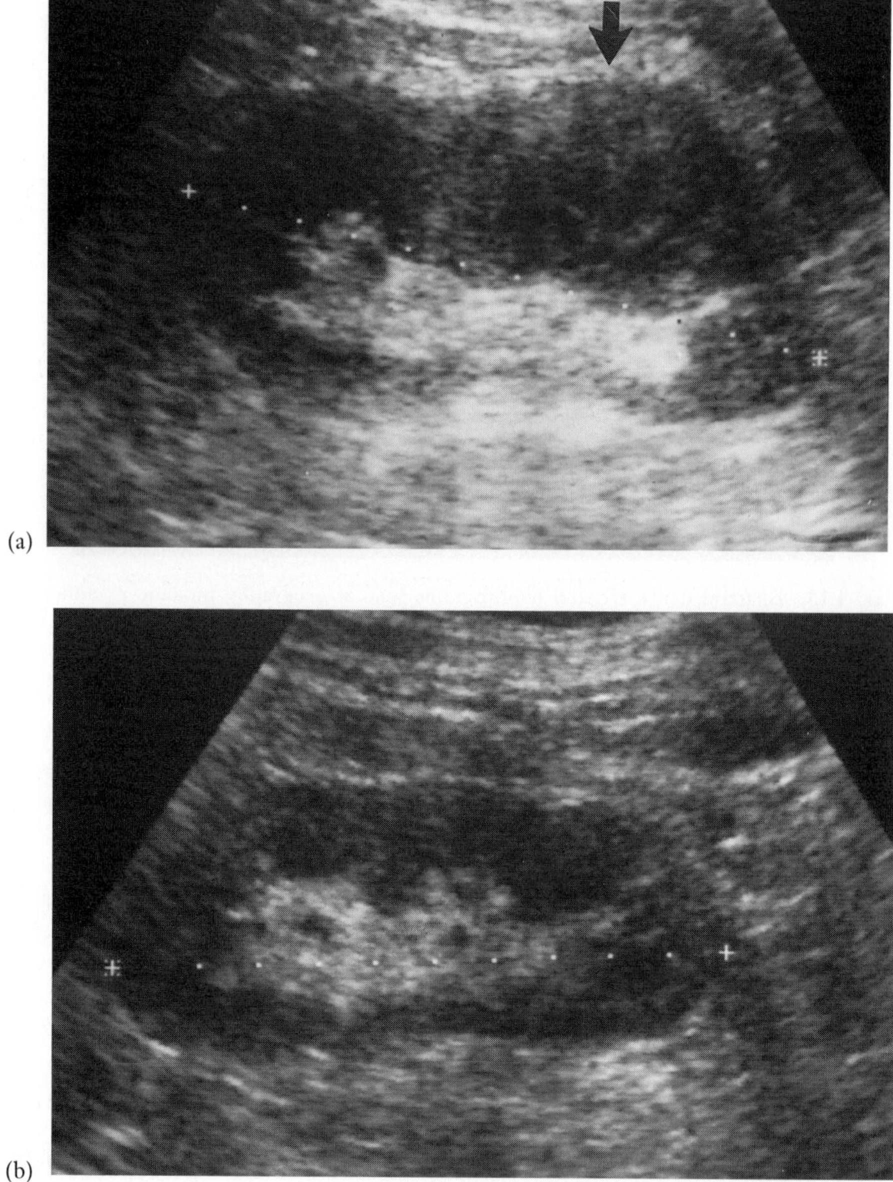

Fig. 4.14 Focal acute pyelonephritis. Hypoechoic swelling of the lower kidney on a longitudinal US scan, arrowed (a), which had resolved 3 months later (b).

shows the presence and site of the air. Although nephrectomy was previously the only therapeutic option, percutaneous drainage of the infected kidney with imaging guidance is now an alternative possibility (Hall *et al.* 1988).

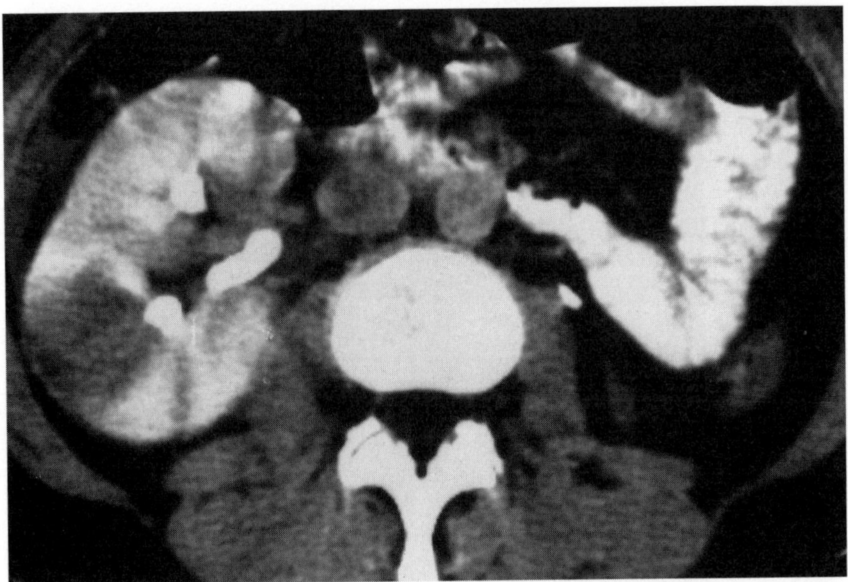

Fig. 4.15 Diffuse acute pyelonephritis. Typical inhomogeneous pattern in the right kidney after contrast medium enhancement at CT. The left kidney was atrophic. (Reproduced by permission of B. C. Decker.)

Acute renal and perinephric suppuration

Renal abscess

Renal imaging cannot distinguish established abscesses secondary to ascending infection from those due to haematogenous spread. However, serial CT can show the progression from severe interstitial nephritis to micro-abscess formation with the development of small collections of fluid density which do not enhance after intravenous contrast medium. These collections may later coalesce to form an abscess.

Urography An abscess appears as a mass which, if peripheral, distorts the renal outline and, if central, displaces the pelvicalyceal system. Nephrotomography may demonstrate that the mass is lucent centrally and that it has a thick wall, but the findings are non-specific (Fig. 4.17a).

Ultrasonography US demonstrates a renal abscess as a fluid collection that may appear simple and indistinguishable from a simple cyst, or may show complex features such as a thick wall or contained echoes (Fig. 4.17b) (Hoddick *et al.* 1983). The contained echoes may be distributed diffusely throughout the abscess or may form a layer. Air within the abscess is seen as a bright echogenicity with an associated acoustic shadow.

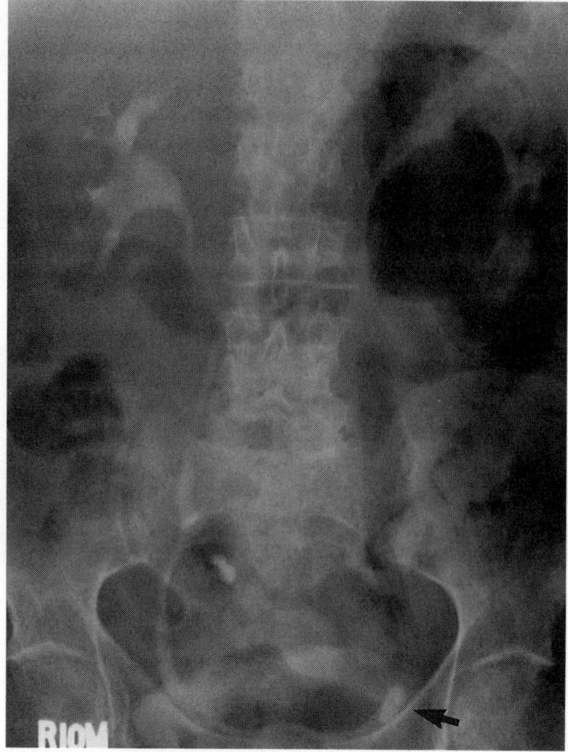

Fig. 4.16 Emphysematous pyelonephritis. Air is present in the left renal parenchyma, pelvicalyceal system, and ureter to the level of an obstructing ureteric calculus (arrowed) and there is no contrast medium excretion. (Reproduced by permission of Churchill Livingstone.)

Computed tomography CT is more sensitive in detecting both micro-abscesses and established abscesses than ultrasound (Hoddick *et al.* 1983; Soulen *et al.* 1989*a*). Abscesses are seen as masses of fluid density, often with a thickened wall which may enhance (Fig. 4.17c). They may contain air.

The appearances of an abscess both on US and CT are non-specific and may also occur with necrotic tumours, haematomas, and some infarcts. The finding of a fluid collection in the kidney of a patient in the appropriate clinical setting is highly suggestive of the diagnosis. This can be established conclusively by needle aspiration guided by US or CT. Small abscesses can often be aspirated completely, and with large abscesses, a drainage catheter can be placed percutaneously under US or CT guidance.

Infected renal cysts

These cysts have features identical to renal abscesses at US and CT. Cyst infection in autosomal-dominant polycystic kidney disease may be difficult to localize among the myriad of other cysts in the enlarged kidney. To date, no

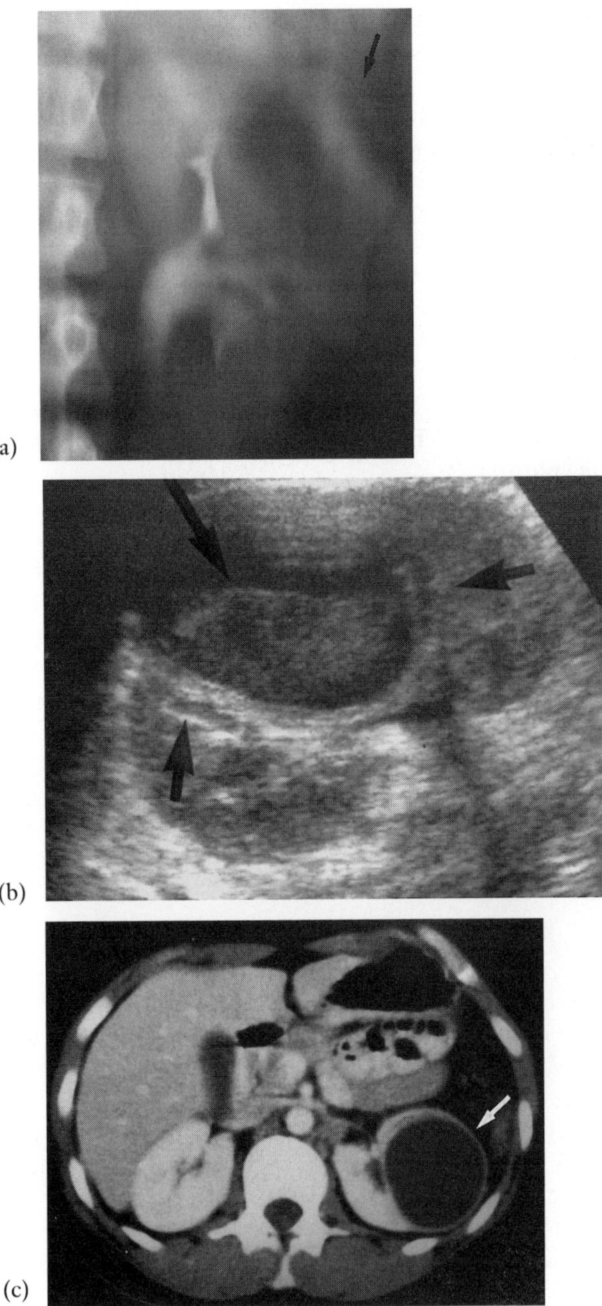

Fig. 4.17 Left renal abscess (a) Urogram shows lucent mass with thick wall (arrowed). (b) Longitudinal US scan shows fluid collection with thick walls (short arrows) and echoes in a layer (long arrow). (c) CT scan after contrast medium shows mass of fluid density with an enhancing wall (arrowed). Figure 4.17b is reproduced by permission of John Wiley & Sons.)

imaging method appears capable of detecting all such infected cysts and when cyst infection is suspected, it may be necessary to use a series of techniques. One cyst larger than the rest (a 'dominant cyst') is a suspicious finding. More specific findings at ultrasonography are a thickened wall or echoes, which may layer, in the cyst fluid. At CT again the cyst may appear thick-walled and may contain air or fluid of increased density. Gallium scanning may be helpful with uptake of ^{67}Ga by the infected cyst. However, in one series this only occurred in half the patients with infected cysts (Schwab *et al.* 1987). Once the infected cyst has been localized, percutaneous puncture and drainage or placement of a drainage catheter can be guided either by US or CT (Chapman *et al.* 1990).

Perinephric abscess

These usually arise by direct extension from either acute renal suppuration (abscess or pyonephrosis) or from chronic suppuration (tuberculosis or xanthogranulomatous pyelonephritis).

The urographic features of perinephric abscess are non-specific with a soft tissue mass which may obscure the psoas outline and displaces the kidney anteriorly and superiorly. The renal displacement may lead to distortion of the pelvicalyceal system. The kidney loses its normal mobility with respiration (Lee and Knific 1990).

US demonstrates the perinephric fluid collection that usually lies posterior or inferior to the kidney. It may appear as simple fluid or may show contained

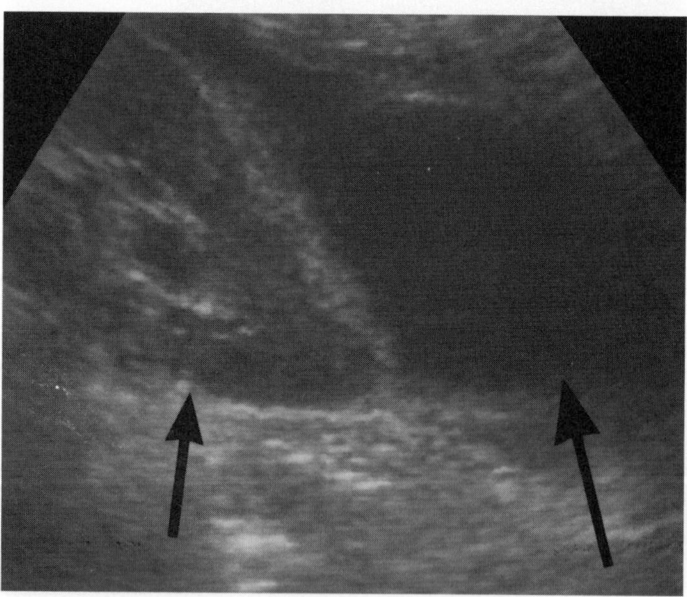

Fig. 4.18 Perinephric abscess. Longitudinal US scan shows fluid collection (long arrow) postero-inferior to the lower pole of the kidney (short arrow). (Reproduced by permission of B. C. Decker.)

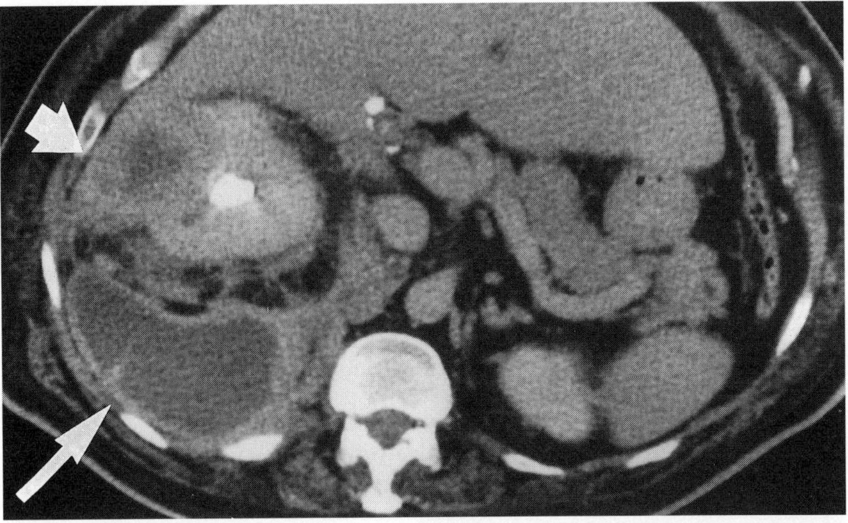

Fig. 4.19 Right perinephric abscess. CT scan after contrast medium shows lateral renal abscess with spread into the perinephric (short arrow) and posterior paranephric (long arrow) spaces.

echoes (Fig. 4.18). CT also shows the perinephric fluid collection and because of its excellent demonstration of the retroperitoneal fascial planes demonstrates the full extent of the inflammatory process better than US (Fig. 4.19) (Hoddick *et al.* 1983). Either US or CT may show contained air and either may be used to guide percutaneous drainage of the collection.

Pyonephrosis

In pyonephrosis there is suppuration in an obstructed collecting system. At urography the pelvicalyceal system fails to fill with contrast medium. The dilated obstructed collecting system may be shown either with US or CT. At US, the content of the collecting system may have the characteristics of simple fluid or may show contained echoes, either diffuse or layered (Fig. 4.20) (Coleman *et al.* 1981; Jeffrey *et al.* 1985). At CT, the collecting system content may either be of water density or of increased density similar to that of the adjacent renal parenchyma (Morehouse *et al.* 1984). Either US or CT may be used to guide percutaneous aspiration to make the diagnosis and subsequent percutaneous catheter drainage. CT is usually more successful than US at demonstrating the cause of obstruction especially if this is in the retroperitoneum. Antegrade contrast medium injection through the draining catheter provides helpful diagnostic information about the site and nature of ureteric obstruction.

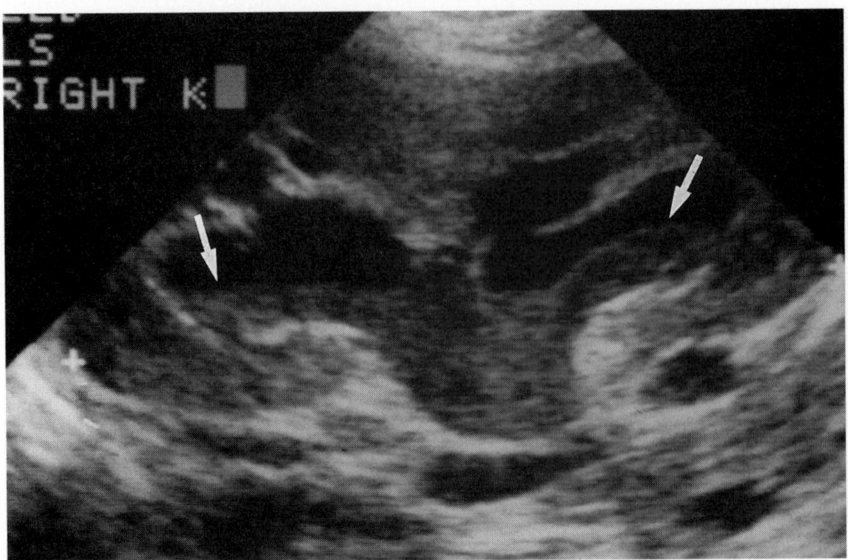

Fig. 4.20 Pyonephrosis in an obstructed kidney. Longitudinal US scan shows dilated pelvicalyceal system with echoes layering in the dependent part (arrowed).

Imaging in adults following acute urinary tract infection

It is generally accepted that all males should have renal imaging following a documented episode of UTI. In females, the criteria for recommending renal imaging following UTI are more controversial. This relates to the low yield of abnormality when imaging is performed in *all* women after UTI, with only approximately 5 per cent of urograms showing abnormality (Fair *et al.* 1979; Fairchild *et al.* 1982). A reasonable recommendation is that imaging is indicated in females when there are two or three recurrent documented attacks of UTI in 12 months (Cattell 1985).

The aims of the investigation are to identify factors which predispose to renal damage and factors which predispose either to relapsing infection or to re-infection (Table 4.1). Although ultrasonography and plain films are adequate during an acute infection to check for most calculi, or for evidence of obstruction or suppuration, they do not demonstrate the detailed anatomy of the urinary tract sufficiently well to make many of the diagnoses shown in Table 4.1. Urography is therefore the method of choice to evaluate adults following acute UTI.

Intravenous urography Detection of *calculi* necessitates a careful plain film technique supplemented by plain renal tomography if the renal areas are hidden by overlying bowel or if low density calculi are suspected, for example in Proteus UTI (Fig. 4.21).

Most of the conditions in Table 4.1 can be identified by urography. *Obstruction* is evidenced by delayed pelvicalyceal filling with a dilated pelvicalyceal system and ureter to the level of the obstructing lesion. In *papillary*

Table 4.1 Complicating factors in patients with urinary tract intection identified by imaging

1. *Factors predisposing to renal damage*
   Stones
   Obstruction
   Vesicoureteric reflux
   Papillary necrosis
2. *Factors predisposing to relapsing infection*
   Stones
   Scars
   Autosomal dominant polycystic kidney disease
   Medullary sponge kidney
   Calyceal cysts
   Congenital anomalies (e.g. obstructed upper pole moiety) of duplex system
   Renal abscess
   Urinary tract fistulae (e.g. vesicoenteric)
   Prostatitis
   Foreign bodies in the urinary tract
3. *Factors predisposing to re-infection*
   Poor bladder emptying

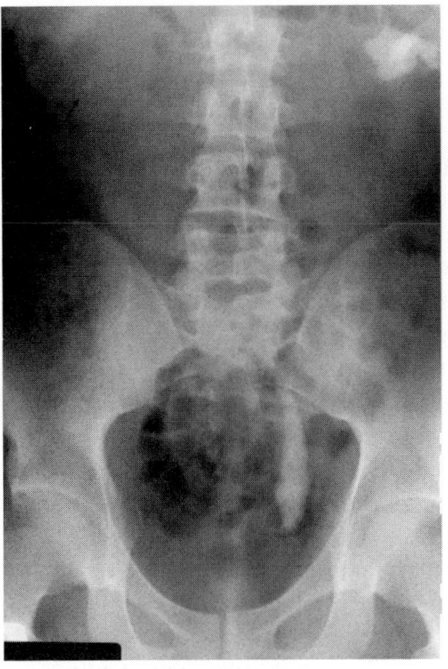

(a)

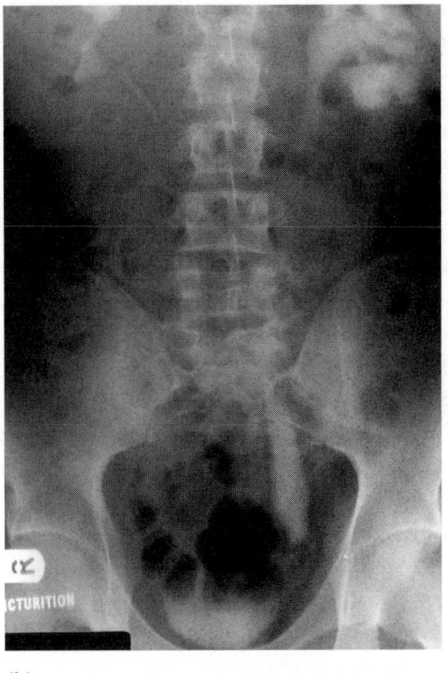

(b)

Fig. 4.21 Multiple calculi in male aged 23 years presenting with Proteus UTI. Note the left staghorn calculus, large calculus in the distal left ureter, and small right lower pole calculus (arrowed) on the plain film (a). After contrast medium (b), there is left pelvicalyceal dilatation. (Reproduced by permission of B. C. Decker.)

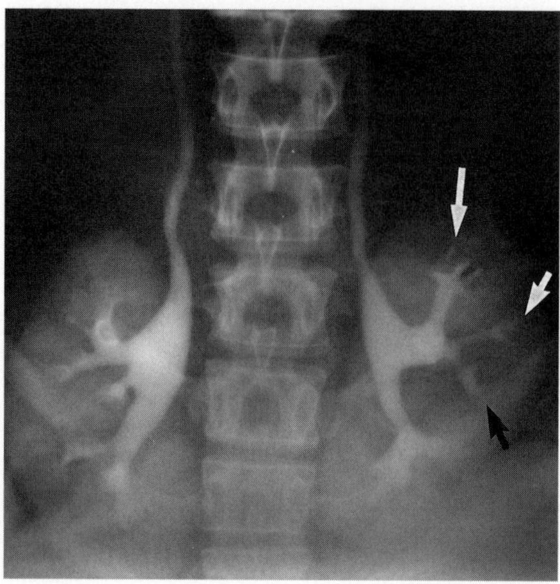

Fig. 4.22 Papillary necrosis in sickle-cell trait. Note the clubbed calyx (black arrow), 'egg in a cup' (short white arrow), and contrast track (long white arrow). (Reproduced by permission of John Wiley & Sons.)

necrosis, cavitation may occur in the centre of papillae ('egg in a cup') or at the margins of the papillae with tracks and horns of contrast medium extending out from the calyceal fornices (Fig. 4.22) (Hare and Poynter 1974). The necrotic tracks may amputate the papilla, with resultant papillary sloughing. The affected calyces appear blunted, and lucent filling defects may be seen in the collecting system. In *medullary sponge kidney* there are commonly punctate calcifications in the affected papillae. Following intravenous contrast medium, these are seen to lie in pools of contrast medium, and there may be further contrast pools and streaks representing the dilated collecting ducts (Fig. 4.23) (Palubinskas 1961). *Calyceal cysts* are usually polar, lying close to the corticomedullary junction. They are seen as smooth-walled cavities communicating with the collecting system and may contain calculi (Wulfsohn 1980). The dilated calyces of an *obstructed upper pole moiety of a duplex kidney* produce an upper pole mass lesion at urography and either fail to fill with contrast medium or show delayed filling (Fig. 4.24). The dilated ureter often displaces the lower pole moiety ureter laterally, and an obstructed ureterocoele at the lower end of the ureter may be seen as a filling defect within the bladder. *Impaired bladder emptying* can be assessed by carefully conducted urography (Cattell *et al.* 1970) or by ultrasonography.

Some women with recurrent UTI have abnormally distensible urinary tracts. This occurs especially if there has previously been UTI during pregnancy. The pelvicalyceal systems and ureters to pelvic brim level are markedly dilated on the films obtained with ureteric compression applied and immediately after release of

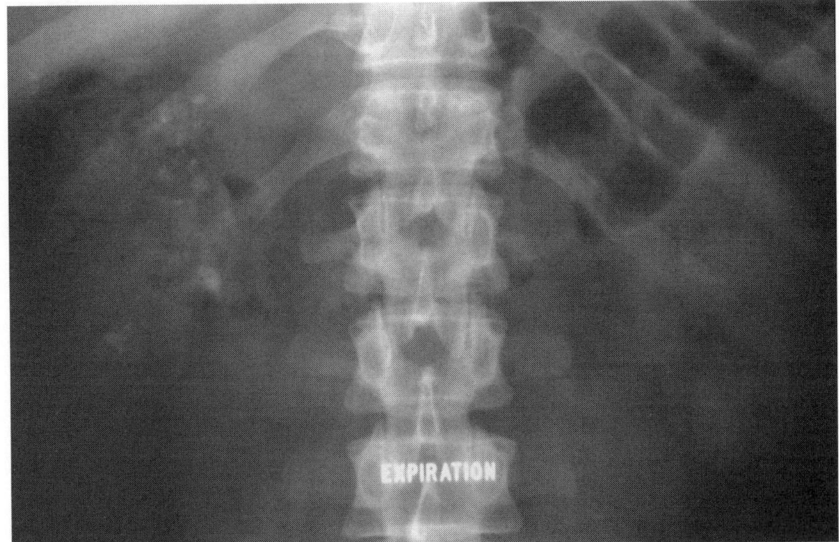

(a)

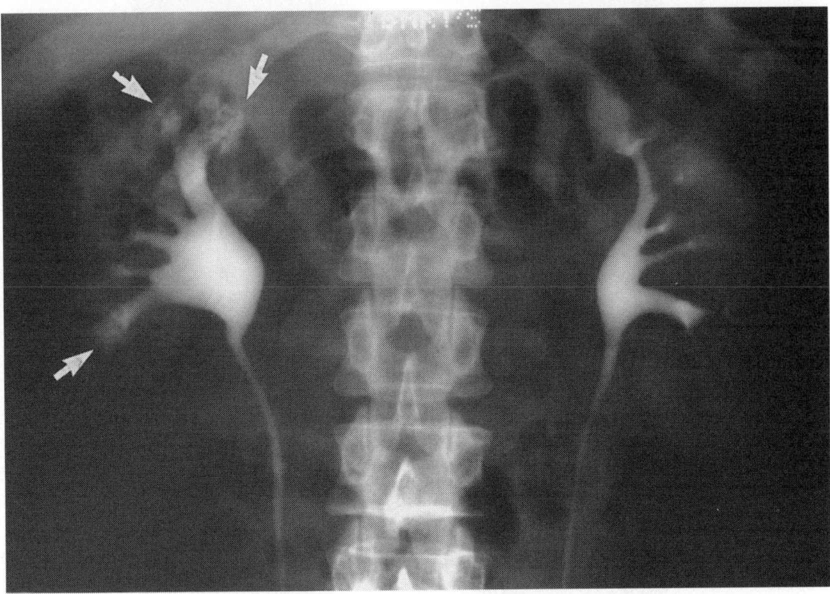

(b)

Fig. 4.23 Medullary sponge kidney. Multiple calcifications on the plain film (a). After contrast medium (b), calcifications are seen to lie in the papillae where there are also pools of contrast (arrowed).

ureteric compression, but then drain normally on the full-length post-micturition film (Fig. 4.25) (Spiro and Fry 1970). This appearance may be associated with persistent loin pain but does not appear to hamper the eradication of infection.

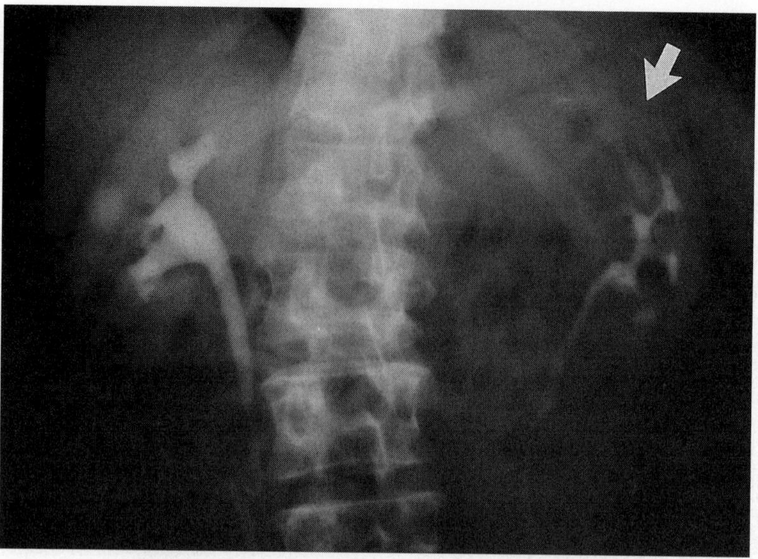

(a)

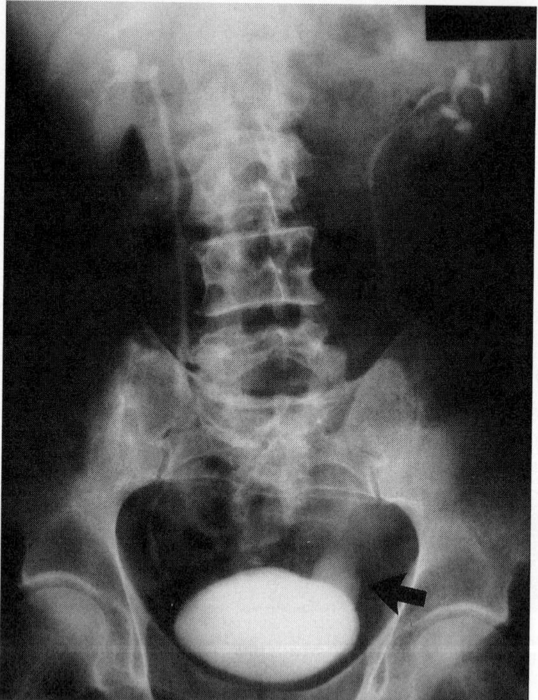

(b)

Fig. 4.24 Obstructed upper pole moiety of left duplex kidney. Note (a) mass effect at the upper pole (arrowed), changes of reflux nephropathy at the lower pole with lateral displacement of the lower pole moiety ureter by the obstructed non-pacified upper pole moiety ureter. (b) Reflux of contrast into the dilated upper pole moiety ureter (arrowed). Opacity overlying right kidney is a gallstone. (Reproduced by permission of B. C. Decker.)

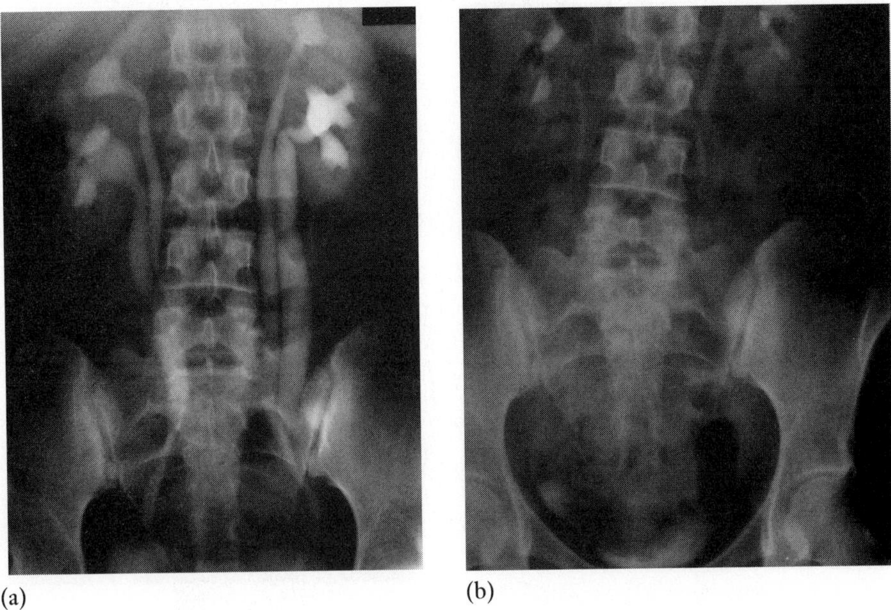

Fig. 4.25 Distensible upper tracts following UTI in pregnancy. (a) Dilated bilateral duplex pelvicalyceal systems and ureters to pelvic brim level after ureteric compression is removed. (b) Drainage of the systems on full-length post-micturition film.

Micturating cystography, videocystometrography, and urethrography In women, micturating cystography is rarely indicated in the evaluation following acute UTI. Vesicoureteric reflux is unlikely if there is no indirect evidence of it at urography (p. 73). To evaluate impaired bladder emptying in females, video-cystometrography will usually be required.

In males with impaired bladder emptying, urethrography may be necessary to check for urethral strictures or video-cystometrography may be indicated to check for impaired bladder function.

Chronic urinary tract infections

Tuberculosis

Intravenous urography This is a good diagnostic technique for diagnosing urinary tract TB because of its ability to detect calcification, to provide a detailed image of anatomy, and to show the multiple lesions which commonly occur (Figs 4.26–4.30, 4.32).

Renal TB may be uni- or bilateral. Calcification is seen in about 30 per cent of cases (Roylance *et al.* 1970). It may have a variety of patterns—punctate,

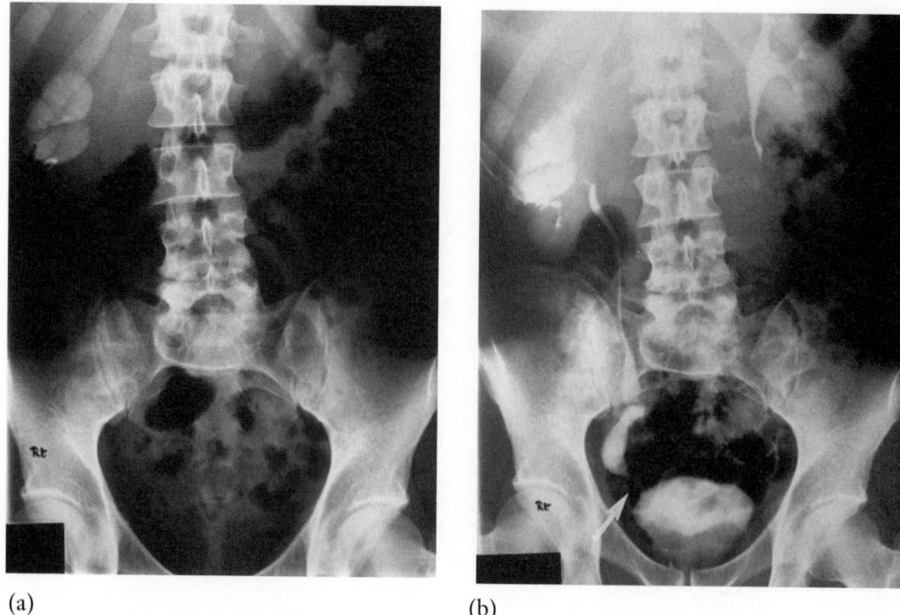

(a) (b)

Fig. 4.26 Right renal and ureteric TB. (a) Hazy calcification in the mid kidney with no calyceal filling (b). Lower ureteric stricture is arrowed. (By permission of Dr A. G. Wilson.)

speckled, or hazy (Fig. 4.26). In advanced TB the whole pelvicalyceal system and ureter may be outlined by calcification—the so-called TB autonephrectomy. (Fig. 4.27).

Early TB is seen as irregularity of the papillary margins with reduced contrast medium density in the affected areas. Cavities, either smooth or irregular, then develop and communicate with pelvicalyceal system (Figs 4.28 and 4.29). As destruction progresses there is associated parenchymal loss. Fibrosis leads to strictures. When these affect the calyceal infundibula there is no calyceal filling at urography and the infundibulum shows a typical 'pinched-off' appearance. Fibrosis at the pelviureteric junction causes obstruction at this level. Local granuloma formation or dilated obstructed calyces, which do not fill with contrast medium, may produce a mass effect (Fig. 4.30). Extension of infection into the perinephric space with abscess formation may occur (p. 88). Fistulae may develop, particularly to the skin and gut, and to show them fully retrograde ureterography or sinography may be required.

In the relatively rare condition of diffuse interstitial renal TB no urographic abnormality is detected and the diagnosis necessitates renal biopsy (Mallinson *et al.* 1981).

Ureteric and bladder TB are usually secondary to renal TB and signs of renal abnormality are therefore present. The earliest ureteric change is ulceration but this is rarely demonstrated radiologically. Stricturing then occurs (Fig. 4.26) and

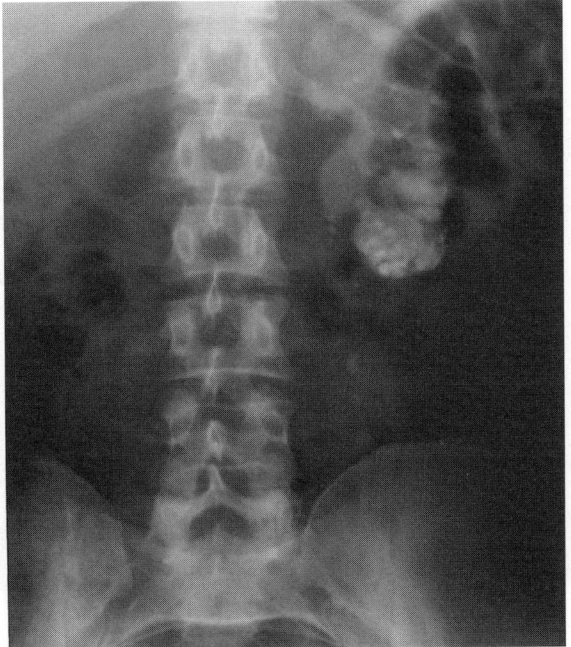

Fig. 4.27 Left TB autonephrectomy. (Reproduced by permission of John Wiley & Sons.)

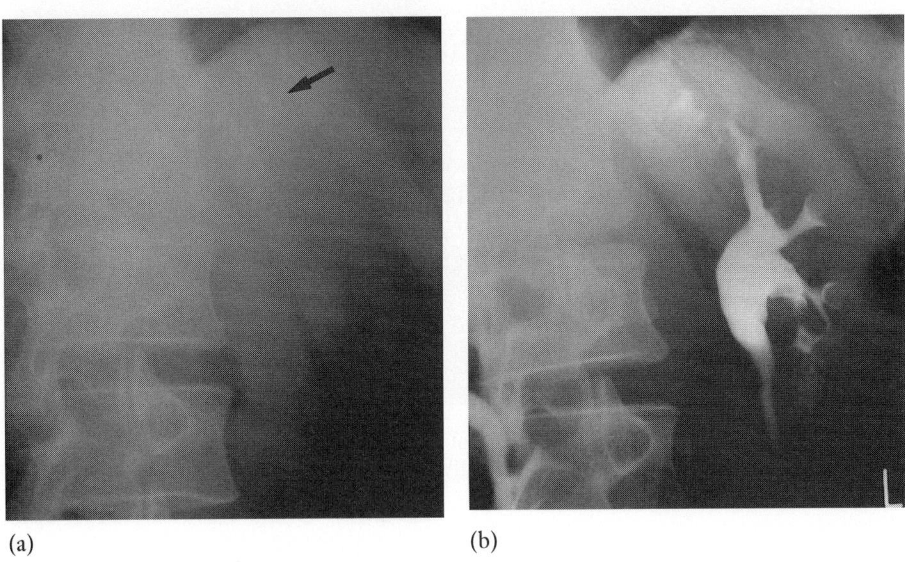

(a) (b)

Fig. 4.28 Early TB. (a) Upper pole calcification (arrowed) lies in an irregular contrast pool. (b) Contrast pool at the lower pole adjacent to abnormal calyx. (Reproduced by permission of John Wiley & Sons.)

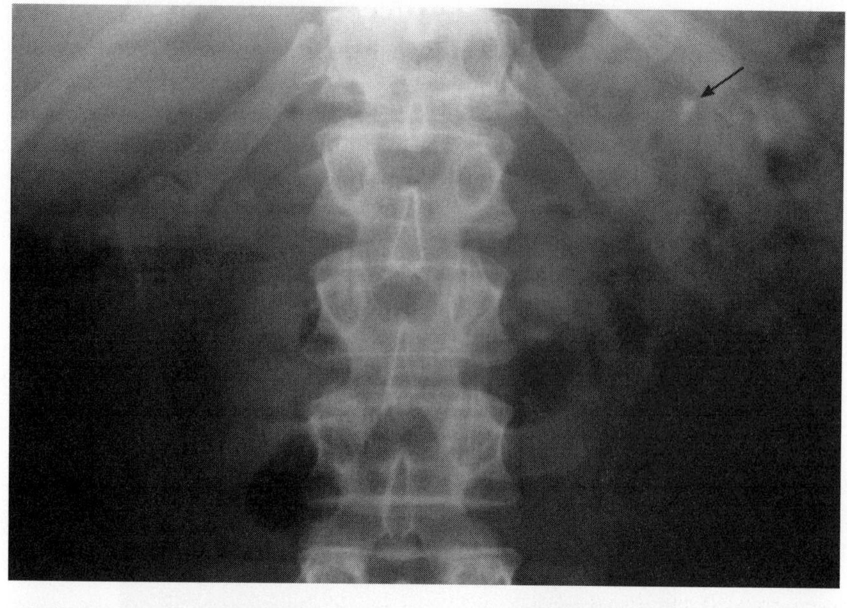

(a)

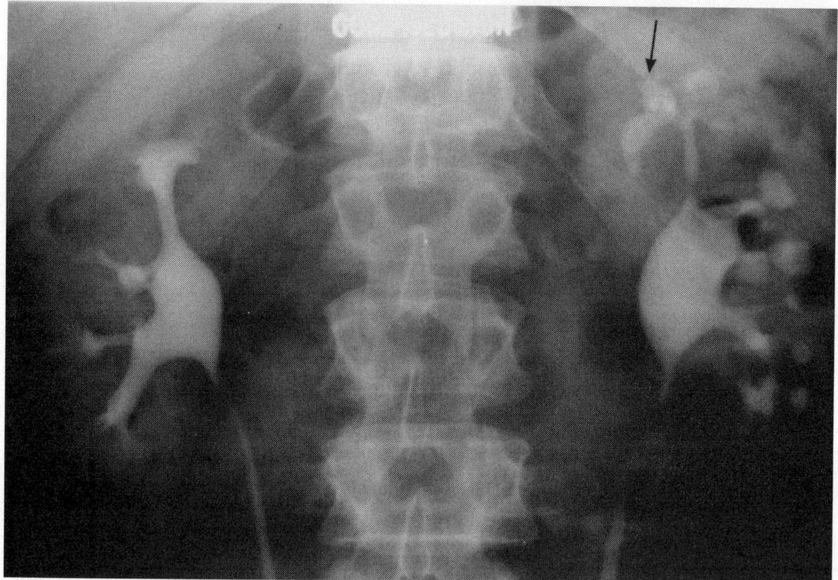

(b)

Fig. 4.29 Left renal (TB). (a) Upper pole calcification (arrowed). (b) After contrast medium, irregular cavity at upper pole fills (arrowed) and there are multiple blunted calyces.

there may be associated filling defects if there is florid granuloma formation. As fibrosis progresses the ureter shortens and becomes thick-walled. Vesicoureteric junction incompetence may occur and lead to vesicoureteric reflux. The bladder

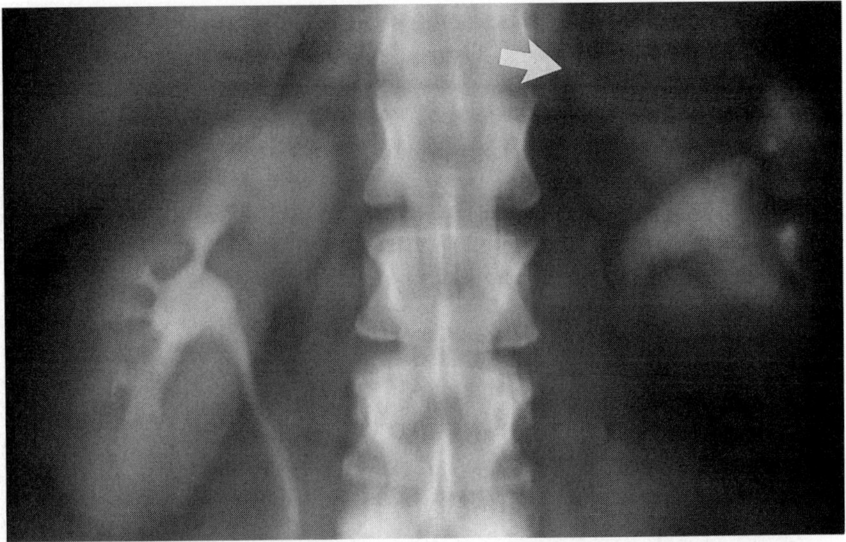

Fig. 4.30 Left renal TB. Tomogram shows mass effect with no calyceal filling at upper pole (arrowed) and dilated calyces and pelvis in remaining kidney.

wall thickens and granulomas may cause filling defects. With generalized involvement, bladder capacity is reduced. Calcification in the ureter and bladder only occur with fairly advance disease. Calcification may also occur in the seminal vesicles, vas, and prostate if these are involved.

Ultrasonography US shows many of the changes of advanced disease, such as pelvicalyceal dilatation, local collections, and calcification (Schaffer *et al.* 1983). However, it is a less sensitive detector, even of advanced disease, than urography (Premkumar *et al.* 1987).

Computed tomography CT is a good method for demonstrating the many changes in advanced disease: calcification, pelvicalyceal dilatation, scars, strictures, and extra-renal spread (Fig. 4.31) (Goldman *et al.* 1985; Premkumar *et al.* 1987). Its sensitivity in early disease has not been assessed but is likely to be less than that of urography because it shows less detailed pelvicalyceal anatomy.

Follow-up studies on chemotherapy During drug treatment of urinary tract TB, ureteric strictures may develop. This may occur at sites apparently normal on the urogram obtained at presentation, presumably because mucosal ulceration at the affected site was not visualized. A limited urogram is the best method to check for ureteric strictures and their effects on the upper tracts (Fig. 4.32).

Xanthogranulomatous pyelonephritis (XGPN)

Xanthogranulomatous pyelonephritis (XGPN) is a relatively unusual form of chronic renal infection in which the renal parenchyma is replaced by lipid-

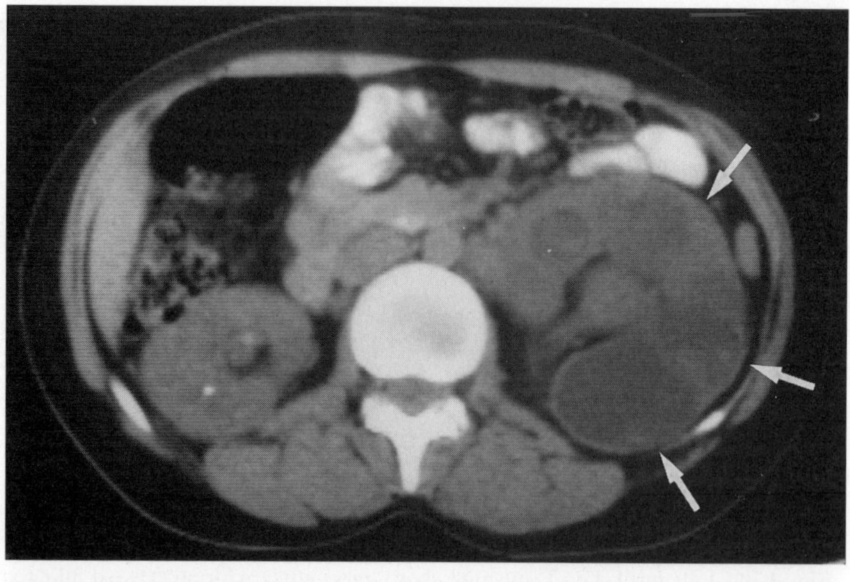

(a)

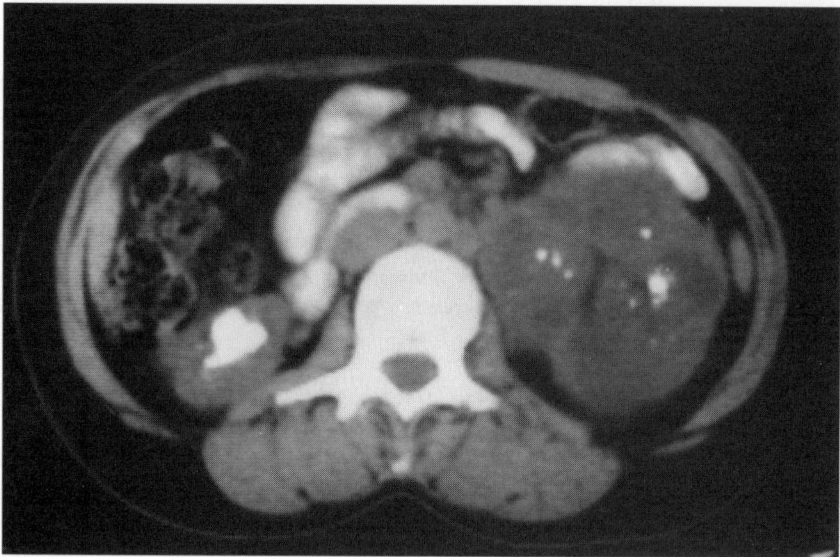

(b)

Fig. 4.31 CT scan in advanced renal TB. Unenhanced scans show bilateral renal calcification. Note (a) dilated calyces in the left mid kidney (arrowed) and (b), mixed attenuation left lower pole mass containing calcification. (By permission of Dr I. Mootoosamy.)

containing macrophages (foam cells). There are strong associations with calculus disease and obstruction, and Proteus is the commonest infecting organism. Involvement is usually unilateral and typically diffuse, involving the whole kidney. More rarely involvement may be focal and produce a mass lesion.

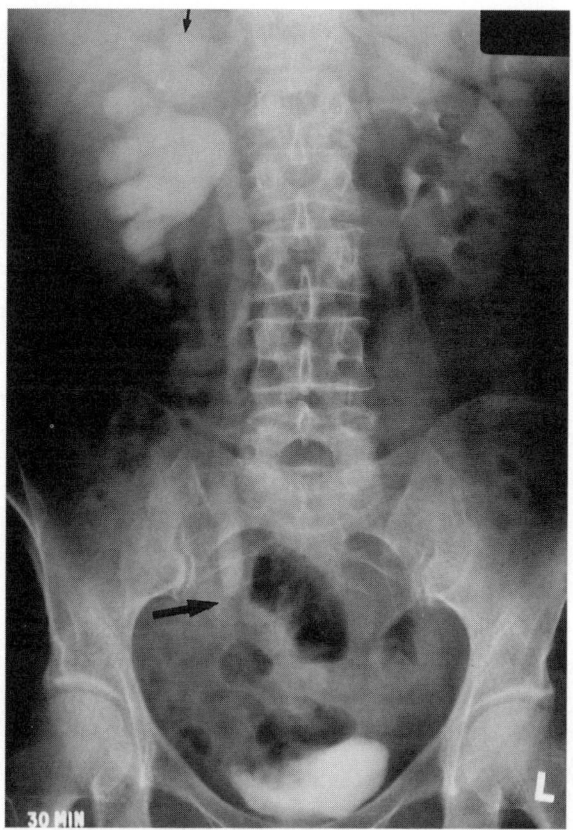

Fig. 4.32 Right ureteric stricture (large arrow) which developed during drug treatment. Note right upper pole cavitation (small arrow). (Reproduced by permission of B. C. Decker.)

Intravenous urography Renal calculi are present in over 75 per cent of cases (Davidson 1985) and in the diffuse form a stag-horn calculus is often present. The kidney is enlarged and films after contrast medium usually show impaired excretion. Peripheral parenchymal enhancement may outline multiple lucent masses in a calyceal distribution.

Ultrasonography US shows an enlarged kidney often with a central calculus and multiple surrounding hypoechoic solid masses in a calyceal distribution (Fig. 4.33a). The parenchyma around these is thinned (Subramanyam *et al.* 1982). Where involvement is focal, typically there is a single hypoechoic mass with a calculus central to it. The appearances may be similar to hydronephrosis or pyonephrosis, but the masses are solid rather than fluid and unlike pyonephrosis show no layering of echoes.

Computed tomography CT typically shows multiple peripheral low-attenuation masses around a contracted pelvis containing a calculus. The masses are usually

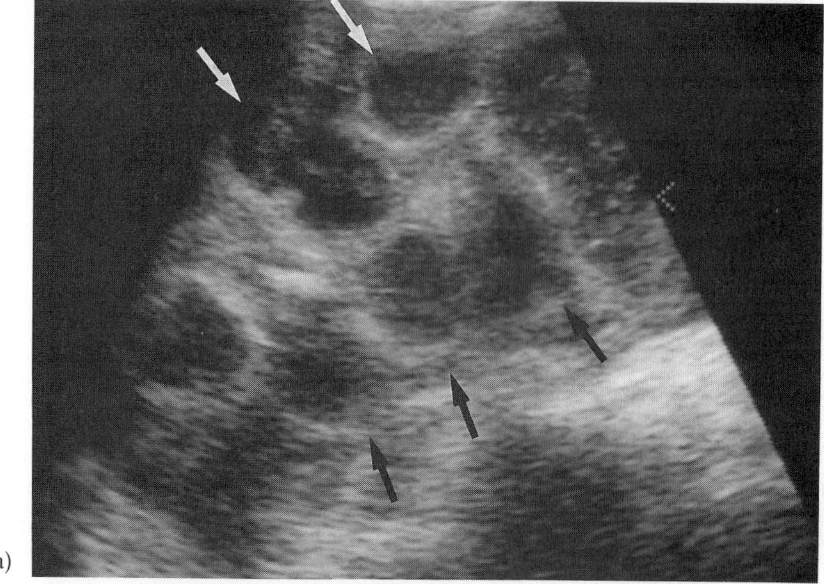

(a)

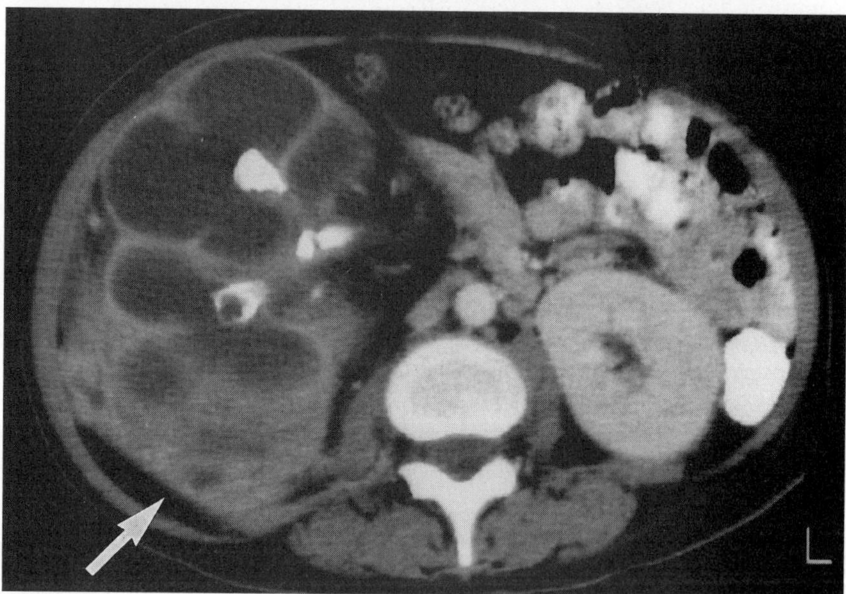

(b)

Fig. 4.33 Diffuse xanthogranulomatous pyelonephritis. (a) Longitudinal US scan shows multiple hypoechoic masses in a calyceal distribution (arrowed). (b) CT scan after contrast medium shows central calculi, dilated calyces, and spread of infection posteriorly producing a perinephric collection (arrowed).

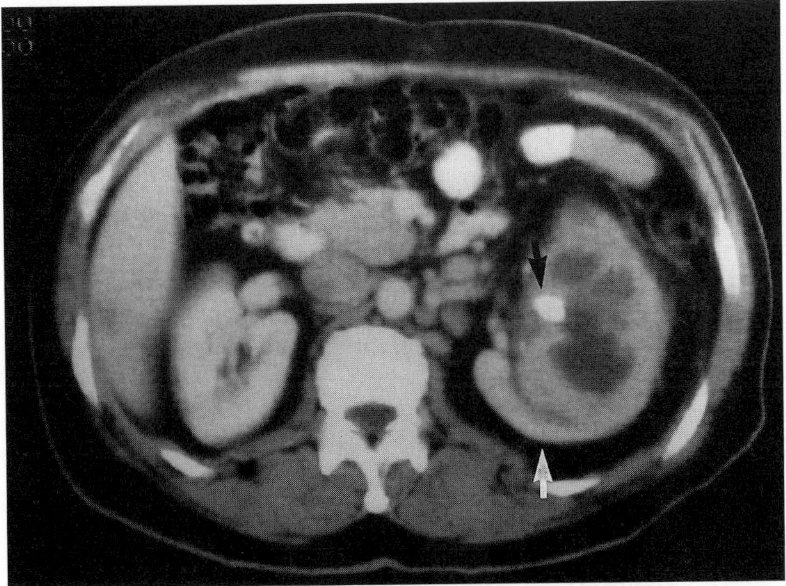

Fig. 4.34 Focal xanthogranulomatous pyelonephritis in the left kidney on CT scan after contrast medium. Note that central calculus (black arrow) and low attenuation masses surrounded by thickened parenchyma, with normal renal parenchyma compressed posteriorly (white arrow).

of water and or soft tissue density and because of their relatively low lipid content are only rarely of fat density (Goldman *et al.* 1984). Following contrast medium, the tissue around the masses enhances (Fig. 4.33b). With focal involvement, appearances are similar but with a single mass localized to one part of the kidney (Fig. 4.34). There is usually thickening of the renal fascia. Spread into the perinephric space, with perinephric abscess, and into adjacent retroperitoneal structures is common (Goldman *et al.* 1984).

None of the imaging findings is specific but in the appropriate clinical setting the combination of imaging signs is highly suggestive of XGPN.

Leukoplakia

Leukoplakia describes squamous metaplasia of the transitional epithelium that occurs in association with chronic or recurrent renal infection and stone disease. This results in keratin debris which accumulate in large masses, usually mixed with chronic inflammatory tissue to form a cholesteatoma.

Intravenous urography IVU shows associated calculi and may show fine-speckled calcification in the keratin mass (Wills *et al.* 1981). Mucosal thickening is an early change and produces linear striations in the contrast medium-filled pelvicalyceal system. With development of a cholesteatoma a lucent mass is seen

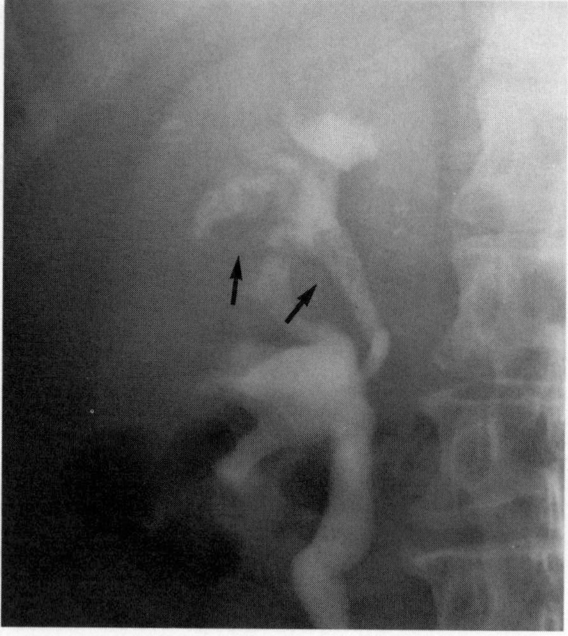

Fig. 4.35 Leukoplakia. Typical urographic appearance of an upper pole mass with a striated surface (arrowed) protruding into the pelvicalyceal system. (Reproduced by permission of Churchill Livingstone.)

with a typical laminar or whorled appearance caused by contrast medium entering the grooves on the surface of the mass (Fig. 4.35). The mass may mimic a large transitional cell tumour or a fungal ball.

Ultrasonography This shows the cholesteatoma as a hypoechoic mass, without specific features (Wills *et al.* 1981).

Computed tomography This will also show the mass and because of the fine calcification it may have a high CT number (110–120 Hounsfield units) (Wills *et al.* 1981). The appearances with US and CT are, however, not specific.

Malacoplakia

Malacoplakia is a rare chronic granulomatous condition associated with long-standing or recurrent *E. coli* infection, apparently secondary to impaired destruction of phagocytosed bacteria by the leucocytes. It most often affects the *bladder* where it gives rise to small masses, indistinguishable from bladder polyps or carcinoma. More rarely, the kidney or ureter are involved. *Renal* involvement is usually multifocal. Urography shows a large kidney containing multiple masses that do not show calcification. The masses may protrude into the collecting system and there may be stricturing at the pelviureteric junction. US and CT both show solid masses with features indistinguishable from neoplasm.

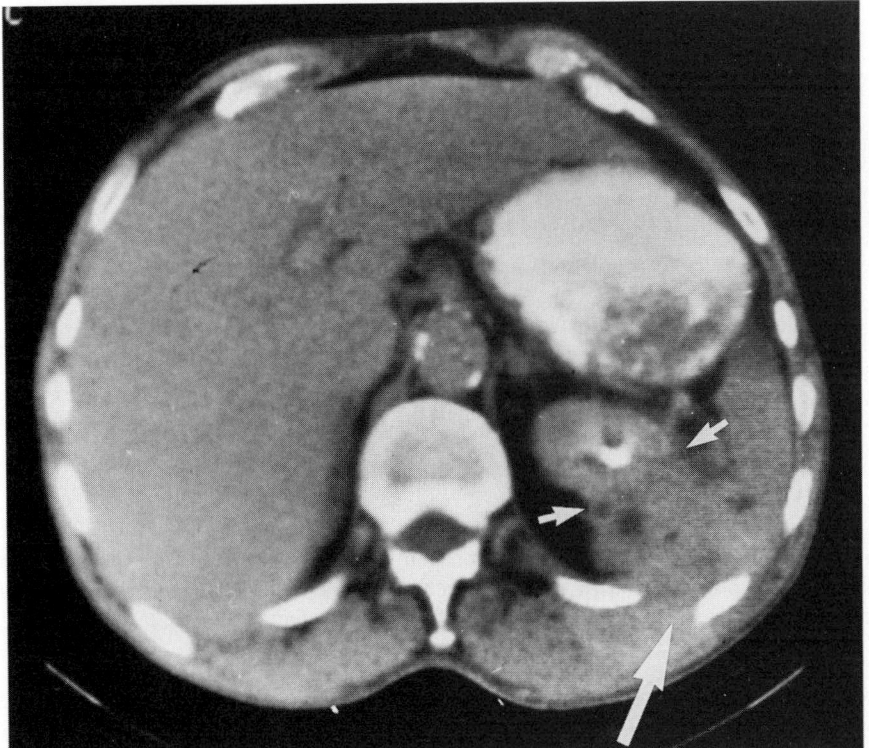

Fig. 4.36 Malacoplakia. CT scan after contrast medium shows left renal mass (small arrows) extending through the perinephric space into the flank (large arrow). (By permission of The Armed Forces Institute of Pathology, Washington DC, and Dr David S. Hartman.)

Perinephric extension may be shown at CT (Fig. 4.36) (Hartman *et al.* 1980). *Ureteric involvement* produces filling defects which may be associated with stricturing of the ureter.

Candidiasis

Candida infection of the urinary tract occurs in a variety of predisposed individuals, especially diabetics, immune suppressed patients, and premature infants, and in association with 'foreign bodies' such as long-standing bladder catheters or urinary tract stents which become colonized with the fungus. Involvement of the kidney usually starts with parenchymal involvement following a systemic candidaemia.

Kidney and ureter

Parenchymal changes caused by Candida can be detected by US in premature infants. Diffuse or focal increase in parenchymal echogenicity, and increased

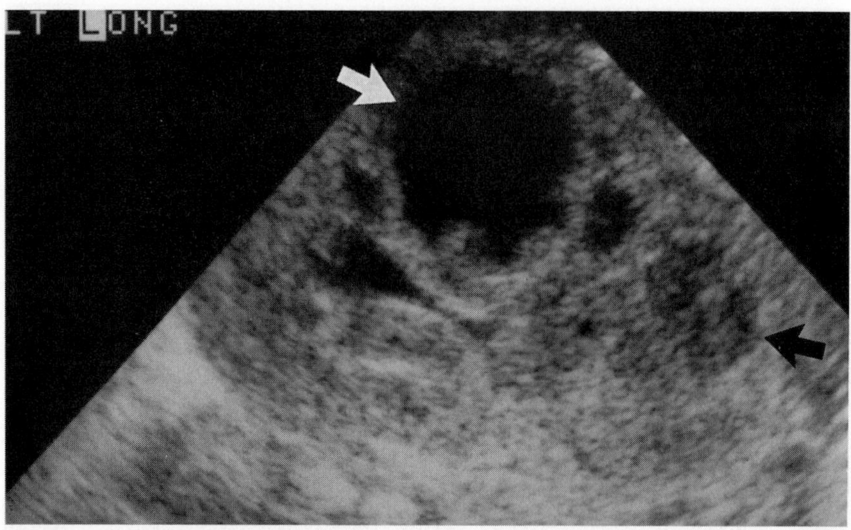

Fig. 4.37 Renal candidiasis in a neonate seen at US. Note the abscess (white arrow), dilated lower pole calyx with contained echoes (black arrow) and generally increased parenchymal echogenicity. (By permission of Dr A. J. S. Saunders.)

echogenicity at the tips of the papillae due to papillary necrosis have been described (Kintanar *et al.* 1986; Berman *et al.* 1989). These changes may progress to abscess formation seen as fluid collections at US (Fig. 4.37), or low attenuation areas at CT. The appearances are indistinguishable from bacterial abscesses. Subsequent invasion of the pelvicalyceal system and ureter may lead to a fungal cast that appears brightly echogenic at US, and does not shadow (Kintanar *et al.* 1986). Contraction of the cast may produce discrete echogenic fungal balls (Fig. 4.38) that do not produce shadows at US (Stuck *et al.* 1981). Fungal balls may also be detected either by urography or on retrograde ureterograms as filling defects (Clark *et al.* 1971). Dilatation of the collecting system and ureter, often with obstruction, are frequent.

Bladder

Candidal involvement causes bladder-wall thickening and fungal balls, identical in character to those in the kidney, may develop. The changes are well shown at US and the filling defects produced by the fungal balls may also be demonstrated with urography or cystography.

Inflammatory disease of the prostate

Acute prostatitis

A variety of changes have been described at transrectal ultrasonography (TRUS) in patients with acute prostatitis. The prostate is slightly and symmetrically en-

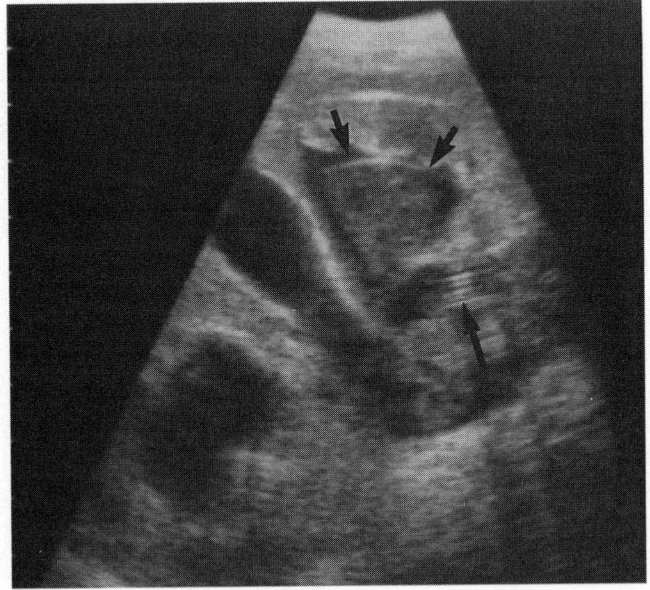

Fig. 4.38 Candida in a transplant kidney with a stent *in situ* seen at US. Note the fungal ball in a dilated lower pole calyx (short arrows) and the stent (long arrow). (By permission of Churchill Livingstone and Dr A. J. S. Saunders.)

larged and shows a heterogeneous echo pattern with multiple echo-poor areas. A prominent periurethral halo extending inferiorly to the level of the verumontanum and prominent periprostatic veins are also seen (Griffiths *et al.* 1984).

Prostatic abscess

Prostatic abscesses are a relatively rare sequel to acute prostatitis and are shown well both by TRUS and CT. TRUS shows a hypoechoic mass often with contained echoes, crossing septa or a thick wall (Fig. 4.39) (Thornhill *et al.* 1987). At CT, the abscess is seen as a low-density collection which may be crossed by septa and may have an enhancing rim (Thornhill *et al.* 1987). Drainage of a prostatic abscess may be guided by US using the transperineal route to avoid further sepsis.

Chronic prostatitis

In chronic prostatitis diffuse symmetrical enlargement of the prostate occurs with a heterogeneous echo pattern at TRUS. Focal areas of increased or decreased echogenicity are seen, especially in the peripheral gland (Fig. 4.40). (Griffiths *et al.* 1990). Prostatic calcification is common.

Unfortunately, none of these changes is specific to chronic prostatitis. Prostatic adenocarcinoma may cause focal lesions in the peripheral gland identical to those caused by prostatitis (Rifkin and Choi 1988). Peripheral focal masses are therefore usually biopsied transrectally with US guidance to determine their nature.

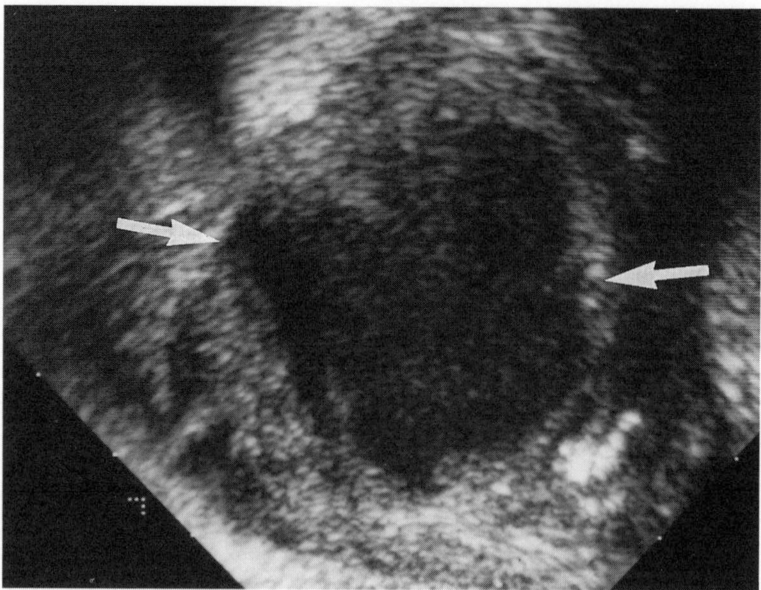

Fig. 4.39 Prostate abscess on a traverse US scan obtained with a transrectal transducer. Note the irregular central fluid collection containing echoes (arrowed). (By permission of Dr D. Rickards.)

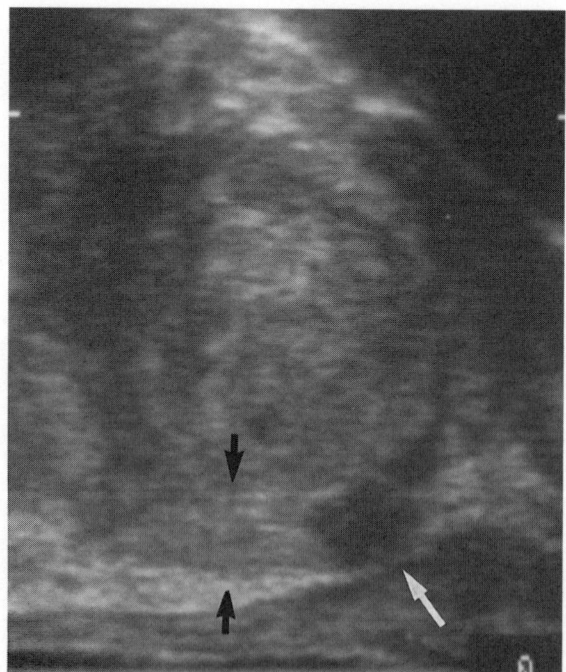

Fig. 4.40 Chronic prostatitis. Small granuloma seen as a hypoechoic mass (white arrow) in the peripheral gland (black arrows) on a longitudinal transrectal US scan. (Patient's head to the left of the image.)

The use of colour flow Doppler increases the sensitivity of TRUS, allowing more abnormalities to be detected. However, it does not help to distinguish inflammatory and neoplastic masses since both may show normal or increased flow (Rifkin *et al.* 1993).

Prostatic calcification is also a non-specific finding. Although it is almost always present in chronic granulomatous prostatitis (Griffiths *et al.* 1990), it can also be seen in 48 per cent of 'normal' prostates at TRUS (Fornage 1988).

Diagnosis of prostatitis with TRUS is also made more difficult because in the male population, from age 50 onwards, the changes of benign prostatic hypertrophy are often seen. This causes enlargement of the periurethral transition zone which is often inhomogeneous and these changes make it difficult to detect focal abnormalities produced by inflammatory disease in the central gland. When TRUS was introduced it was hoped that the detection of a normal gland in a patient with prostatic pain would allow a diagnosis of prostatodynia rather prostatitis. In practice, this is only possible in men who have not yet developed changes of benign prostatic hypertrophy.

References

Ansell, G. (1970). Adverse reactions to contrast agents. *Investigative Radiology*, **5**, 374–84.

Ansell, G., Tweedie, M. C. K., West, C. R., Price Evans, D. A., and Couch, L. (1980). The current status of reactions to intravenous contrast media. *Investigative Radiology*, **15**, S32–9.

Bailey, R. R. (1973). The relationship of vesico-ureteric reflux to urinary tract infection and chronic pyelonephritis—reflux nephropathy. *Clinical Nephrology*, **1**, 132–41.

Berman, L. H., Stringer, D. A., Onge, O. S., Daneman, A., and Whyte, H. (1989). An assessment of sonography in the diagnosis and management of neonatal renal candidiasis. *Clinical Radiology*, **40**, 577–81.

Berns, A. S. (1989). Nephrotoxicity of contrast media. *Kidney International*, **36**, 730–40.

Blickman, J. G., Taylor, G. A. and Lebowitz, R. L. (1985). Voiding cystourethrography: the initial radiologic study in children with urinary tract infection. *Radiology*, **156**, 659–62.

Byrd, L. and Sherman, R. L. (1979). Radiocontrast-induced acute renal failure. *Medicine*, **58**, 270–9.

Cattell, W. R. (1985). Urinary infection in adults—1985. *Postgraduate Medical Journal*, **61**, 907–13.

Cattell, W. R., Fry, I. K., Spiro, F. I., Sardeson, J. M., Sutcliffe, M. B., and O'Grady, F. (1970). Effect of diuresis and frequent micturition on the bacterial content of infected urine: a measure of competence of intrinsic hydrokinetic clearance mechanisms. *British Journal of Urology*, **42**, 290–5.

Cattell, W. R., McIntosh, C. S., Moseley, I. F., and Fry, I. K. (1973). Excretion urography in acute renal failure. *British Medical Journal*, **2**, 575–8.

Cavanagh, P. M. and Sherwood, T. (1983). Too many cystograms in the investigation of urinary tract infection in children? *British Journal of Urology*, **55**, 217–9.

Chapman, A. B., Thickman, D., and Gabow, P. A. (1990). Percutaneous puncture in the treatment of cyst infection in autosomal dominant polycystic kidney disease. *American Journal of Kidney Diseases*, **16**, 252–5.

Chapman, S. J., Chantler, C., Haycock, G. B., Maisey, M. N., and Saxton, H. M. (1988). Radionuclide cystography in vesicoureteric reflux. *Archives of Disease in Childhood*, **63**, 650–71.

Clark, R. E., Minagi, H., and Palubinskas, A. J. (1971). Renal candidiasis. *Radiology*, **101**, 567–72.

Coleman, B. G., Arger, P. H., Mulhern, C. B., Pollack, H. M., and Banner, M. P. (1981). Pyonephrosis: sonography in the diagnosis and management. *American Journal of Roentgenology*, **137**, 939–43.

Cremin, B. J. (1979). Observations on vesico-ureteric reflux and intrarenal reflux: a review and survey of material. *Clinical Radiology*, **30**, 607–21.

Davidson, A. J. (1985). *Radiology of the kidney*, p. 315. W. B. Saunders, Philadelphia.

Davidson, A. J. and Talner, L. B. (1973). Urographic and angiographic abnormalities in adult-onset acute bacterial nephritis. *Radiology*, **106**, 249–56.

Dinkel, E., Ertel, M., Dittrich, M., Peters, H., Berres, M., and Schulte-Wisserman, H. (1985). Kidney size in childhood. Sonographical growth charts for kidney length and volume. *Paediatric Radiology*, **15**, 38–43.

Eklof, O. and Ringertz, H. (1976). Kidney size in children. A method of assessment. *Acta Radiologica*, **17**, 617–625.

Fair, W. R., McClennan, B. L., and Jost, R. G. (1979). Are excretory urograms necessary in evaluating women with urinary tract infection? *Journal of Urology*, **121**, 313–5.

Fairchild, T. N., Shuman, W., and Berger, R. E. (1982). Radiographic studies for women with recurrent urinary tract infection. *Journal of Urology*, **128**, 344–5.

Fornage, B. D. (1988). *Ultrasound of the prostate*, p. 185. Wiley, Chichester.

Fotter, R., Kopp, W., Klein, E., Hollwarth, M., and Uray, E. (1986). Unstable bladder in children: functional evaluation by modified voiding cystourethrography. *Radiology*, **161**, 811–3.

Fraser, I., *et al.* (1989). Parenchymal involvement in cases of acute pyelonephritis in patients with normal IVP. *Kidney International*, **36**, 1178.

Friedland, G. W. and Forsberg, L. (1972). Striation of the renal pelvis in children. *Clinical Radiology*, **23**, 58–60.

Friedland, G. W., Filly, R., and Brown, B. W. (1974). Distance of upper pole calyx to spine and lower pole calyx to ureter as indicators of parenchymal loss in children. *Paediatric Radiology*, **2**, 29–38.

Gedroyc, W. M. W., Chaudhuri, R., and Saxton, H. M. (1988). Normal and near normal calyceal patterns in reflux nephropathy. *Clinical Radiology*, **39**, 615–9.

Gold, R. P., McClennan, B. L., and Rottenberg, R. R. (1983). CT appearance of acute inflammatory disease of the renal interstitium. *American Journal of Roentgenology*, **141**, 343–9.

Goldman, S. M., Hartman, D. S., Fishman, E. K., Finizio, J. P., Gatewood, O. M. B., and Siegelman, S. S. (1984). CT of xanthogranulomatous pyelonephritis, radiologic-pathologic correlation. *American Journal of Roentgenology*, **141**, 963–9.

Goldman, S. M., Fishman, E. K., Hartman, D. S., Kim, Y. C., and Siegelman, S. S. (1985). Computed tomography of renal tuberculosis and its pathological correlates. *Journal of Computer Assisted Tomography*, **9**, 771–6.

Griffiths, G. J., *et al.* (1984). Ultrasonic appearances associated with prostatic inflammation: a preliminary study. *Clinical Radiology*, **35**, 343–5.

Griffiths, G. J., Clements, R., and Peeling, W. B. (1990). Inflammatory disease and calculi. In *Prostatic ultrasonography*, (ed. M. I. Resnick), pp. 123–52. Decker, Philadelphia.

Hall, J. R. W., Choa, R. G., and Wells I. P. (1988). Percutaneous drainage in emphysematous pyelonephritis—an alternative to major surgery. *Clinical Radiology*, **39**, 622–4.

Hampel, N., Class, R. N., and Persky, L. (1980). Value of ^{67}gallium scintigraphy in the diagnosis of localized renal and perirenal inflammation. *Journal of Urology*, **124**, 311–4.

Han, B. K. and Babcock, D. S. (1985). Sonographic measurements and appearance of normal kidneys in children. *American Journal of Roentgenology*, **145**, 611–6.

Hare, W. S. C. and Poynter, J. D. (1974). The radiology of renal papillary necrosis as seen in analgesic nephropathy. *Clinical Radiology*, **25**, 423–43.

Hartman, D. S., Davis, C. J., Lichtenstein, J. E., and Goldman, S. M. (1980). Renal parenchymal malacoplakia. *Radiology*, **136**, 33–42.

Hartman, G. W., Hattery, R. R., Witten, D. M., and Williamson, B. (1982). Mortality during excretory urography: Mayo Clinic experience. *American Journal of Roentgenology*, **139**, 919–22.

Hoddick, W., Jeffrey, R. B., Goldberg, H. I., Federle, M. P., and Laing, F. C. (1983). CT and sonography of severe renal and perirenal infections. *American Journal of Roentgenology*, **140**, 517–20.

Hodson, C. J. (1967). The radiological contribution toward the diagnosis of chronic pyelonephritis. *Radiology*, **88**, 857–71.

Hodson, C. J. (1979). Reflux nephropathy: scoring the damage. In *Reflux nephropathy*, (ed. J. Hodson and P. Kincaid-Smith), pp. 29–47. Masson, New York.

Hodson, C. J. and Wilson, S. (1965). Natural history of chronic pyelonephritic scarring. *British Medical Journal*, **2**, 191–4.

Hodson, C. J., Davies, Z., and Prescod, A. (1975). Renal parenchymal radiographic measurements in infants and children. *Paediatric Radiology*, **3**, 16–9.

Ishikawa, I., *et al.* (1985). Delayed contrast enhancement in acute focal bacterial nephritis: CT features. *Journal of Computed Assisted Tomography*, **9**, 894–7.

Jeffrey, R. B., Laing, F. C., Wing, V. W., and Hoddick, W. (1985). Sensitivity of sonography in pyonephrosis: a reevaluation. *American Journal of Roentgenology*, **144**, 71–3.

Jequier, S. and Jequier, J. C. (1989). Reliability of voiding cystourethrography to detect reflux. *American Journal of Roentgenology*, **153**, 807–10.

June, C. H., *et al.* (1985). Ultrasonography and computed tomography in severe urinary tract infection. *Archives of Internal Medicine*, **145**, 841–5.

Kangarloo, H., Gold, R. H., Fine, R. N., Diament, M. J. and Boechet, M. I. (1985). Urinary tract infection in infants and children evaluated by ultrasound. *Radiology*, **154**, 367–73.

Kass, E. J., Fink-Bennett, D., Cacciarelli, A. A., Balon, H., and Parlock, S. (1992). The sensitivity of renal scintigraphy and sonography in detecting nonobstructive acute pyelonephritis. *Journal of Urology*, **148**, 606–8.

Katayama, H., Yamaguchi, K., Kozuka, T., Takashima, T., Seez, P., and Matsuura, K. (1990). Adverse reaction to ionic and non-ionic contrast media. *Radiology*, **175**, 621–8.

Kintanar, C., Cramer, B. C., Reid, W. D., and Andrews, W. L. (1986). Neonatal renal candidiasis: sonographic diagnosis. *American Journal of Roentgenology*, **147**, 801–5.

Lanning, P., Sepannen, U., Huttunen, N-P., and Uhari, M. (1979). Prediction of vesicoureteral reflux in children from intravenous urography films. *Clinical Radiology*, **30**, 67–70.

Lasser, E. C., Lang, J. H., Hamblin, A. E., Lyon, S. G., and Howard, M. (1980). Activation systems in contrast idiosyncrasy. *Investigative Radiology*, **15**, S2–5.

Lebowitz, R. L. (1986). The detection of vesicoureteral reflux in the child. *Investigative Radiology*, **21**, 519–31.

Lebowitz, R. L., Olbing, H., Parkkulainen, K. V., Smellie, J. M., and Tamminen-Mobius, T. E. (1985). International system of radiographic grading of vesicoureteric reflux. *Paediatric Radiology*, **15**, 105–9.

Lee, J. K. T. and Knific, R. J. (1990). In *Clinical urography*, (ed. H. M. Pollack), pp. 863–83. W. B. Saunders, Philadelphia.

Lee, J. K. T., McClennan, B. L., Melson, G. L., and Stanley, R. J. (1980). Acute focal bacterial nephritis: emphasis on gray scale sonography and computed tomography. *American Journal of Roentgenology*, **135**, 87–92.

Leonidas, J. C., McCauley, R. G. K., Klauber, G. C., and Fretzayas, A. M. (1985). Sonography as a substitute for excretory urography in children with urinary tract infection. *American Journal of Roentgenology*, **144**, 815–9.

Little, P. J., McPherson, D. R., and de Wardener, H. E. (1965). The appearance of the intravenous pyelogram during and after acute pyelonephritis. *Lancet*, **1**, 1186–8.

Mallinson, W. J. W., Fuller, R. W., Levison, D. A., Baker, L. R. I., and Cattell, W. R. (1981). Diffuse interstitial renal tuberculosis—an unusual cause of renal failure. *Quarterly Journal of Medicine*, **198**, 137–48.

Merrick. M. V., Uttley, W. S., and Wild, R. (1977). A comparison of two techniques of detecting vesico-ureteric reflux. *British Journal of Radiology*, **50**, 792–5.

Merrick, M. V., Uttley, W. S., and Wild, S. R. (1980). The detection of pyelonephritic scarring in children by radioisotope imaging. *British Journal of Radiology*, **53**, 544–56.

Meyrier, A. *et al.* (1989). Frequency of development of early cortical scarring in acute primary pyelonephritis. *Kidney International*, **35**, 696–703.

Michaeli, P., Mogle, P., Pelberg, S., Heiman, S., and Caine, M. (1984). Emphysematous pyelonephritis. *Journal of Urology*, **131**, 203–8.

Middleton, W. D., Dodds, W. J., Lawson, T. L., and Foley, W. D. (1988). Renal calculi: sensitivity for detection with US. *Radiology*, **167**, 239–44.

Monsour, M., Azmy, A. F., and Mackenzie, J. R. (1987). Renal scarring secondary to vesicoureteric reflux. Critical assessment and new grading. *British Journal of Urology*, **60**, 320–4.

Morehouse, H. T., Weiner, S. N., and Hoffman, J. C. (1984). Imaging in inflammatory disease of the kidney. *American Journal of Roentgenology*, **143**, 135–41.

Owen, J. P., *et al.* (1985). Urographic findings in adults with chronic pyelonephritis. *Clinical Radiology*, **36**, 81–7.

Palmer, F. J. (1988). The RACR survey of intravenous contrast media reactions. Final report. *Australasian Radiology*, **32**, 426–8.

Palubinskas, A. J. (1961). Medullary sponge kidney. *Radiology*, **76**, 911–9.

Poston, G. J., Joseph, A. E. A., and Riddle, P. R. (1983). The accuracy of ultrasound in the measurement of changes in bladder volume. *British Journal of Urology*, **55**, 361–3.

Premkumar, A., Latimer, M., and Newhouse, J. H. (1987). CT and sonography of advanced urinary tract tuberculosis. *American Journal of Roentgenology*, **148**, 65–9.

Ransley, P. G. and Risdon, R. A. (1975*a*). Renal papillary morphology and intrarenal reflux in the young pig. *Urology Research*, **3**, 105–9.

Ransley, P. G. and Risdon, R. A. (1975*b*). Renal papillary morphology in infants and young children. *Urological Research*, **3**, 111–5.

Rickwood, A. M. K., *et al.* (1992). Current imaging of childhood urinary infections: prospective survey. *British Medical Journal*, **304**, 663–5.

Rifkin, M. D. and Choi, H. (1988). Implications of small, peripheral hypoechoic lesions in endorectal US of the prostate. *Radiology*, **166**, 619–22.

Rifkin, M. D., Sudakoff, G. S., and Alexander, A. A. (1993). Prostate: technique, results and potential applications of colour Doppler US scanning. *Radiology*, **186**, 509–13.

Rigsby, C. M., Rosenfield, A. T., Glickman, M. G., and Hodson, J. (1986). Haemorrhagic focal bacterial nephritis: findings on gray-scale sonography and CT. *American Journal of Roentgenology*, **146**, 1173–7.

Rolleston, G. L. and Maling, T. M. J., and Hodson, C. J. (1974). Intrarenal reflux and the scarred kidney. *Archives of Disease in Childhood*, **49**, 531–9.

Rosenbaum, D. M., Korngold, E., and Teele, R. L. (1984). Sonographic assessment of renal length in normal children. *American Journal of Roentgenology*, **142**, 467–9.

Rosenfield, A. T., Glickman, M. G., Taylor, K. J. W., Grade, M., and Hodson, J. (1979). Acute focal bacterial nephritis (acute lobar nephronia). *Radiology*, **132**, 553–61.

Roylance, J., Penry, J. B., Davies, E. R., and Roberts, M. (1970). The radiology of tuberculosis of the urinary tract. *Clinical Radiology*, **21**, 163–70.

Rushton, H. G. and Majd, M. (1992). Dimercaptosuccinic acid renal scintigraphy for the evaluation of pyelonephritis and scarring: a review of clinical and experimental studies. *Journal of Urology*, **148**, 1726–32.

Sargent, M. A. and Wilson, B. P. M. (1992). Observer variability in the sonographic measurement of renal length in childhood. *Clinical Radiology*, **46**, 344–7.

Schaffer, R., Becker, J. A., and Goodman, J. (1983). Sonography of tuberculous kidney. *Urology*, **22**, 209–11.

Schlesinger, A. E., Hernandez, R. J., Zerin, J. M., Marks, T. I., and Kelsch, R. C. (1991). Interobserver and intraobserver variations in sonographic renal length measurements in children. *American Journal of Roentgenology*, **156**, 1029–32.

Schrott, K. M., Behrends, B., Clauss, W., Kaufmann, J., and Lehnert, J. (1986). Iohexol in excretory urography. *Fortschritte der Medizin*, **104**, 153–6.

Schwab, S. J., Bander, S. J., and Klahr, S. (1987). Renal infection in autosomal dominant polycystic kidney disease. *American Journal of Medicine*, **82**, 714–18.

Schwartz, G., Lipschitz, S., and Becker, J. A. (1984). Detection of renal calculi: the value of tomography. *American Journal of Roentgenology*, **143**, 143–5.

Seruca, H. (1989). Vesicoureteral reflux and voiding dysfunction: a prospective study. *Journal of Urology*, **142**, 494–8.

Shah, K. J., Robins, D. G., and White, R. H. R. (1978). Renal scarring and vesicoureteric reflux. *Archives of Disease in Childhood*, **53**, 210–7.

Shehadi, W. H. (1975). Adverse reactions to intravascularly administered contrast media. *American Journal of Roentgenology*, **124**, 145–52.

Silver, T. M., Kass, E. J., Thornbury, J. R., Konnak, J. W., and Wolfman, M. G. (1976). The radiological spectrum of acute pyelonephritis in adults and adolescents. *Radiology*, **118**, 65–71.

Smellie, J. M., Edwards, D., Hunter, N. Normand, I. C. S., and Prescod, N. (1975). Vesico-ureteric reflux and renal scarring. *Kidney International*, **8**, S65–72.

Smellie, J. M., Shaw, P. J., Prescord, N. P., and Bantock, H. M. (1988). ^{99m}Tc dimercaptosuccinic acid (DMSA) scan in patients with established radiological renal scarring. *Archives of Disease in Childhood*, **63**, 1315–9.

Soulen, M. C., Fishman, E. K., Goldman, S. M., and Gatewood, O. M. B. (1989*a*). Bacterial renal infection: role of CT. *Radiology*, **171**, 703–7.

Soulen, M. C., Fishman, E. K., and Goldman, S. M. (1989*b*). Sequelae of acute renal infections: CT evaluation. *Radiology*, **173**, 423–6.

Spiro, F. I. and Fry, I. K. (1970). Ureteric dilatation in non-pregnant women. *Proceedings of the Royal Society of Medicine*, **63**, 462–4.

Stuck, K. J., Silver, T. M., Jaffe, M. H., and Bowerman, R. A. (1981). Sonographic demonstration of renal fungus balls. *Radiology*, **142**, 473–4.

Subramanyam, B. R., Megibow, A. J., Raghavendra, B. N., and Bosniak, M. A. (1982). Diffuse xanthogranulomatous pyelonephritis: analysis by computed tomography and sonography. *Urologic Radiology*, **4**, 5–9.

Talner, L. B., Davidson, A. J., Lebowitz, R., dalla Palma, L., and Goldman, S. (1994). Acute pyelonephritis: can we agree on terminology? *Radiology*, **192**, 297–305.

Tasker, A. D., Lindsell, D. R. M., and Moncrieff, M. (1993). Can ultrasound reliably detect renal scarring in children with urinary tract infection? *Clinical Radiology*, **47**, 177–9.

Teplick, J. G., Teplick, S. K., Berinson, H., and Haskin, M. E. (1979). Urographic and angiographic changes in acute unilateral pyelonephritis. *Clinical Radiology*, **30**, 59–66.

Thompson, P. M., *et al.* (1982). The problem of infection after prostatic biopsy: the case for the transperineal approach. *British Journal of Urology*, **54**, 736–40.

Thomsen, H. S. (1985). Vesicoureteral reflux and reflux nephropathy. *Acta radiologica diagnosis*, **26**, 3–13.

Thornhill, B. A., Morehouse, H. T., Coleman, P., and Hoffman-Trehn, J. C. (1987). Prostatic abscess: CT and sonographic findings. *American Journal of Roentgenology*, **148**, 899–900.

Tsugaya, M., *et al.* (1990). Computerized tomography in acute pyelonephritis: the clinical correlations. *Journal of Urology*, **144**, 611–3.

Verber, I. G. and Meller, S. T. (1989). Serial ^{99m}Tc dimercaptosuccinic acid (DMSA) scans after urinary infections presenting before the age of 5 years. *Archives of Disease in Childhood*, **64**, 1533–7.

Webb, J. A. W., Reznek, R. H., White, F. E., Cattell, W. R., Fry, I. K., and Baker, L. R. I. (1984). Can ultrasound and computed tomography replace high-dose urography in patients with impaired renal function? *Quarterly Journal of Medicine*, **53**, 411–25.

Whitear, P., Shaw, P., and Gordon, I. (1990). Comparison of ^{99m}Tc dimercaptosuccinic acid scans and intravenous urography in children. *British Journal of Radiology*, **63**, 438–43.

Willi, U. and Treves, S. (1983). Radionuclide voiding cystography. *Urologic Radiology*, **5**, 161–73.

Wills, J. S., Pollack, H. M., and Curtis, J. A. (1981). Cholesteatoma of the upper urinary tract. *American Journal of Roentgenology*, **136**, 941–4.

Wulfsohn, M. A. (1980). Pyelocalyceal diverticula. *Journal of Urology*, **123**, 1–8.

5

Uncomplicated urinary tract infection in women

L. E. Nicolle

Introduction

Uncomplicated urinary tract infection (UTI) occurs in individuals with structurally and functionally normal genitourinary tracts. It is the most common bacterial infection that occurs in women; but is uncommon in men. Thus, discussion of uncomplicated urinary infection primarily relates to a condition affecting women. It has been estimated that most women will experience at least one urinary tract infection during their lifetime. In addition, a substantial subset of women, from 5 to 10 per cent, will have recurrent symptomatic episodes of urinary infection. Uncomplicated UTI may involve the bladder or the kidneys and may be symptomatic or asymptomatic.

Clinical presentations

Acute uncomplicated urinary infection

Acute uncomplicated urinary infection, also called acute cystitis, is characterized by lower tract irritative symptoms. These include dysuria, frequency, urgency, hesitancy, suprapubic, and pelvic discomfort, as well as associated complaints of bad odour to the urine and cloudy urine. Dysuria is usually a prominent symptom, and presents as internal, or urethral, dysuria rather than external dysuria more characteristic of vulvovaginal complaints (Komaroff 1984). Hemorrhagic cystitis is a frequent manifestation of symptomatic lower tract infection (Stamm *et al.* 1980). There is wide variability in symptoms reported by women presenting with acute infection but, generally, symptoms are consistent from one infection to the next for an individual woman. The majority of women who present acutely with these symptoms will have UTI involving the bladder (Stamm *et al.* 1980).

Many of the symptoms associated with lower tract infection may be due to causes other than UTI. Sexually transmitted diseases including *Neisseria gonorrhea, Chlamydia trachomatis, Trichomonas vaginalis*, and *Herpes simplex* may present with dysuria (Komaroff 1984). Vulvovaginal candidiasis is common, especially in women who have received antimicrobial therapy, and vaginitis from irritative or hypersensitivity reactions, the entity of vestibulitis (Peckham *et al.*

1986), and other non-infectious causes must be considered. Interstitial cystitis is uncommon but may present with similar symptoms. A history with careful attention to aspects which may suggest an increased risk of sexually transmitted diseases will help to identify other aetiological possibilities. A history of previous similar episodes, including response to prior antimicrobial therapy, will also assist in determining the likelihood of urinary infection compared with other causes of acute dysuria.

The term 'acute urethral syndrome', previously used to describe women who presented with symptoms consistent with acute cystitis but without positive urine cultures, is no longer considered a useful clinical designation. From 30 to 50 per cent of women with acute uncomplicated UTI will have low quantitative counts ($< 10^5$ colony-forming units per ml) in their urine, and, thus, most women presenting with what was previously known as the acute urethral syndrome do have urinary infection (Stamm *et al.* 1982). Any constellation of symptoms in association with pyuria should make the diagnosis of UTI most likely, regardless of the quantitative counts of bacteria.

Acute non-obstructive pyelonephritis

Acute non-obstructive pyelonephritis classically presents with costovertebral angle pain and tenderness, fever, and commonly, associated irritative lower urinary symptoms. It is characteristic and not usually confused with other diagnoses. It may, however, present with less characteristic manifestations. The clinical presentation is a continuum ranging from low-grade symptoms, such as mild or absent fever with slight costovertebral angle tenderness, to acute septic shock. Some subjects with upper tract infection will present with only lower tract symptoms. This has been referred to as occult pyelonephritis (Komaroff 1986).

Prevalence

Asymptomatic bacteriuria

Extensive epidemiological studies performed in community populations have documented the prevalence of asymptomatic urinary infection. A summary of studies in adult women is provided in Table 5.1. The observations reported from these different populations are remarkably consistent, and support several conclusions. First, the prevalence of bacteriuria in adult women increases with age and, within age groups, is consistent among the different studies. Secondly, sexually active women have a higher prevalence of bacteriuria than those who are not. Several of these studies also examined the association between parity and prevalence of bacteriuria. Kunin and McCormack (1968) reported no association. Evans *et al.* (1978), however, found an increased occurrence of asymptomatic bacteriuria with increased parity for all ages. This association was no longer present when analysis was restricted to married women. Thus, the

Table 5.1 Prevalence of asymptomatic bacteriuria in selected populations of adult women

Study	Population	No. of women studied	Age (yrs)	Prevalence of bacteriuria (%)
Miall *et al.* (1962)	Jamaican women	2365	15–24	1.4
			25–34	2.4
			35–44	3.6
			45–54	4.1
			55–64	8.6
Freedman *et al.* (1964–5)	Hiroshima survivors	3191	< 20	0.8
			20–39	1.6
			40–49	3.1
			50–59	2.8
			60–69	7.4
			≥ 70	10.8
Kunin & McCormack (1968)	US working women	2698	15–34	4.8
			35–54	4.5
			≥ 55	6.4
	US nuns	3304	15–34	.3
			35–54	1.5
			≥ 55	4.7
Evans *et al.* (1978)	Working class community population, Boston, USA	7834	16–19	1.1
			20–29	1.7
			30–39	3.7
			40–49	2.5
			50–59	4.3
			60–69	5.8
Takala *et al.* (1977)	Middle-aged Finnish population	1223	40–49	2.5
			50–59	5.1
			60–64	8.5
Bengtsson *et al.* (1980)	Community population, Göteborg, Sweden	1462	38	2.7
			46	3.9
			50	4.3
			54	3.9
			60	8.6

apparent association with parity may have been due to the level of sexual activity.

Symptomatic bacteriuria

Some community studies have reported the prevalence of symptoms consistent with cystitis, principally dysuria and frequency, in bacteriuric and non-bacteriuric women. Takala *et al.* (1977) found that 6.4 per cent of 1223 women reported symptoms. Of these symptomatic women, 78 per cent were not bacteriuric. In the study of Evans *et al.* (1978), 5.8 per cent of women reported symptoms; 95 per cent of those with symptoms did not have bacteriuria. The lack of specificity of these lower tract irritative symptoms for urinary infection in the general population means meaningful information with respect to the prevalence of symptomatic infection cannot really be derived. These studies do, however, convincingly document that the majority of women complaining of such symptoms in these population-based prevalence surveys do not have bacteriuria.

Incidence

Symptomatic uncomplicated urinary infection

The incidence of symptomatic and asymptomatic bacteriuria documented for different female populations in several prospective studies is summarized in Table 5.2. There are no population-based studies with appropriate bacteriological evaluation and long-term follow-up documenting the occurrence of symptomatic or asymptomatic infection in unselected female populations. Generally, women included in prospective studies have been recruited from populations experiencing recurrent infection, although for some studies controls with no history of infection were also included. These studies consistently document episodes of symptomatic infection occurring at a rate of about two infections per patient year for women with a prior history of frequent symptomatic urinary infection. This is consistent with the reported rates of symptomatic infection in the placebo-comparative arms of studies of antimicrobial prophylaxis (Nicolle and Ronald 1987).

Table 5.2 The incidence of symptomatic lower tract infection and asymptomatic bacteriuria in female populations without identified genitourinary abnormalities

Study	Population (*N*)	Follow-up	Incidence of infection (patient yr)	
			Symptomatic	Asymptomatic
Kraft & Stamey (1977)	2 symptomatic infections over 12 mos (23)	Mean 36.3 mos (15–110) mos)	2.1	
Kunin *et al.* (1980)	Prior UTI* (13)	Mean 245.2 days	1.8	1.9
	Control (18)	Mean 276.3 days	0.07	0.44
Nicolle *et al.* (1982)	Prior UTI* (15)	Mean 66 days	2.6	3.3
	control (13)	Mean 90 days	0	0.94
Wong *et al.* (1985)	2 infections past 12 mos (38)	6 mos	2.2	
Stamm *et al.* (1991)	Infection-prone (51)	Median 9 yrs	1.9	0.7

* UTI, urinary tract infection; mos, months.

A feature of recurrent acute uncomplicated urinary infection in women is a changing frequency of attacks (Stamm *et al.* 1991; Kraft and Stamey 1977). Thus, there will be periods during which multiple closely spaced infections occur and extended periods of months or years free of symptoms. The majority of these episodes of recurrence are re-infections, although relapsing infection following antimicrobial therapy which does not eradicate the infection from an upper tract focus will sometimes occur. Kraft and Stamey (1977) reported an overall infection rate of 0.17 infection per month in 23 women, but a rate of 0.47 per month when these women were not in 'a six month or longer remission'. Stamm *et al.* (1991) reported similar observations, with a declining frequency of infection the longer the time since the previous episode. If a patient experienced recurrence of cystitis, the most likely time for recurrence was between days 30 and 60 after the onset of the last episode. The predictors of episodes of increased frequency of symptomatic infection are not fully clarified.

Asymptomatic bacteriuria

In the studies summarized in Table 5.2, the frequency with which urine cultures were obtained and, hence, the sensitivity for identification of asymptomatic bacteriuria varied widely. For instance, the studies of Kunin *et al.* (1980) and Nicolle *et al.* (1982) involved daily or every other day urine cultures, whereas Kraft and Stamey (1977) obtained cultures monthly, and Stamm *et al.* (1991) obtained routine cultures every third month. These studies suggest that asymptomatic urinary infection occurs with a frequency similar to symptomatic infection in women with a history of recurrent symptomatic infection.

For women identified initially with asymptomatic bacteriuria, Bengtsson *et al.* (1980) reported that 52 per cent of women who became non-bacteriuric with treatment had recurrence of bacteriuria on at least one occasion in up to two years of follow-up. The frequency of obtaining urine cultures was not stated. They also reported that six years after initial screening, 23 per cent of initially bacteriuric and 5 per cent of initially non-bacteriuric women had bacteriuria. Asscher *et al.* (1969) also reported a prevalence of 5 per cent of women developing bacteriuria over one year who were free of bacteriuria when initially screened. In women with no history of symptomatic urinary infection, episodes of asymptomatic bacteriuria also occur with considerable frequency. Reported rates (Table 5.2) have been 0.44 per patient year (Kunin *et al.* 1980) and 0.94 per patient year (Nicolle *et al.* 1982). This is less common than asymptomatic bacteriuria in women with a history of frequent recurrent symptomatic infection. Episodes of asymptomatic bacteriuria in women without a history of symptomatic infection generally resolve spontaneously in a few days.

Pyelonephritis

There are no population-based studies of the incidence of pyelonephritis in the general population. Women who experience acute uncomplicated UTI are, however, also at increased risk of acute non-obstructive pyelonephritis. Stamm *et al.* (1991) reported a rate of pyelonephritis of 0.1 ± 0.3 per patient year in their group of 51 infection-prone women. The estimated ratio of episodes of symptomatic cystitis to episodes of acute non-obstructive pyelonephritis was 18 to 1 in these women. In a group of 74 women between the ages of 15 and 35 years with hospital admission for acute pyelonephritis, reviewed at a mean of 15.5 years after admission, Parker and Kunin (1973) reported that 12 (17 per cent) had no further symptomatic infections. However, 16 (23 per cent) had had recurrent infection within the six months prior to the date of follow-up (mean 15.5 years) and 29 (40 per cent) within three years. A substantial proportion of these patients with recurrent urinary infection, however, had underlying genitourinary abnormalities such as urolithiasis. Finally, Asscher *et al.* (1973) reported that two (2.2 per cent) of 93 women with asymptomatic bacteriuria identified at an outpatient clinic had developed symptomatic pyelonephritis on review three to five years later. None of 57 control subjects had developed upper tract infection. Thus, although there are few data documenting the incidence or recurrence of acute pyelonephritis in the general female population, the information available does suggest that women with a past history of symptomatic or asymptomatic uncomplicated urinary infection are at increased risk for developing acute pyelonephritis.

Microbiology

Escherichia coli is the organism isolated in the overwhelming majority of symptomatic or asymptomatic uncomplicated urinary infections. In many studies this organism was consistently isolated in 75–90 per cent of infections (Kunin and McCormack 1968; Bengtsson *et al.* 1980; Evans *et al.* 1978; Kraft and Stamey 1977; Stamm *et al.* 1991). *Escherichia coli* is the most common Gram-negative bacterium in the human gut, the reservoir for bacteria causing UTI. Bacterial factors associated with symptomatic infection are better characterized for pyelonephritis than for cystitis. In particular, acute non-obstructive pyelonephritis is virtually always caused by *E. coli* which express one particular adhesin, the P-pilus (fimbria). *Escherichia coli* isolated from women with asymptomatic bacteriuria is characterized by decreased frequency of potential virulence factors, including adhesins, haemolysin, aerobactin, and lipopolysaccharide (Svanborg-Edén and de Man 1987). Potential virulence factors of *E. coli* are discussed in greater detail elsewhere in this monograph.

The second most frequent organism isolated in symptomatic uncomplicated urinary infection is *Staphylococcus saprophyticus*. The frequency of isolation of this organism has varied in different populations, with some authors reporting it as the aetiological agent in up to 22 per cent (Wallmark *et al.* 1978) and 30 per cent (Gillespie *et al.* 1978) of symptomatic episodes. Most studies, however, report its isolation from 5 to 10 per cent of symptomatic infections. (Latham *et al.* 1983; Saginur *et al.* 1992). Urinary infection with *Staph. saprophyticus* has been repeatedly shown to occur with increased frequency in summer and autumn

(Wallmark *et al.* 1978; Latham *et al.* 1983; Pead *et al.* 1985). An explanation for this consistent seasonal variation is not apparent.

Klebsiella pneumoniae and *Proteus mirabilis* are the most frequently isolated Enterobacteriaceae other than *E. coli*, although each occurs in less than 5 per cent of infections. The infrequency with which Enterococcus spp. are isolated from uncomplicated urinary infection is noteworthy. Stamm *et al.* (1991) reported isolating these species from 4 per cent of episodes of cystitis and none of acute pyelonephritis, and Kraft and Stamey (1977) from 2 per cent of infections. Population-based studies of asymptomatic bacteriuria have generally failed to report any isolation of Enterococcus spp.

Demographic characteristics

Women who experience recurrent acute uncomplicated urinary infection are characterized by both a genetic predisposition and selected behavioral factors. The most convincing associations documented are listed in Table 5.3. A genetic predisposition is suggested by the observation that first-degree relatives of women with recurrent urinary infection have a higher frequency of infection than the relatives of controls without recurrent infection (Leibovici *et al.* 1987). In addition, women with recurrent symptomatic urinary infection are more likely to be non-secretors of the ABO blood group substances (Kinane *et al.* 1982)

Sexually active women have a much greater frequency of both symptomatic and asymptomatic urinary infection (Kunin and McCormack 1968; Foxman and Frerichs 1985*a*; Remis *et al.* 1987; Leibovici *et al.* 1987). Several studies have documented a relationship between increasing frequency of intercourse and increased frequency of infection (Nicolle *et al.* 1982; Foxman and Frerichs 1985*a*; Remis *et al.* 1987). Additional factors independently associated with recurrent urinary infection are diaphragm use (Fihn *et al.* 1985; Foxman and Frerichs 1985*a*; Remis *et al.* 1987; Hooton *et al* . 1991) and spermicide use independently of diaphragm use (Hooton *et al.* 1991; Foxman and Frerichs 1985*a*). Other purported behavioural factors, including frequency of urination, aspects of personal hygiene, or use of the birth control pill, have not been convincingly associated with recurrent infection (Remis *et al.* 1987).

Table 5.3 Factors associated with an increased risk of recurrent urinary tract infection in women

Genetic
Non-secretor of blood group substance.
First-degree female relative with recurrent urinary infection
Behavioural
Sexual activity
Spermicide use
Diaphragm use

The source of uropathogens isolated from uncomplicated urinary infection is the gut. It has been proposed that introital colonization with a potential uropathogen from the gut is a necessary prerequisite for uncomplicated urinary tract infection, and that women with recurrent infection have a longer duration and higher degree of introital carriage than women who do not experience recurrent infection (Stamey *et al.* 1971). Other investigators have reported that the duration of periurethral colonization does not differ for women with recurrent infection and controls (Kunin *et al.* 1980). From the available data, it seems reasonable to conclude that most women with acute uncomplicated urinary infection have concomitant vaginal or introital carriage of Enterobacteriaceae, primarily *E. coli* (Kunin *et al.* 1980; Brumfit *et al.* 1987), and that women who use spermicide methods of birth control have a higher prevalence and intensity of *E. coli* vaginal colonization (Hooton *et al.* 1991).The question as to whether women who experience recurrent urinary infection, independent of spermicide use, have an increased frequency or duration of *E. coli* introital colonization, has not been fully answered.

Short-term morbidity

The short-term morbidity of acute uncomplicated UTI is primarily disruption of normal activities due to urinary frequency and discomfort. However, since symptoms vary, morbidity will range from none in asymptomatic non-pregnant women to hospitalization for those with severe pyelonephritis. The majority of women with symptomatic infection will have acute cystitis. This may require a physician visit, and in some cases will be associated with work absence or inability to perform usual activities. In one American study (Foxman and Frerichs 1985*b*), women reported a mean of 6.1 symptom days, 2.4 restricted-activity days, and 1.6 office visits and laboratory tests with each episode of cystitis. Thus, there is the opportunity for substantial disruption of a woman's normal activities due to acute episodes of lower tract infection.

Not all women who experience acute uncomplicated UTI will seek medical care. The possible outcomes for women who are not treated early with antibiotics include spontaneous resolution, persistent symptomatic infection, persistent infection which becomes asymptomatic, and progression to acute non-obstructive pyelonephritis. In 53 women presenting with symptoms of acute cystitis who received placebo, 81 per cent had spontaneously cleared their infection by five months, 15 per cent received therapy for persistent symptoms, and 4 per cent had persistent infection at 12 months (Mabeck 1972). The frequency with which women who present with acute lower tract symptoms progress to pyelonephritis is not known. Saginur *et al.* (1992) reported one case (1.4 per cent) in 73 women initially treated with single dose norfloxacin.

Some women with acute pyelonephritis will require hospital admission. In most cases this will be a short-term admission to stabilize the patient and ensure a response to parental therapy, followed by discharge to complete a course of oral therapy. Safrin *et al.* (1988) reported a mean duration of hospitalization of

6.02 ± 4.46 days in 95 women hospitalized for treatment of pyelonephritis, some of whom had underlying renal disease. The costs of acute pyelonephritis or the impact measured as loss of productivity for women who are not hospitalized have not been reported.

Acute non-obstructive pyelonephritis has been reported, rarely, to be associated with acute renal failure in adults. This has recently been reviewed by Jones (1992). He described one woman and identified five others previously reported in the literature. Three of these five had also received non-steroidal anti-inflamatory agents. *Escherichia coli* was the infecting organism in every case and none had a history of prior urinary infections. All but one ultimately recovered renal function. Thus, although acute renal failure may occur due to acute non-obstructive pyelonephritis, it is an extremely rare clinical occurrence.

Screening for asymptomatic bacteriuria might be rational if treatment decreased short- or long-term morbidity due to symptomatic episodes. Asscher *et al.* (1969) reported that 16 (36 per cent) of 45 untreated women with asymptomatic bacteriuria developed symptomatic urinary infection in one year of follow-up, but 18 (37 per cent) patients with treated asymptomatic bacteriuria also developed symptomatic infection. Thus, antimicrobial therapy of asymptomatic bacteriuria did not decrease the high frequency of symptomatic infection in the subsequent year. Symptomatic infection, in fact, occurred more frequently in women with post-therapy re-infections compared to those with persisting or relapsing bacteriuria. This observation is consistent with reports from paediatric populations (Hansson *et al.* 1989) and suggests treatment of asymptomatic bacteriuria in non-pregnant female populations increases short-term morbidity and is, thus, detrimental. The explanation for this observation may be replacement of a non-virulent organism in a stable host–organism relationship in a patient with a genetic predisposition to recurrent infection with an organism of greater virulence more likely to cause symptomatic infection.

Long-term morbidity

The introduction of the quantitative urine culture as a standardized and reproducible means of differentiating infected from non-infected populations allowed the exploration of the association between UTI and selected potential long-term complications of infection. Those which have primarily been studied include hypertension, renal failure, and renal scarring. In addition, an association between bacteriuria and bladder carcinoma has been proposed in at least one study.

Reports of the association of bacteriuria and hypertension are summarized in Table 5.4. Early studies suggested women with asymptomatic bacteriuria more frequently had hypertension or were more likely to develop increased blood pressure on follow-up. Subsequent studies have been unable to confirm such an association. In addition, Parker and Kunin (1973) in their follow-up of 74 women admitted to hospital with pyelonephritis, some of whom had underlying abnormalities, reported an incidence of hypertension in their study population similar

Table 5.4 Studies which have reported the association of hypertension and acute uncomplicated urinary infection in women

Study	Population	Observations
Miall *et al.* (1962)	Jamaican women	Increased occurrence of hypertension with asymptomatic bacteriuria, ages 30–60.
Freedman *et al.* (1964–5)	Hiroshima survivors	No initial difference in blood pressure (BP) between bacteriuric and non-bacteriuric. Greater increase in BP in women with urinary infection at 3-year follow-up.
Kunin & McCormack (1968)	US working women and nuns	Higher systolic BP in bacteriuric women, but the difference was not significant.
Asscher *et al.* (1973)	Hospital outpatients	No difference in initial BP between asymptomatic bacteriuric women and controls. No differences after 4-year follow-up.
Tencer (1988)	Swedish women	No difference in BP in women with or without asymptomatic bacteriuria.

to that reported for the general population. Thus, available information indicates that acute uncomplicated urinary infection, either asymptomatic or presenting as intermittently symptomatic episodes, is not associated with an increased occurrence of hypertension.

Studies of renal scarring due to urinary infection have been primarily performed in paediatric populations. Some subjects have been followed-up into adulthood. In addition, there are some reports of frequency of subsequent renal scarring in women initially presenting with acute pyelonephritis. These studies document that women with progressive scarring or progressive renal impairment consistently had scarring present when initially investigated or had genitourinary abnormalities other than urinary infection to explain progression. Huland and Busch (1984) followed-up 201 girls, aged from 2 to 8 years (some into adulthood), and new pyelonephritic scars formed only in those with both urinary infection and vesicoureteric reflux. The Bristol pyelonephritis registry (Gaches *et al.* 1976) followed-up 84 female subjects with a clinical diagnosis of recurrent pyelonephritis; 48 of these for over five years. Radiological development of renal scars was not observed in any adults. Alwall (1978), however, describes 29 women with follow-up over 20–30 years, with evidence of progressive renal damage and scarring. Two-thirds had a history of acute pyelonephritis and about half had chronic pyelonephritis or interstitial nephritis on biopsy. He suggested renal damage with chronic urinary infection may be identified in some women if the follow-up is prolonged. Other factors that would be important, however, particularly analgesic use, were not reported for the population. Freedman (1975) summarized available data and suggested that, for adults, there was no evidence to support a contribution of urinary infection by itself to progressive renal damage. Thus, evidence is consistent that women with recurrent uncomplicated urinary infection or asymptomatic bacteriuria without genitourinary abnormalities will not develop or have progression of renal scarring on the basis of urinary infection alone. It seems likely, however, that episodes of severe acute non-obstructive pyelonephritis may, rarely, heal with renal scarring in some subjects, particularly if treatment is delayed (Martin *et al.* 1976).

Several recent reports have studied sequelae of acute non-obstructive pyelonephritis with the more sensitive imaging modality of computed tomography (CT). A relatively high proportion of women with acute non-obstructive pyelonephritis have been reported to heal with renal scarring (Meyrier *et al.* 1989). This apparently occurs more frequently in subjects with delayed initiation of therapy. Generalization on the observations from these studies in respect to the larger population of women with acute non-obstructive pyelonephritis is not clear. In addition, most of the 'scars' identified by CT are not visible with the previous standard of excretion urography, nor has any association of observed scars with renal failure been reported. Thus, currently it is not clear whether these observations are clinically meaningful or are simply an interesting but clinically unimportant consequence of the increased sensitivity of imaging techniques.

In one case-control study (Kantor *et al.* 1984), subjects with bladder cancer had an increased reported frequency of UTI for both men and women. The risk was greatest for invasive disease, suggesting urinary infection may have been a concomitant rather than a pre-existing condition. This information is too preliminary, at present, to give convincing support for an association between bladder cancer and acute uncomplicated UTI in women.

Mortality

The long-term mortality associated with asymptomatic bacteriuria in women, the majority of which is presumed to be uncomplicated, has been controversial. Survival outcomes have been primarily explored in elderly populations, and these studies are discussed elsewhere in this monograph. One study in young Jamaican and Welsh women suggested that the mortality in women with asymptomatic bacteriuria was 1.5 to 2.0 times higher than those without bacteriuria (Evans *et al.* 1982). The association was not as strong when adjusted for age and weight, and data with respect to many other possible factors were not collected. In the absence of documentation of differences in long-term morbidity between women with and without bacteriuria, there is no apparent explanation why bacteriuria, *per se*, would affect survival. Large-scale population-based studies in young populations are not available to answer this question fully, but it is reasonable to conclude there is, currently, no convincing evidence that asymptomatic bacteriuria by itself is causally related to mortality.

Summary

Both asymptomatic bacteriuria and acute uncomplicated urinary infection manifest as symptomatic cystitis are common in the female population. Urinary infection, either symptomatic or asymptomatic, increases in frequency with increasing age, with increased sexual activity, and with the use of certain types of birth control. In addition, there appears to be a genetic predisposition that may largely be explained by ABO secretor status. Acute non-obstructive pyelonephritis is a more serious illness which occurs primarily in these same populations of women with urinary infection. Despite the frequency of acute uncomplicated urinary infection, there is little long-term morbidity and, currently, no evidence for mortality attributable to this problem. These women are not at increased risk of developing hypertension or renal failure. Short-term morbidity due to acute symptoms may, however, be substantial, especially for women with frequent recurrent infection.

References

Alwall, N. (1978). On controversial and open questions about the course and complications of non-obstructive urinary tract infection in adult women. *Acta Med. Scand.*, **203**, 369–77.

Asscher, A. W., *et al.* (1969). Asymptomatic significant bacteriuria in the non-pregnant woman. II. Response to treatment and follow-up. *BMJ*, **i**, 804–6.

Asscher, A. W. *et al.* (1973). Natural history of asymptomatic bacteriuria in non-pregnant women. In *Urinary tract infection*, (ed. W. Brumfitt and A. W. Asscher). pp. 51–60. Oxford University Press, London.

Bengtsson, C., Bengtsson, U., and Lincoln, K. (1980). Bacteriuria in a population sample of women. *Acta Med. Scand.* **208**, 417–23.

Brumfitt, W., Gargan, R. A., and Hamilton-Miller, J. M. T. (1987). Periurethral enterobacterial carriage preceding urinary infection. *Lancet*, **i**, 824–6.

Evans, D. A., *et al.* (1978). Bacteriuria in a population-based cohort of women. *J. Infect. Dis.*, **138**, 768–73.

Evans, D. A., *et al.* (1982). Bacteriuria and subsequent mortality in women. *Lancet*, **i**, 156–8.

Fihn, S. D., Latham, R. H., Roberts, P., Running, K., and Stamm, W. E. (1985). Association between diaphragm use and urinary tract infection. *J. Am. Med. Assoc.*, **254**, 240–5.

Foxman, B. and Frerichs, R. R. (1985*a*). Epidemiology of urinary tract infection: I. Diaphragm use and sexual intercourse. *Am. J. Pub. Health.*, **75**, 1308–13.

Foxman, B. and Frerichs, R. R. (1985*b*). Epidemiology of urinary tract infection: II. Diet, clothing and urination habits. *Am. J. Pub. Health*, **75**, 1314–17.

Freedman, L. R. (1975). Natural history of urinary infection in adults. *Kidney Internat.*, **8**, S96–100.

Freedman, L. R., Phair, J. P., Seki, M., Hamilton, H. B., and Nefzger, M. D. (1964–65). The epidemiology of urinary tract infections in Hiroshima. *Yale J. Biol. Med.*, **37**, 262–82.

Gaches, C. G. C., Miller, K. W., Roberts, J. B. M., and Slade, N. (1976). The Bristol Pyelonephritis Registry: 10 years on. *Br. J. Urol.* **47**, 721–5.

Gillespie, W. A., Sellin, M. A., Gill, P., Stephens, M., Tuckwell, I. A., and Hilton, A. L. (1978). Urinary tract infection in young women, with special reference to *Staphylococcus saprophyticus*. *J. Clin. Path.* **31**, 348–50.

Hansson, S., Jodal, U., Lincoln, K., and Svanborg-Eden, C. (1989). Untreated asymptomatic bacteriuria in girls: II. Effect of phenoxymethylpenicillin and erythromycin given for intercurrent infections. *BMJ*, 1, 859–9.

Hooton, T. M., Hillier, S., Johnson, C., Roberts, P. L., and Stamm, W. E., (1991). *Escherichia coli* bacteriuria and contraceptive method. *J. Am. Med. Assoc.*, **265**, 64–9.

Huland, H. and Busch, R. (1984). Pyelonephritis scarring in 213 patients with upper and lower urinary tract infections: Long term follow-up. *J. Urol.* **132**, 936–9.

Jones, S. R. (1992). Acute renal failure in adults with uncomplicated acute pyelonephritis: Case reports and review. *Clin. Infect. Dis.* **14**, 243–6.

Kantor, A. F., Hartge, P., Hoover, R. N., Narayana, A. S., Sullivan, J. W., and Fraumeni, J. F. jun. (1984). Urinary tract infection and risk of bladder cancer. *Am. J. Epidemiol.*, **119**, 510–15.

Kinane, D. F., Blackwell, C., Brettle, R. P., Weir, D. M., Winstanley, F. P., and Elton, R. A. (1982). ABO blood group, secretor state and susceptibility to recurrent urinary tract infection in women. *BMJ*, **285**, 7–9.

Komaroff, A. L. (1984). Acute dysuria in women. *New Engl. J. Med.*, **310**, 368–75.

Komaroff, A. L. (1986). Urinalysis and urine culture in women with dysuria. *Ann. Intern. Med.*, **104**, 212–18.

Kraft, J. K. and Stamey, T. A. (1977). The natural history of symptomatic recurrent bacteriuria in women. *Medicine.* **56**, 55–60.

Kunin, C. M. and McCormack, R. C. (1968). An epidemiology study of bacteriuria and blood pressure among nuns and working women. *New Engl. J. Med.*, **278**, 635–42.

Kunin, C. M., Polyak, F., and Postel, E. (1980). Periurethral bacterial flora in women: Prolonged intermittent colonization with *E. coli. J. Am. Med. Assoc.*, **243**, 134–9.

Latham, R. H., Running, K. and Stamm, W. E. (1983). Urinary tract infections in young adult women caused by *Staphylococcus saprophyticus. J. Am. Med. Assoc.*, **250**, 3063–6.

Leibovici, L., Alpert, G., Laor, A., Kalter-Leibovici, O., and Danon, Y. L. (1987). Urinary tract infections and sexual activity in young women. *Arch. Intern. Med.*, **147**, 345–7.

Mabeck, C. E. (1972). Treatment of uncomplicated urinary tract infection non-pregnant women. *Postgrad. Med. J.* **48**, 69–75.

Martin, M. A., Davies, P., and Knopp, M. S. (1976). Development of renal scarring in an adult with recurrent urinary tract infection. *Clin. Nephrol.*, **5**, 269–74.

Meyrier, A., *et al.* (1989). Frequency of development of early cortical scarring in acute primary pyelonephritis. *Kidney Internat.* **35**, 696–703.

Miall, W. E., Kass, E. H., Ling, J., and Stuart, K. L. (1962). Factors influencing arterial pressure in the general population in Jamaica. *BMJ*, **ii**, 497–506.

Nicolle, L. E. and Ronald, A. R. (1987). Recurrent urinary tract infection in adult women: Diagnosis and treatment. *Infect. Dis. Clin. N. Am.*, **1**, 793–806.

Nicolle, L. E., Harding G. K. M., Preiksaitis, J., and Ronald, A. R. (1982). The association of urinary tract infection with sexual intercourse. *J. Infect. Dis.*, **146**, 579–83.

Parker, J. and Kunin, C. (1973). Pyelonephritis in young women. A 10 to 20 year follow-up. *J. Am. Med. Assoc.*, **224**, 585–90.

Pead, L., Maskell, R., and Morris, J. (1985). *Staphylococcus saprophyticus* as a urinary pathogen: a six year prospective survey. *BMJ*, **291**, 1157–9.

Peckham, B. M., Maki, D. G., Patterson, J. J., and Itafez, G-K. (1986). Focal vulvitis: a characteristic syndrome or cause of dyspareunia: Features, natural history and management. *Am. J. Obstet. Gynecol.*, **154**, 855–64.

Remis, R. S., Gurwith, M. J., Gurwith, D., Hargrett-Bean, N. T., and Layde, P. M. (1987). Risk factors for urinary tract infection. *Am. J. Epidemiol.*, **126**, 685–94.

Safrin, S., Siegal, D., and Black, D. (1988). Pyelonephritis in adult women: Inpatient versus outpatient therapy. *Am. J. Med.*, **85**, 793–8.

Saginur, R., Nicolle, L. E., and the Canadian Infectious Diseases Society Clinical Trials Study Group (1992). Single dose compared with three days norfloxacin for treatment of uncomplicated urinary infection in women. *Arch. Intern. Med.*, **152**, 1233–7.

Stamey, T. A., Timothy, M., Millar, M. and Mihara, G. (1971). Recurrent urinary infections in adult women: The role of introital enterobacteria. *Calif. Med.*, **115**, 1–19.

Stamm, W. E., *et al.* (1980). Causes of the acute urethral syndrome in women. *New Engl. J. Med.*, **303**, 409–15.

Stamm, W. E., Counts, G. W., Running, K. R., Fihns, S., Turck, M. and Holmes, K. K. (1982). Diagnosis of coliform infection in acutely dysuric women. *New Engl. J. Med.*, **307**, 463–8.

Stamm, W. E., McKevitt, M., Roberts, P., and White, N. J. (1991). Natural history of recurrent urinary tract infections in women. *Rev. Infect. Dis.*, **13**, 77–84.

Svanborg-Edén, C. and de man, P. (1987). Bacterial virulence in urinary tract infection. *Infect. Dis. Clin. N. Am.*, **1**, 731–50.

Takala, J., Jousimies, H., and Sievers, K. (1977). Screening for and treatment of bacteruria in a middle-aged female population. *Acta Med. Scand.*, **202**, 69–73.

Tencer, J. (1988). Asymptomatic bacteriuria—A long term study. *Scand. J. Urol. Nephrol.*, **22**, 31–4.

Wallmark, G., Arremark, I., and Telander, B. (1978). *Staphylococcus saprophyticus*: A frequent cause of acute urinary tract infection among female outpatients. *J. Infect. Dis.* **138**, 791–7.

Wong, E. S., McKevitt, M., Running, K., Counts, G. W., Turck, M., and Stamm, W. E. (1985). Management of recurrent urinary tract infections with patient-administered single-dose therapy. *Ann. Intern. Med.*, **102**, 302–7.

6

Management of uncomplicated urinary tract infection in women

Ross R. Bailey

Introduction

The majority of urinary tract infections present as bacterial cystitis or asymptomatic (covert) bacteriuria in otherwise healthy women in the sexually active age group. The commonest infecting pathogen is *Escherichia coli* with most of the remainder being due to *Staphylococcus saprophyticus*. Uncomplicated urinary tract infection (normal urinary tract and normal renal function) in women has a high cure rate when treated with any antimicrobial agent to which the infecting pathogen is sensitive.

It has been widely believed for some time that traditional dosage regimens for uncomplicated urinary tract infections have been extravagant. Although it is still not uncommon for a patient to be treated with an antimicrobial agent for several weeks there is no convincing evidence that this is more effective than a shorter course of treatment.

This chapter will consider the management of women with uncomplicated urinary tract infection (UTI).

Clinical syndromes of uncomplicated urinary tract infection

There are several clinical syndromes of uncomplicated UTI in women (Rubin *et al.* 1992*a*,*b*).

1. Uncomplicated acute UTI, also referred to as cystitis or the frequency–dysuria syndrome.
2. Asymptomatic bacteriuria: the management of this entity in pregnancy and in the elderly is discussed in Chapters 9 and 11, respectively.
3. Abacterial cystitis (urethral syndrome)
4. Uncomplicated acute pyelonephritis (APN).
5. Recurrent UTI, defined as at least three episodes of uncomplicated acute infection in the last 12 months.

Within each of these clinical categories, the results of urine culture, microscopy, and urinalysis are the diagnostic cornerstones for establishing the presence of infection and determining the results of therapy.

General principles of management

If an accurate bacteriological diagnosis is not made at the onset then a patient with urinary tract symptoms may be subjected unnecessarily to expensive treatment with potential side-effects, the anxiety of follow-up examinations, and the high costs and possible risks of invasive investigations of the urinary tract. This is especially true in women with recurrent or persistent symptoms.

Although it may be inconvenient to withhold antimicrobial treatment for a patient with lower urinary tract symptoms until the results of the urine culture and the antibacterial sensitivity tests are known this remains ideal clinical practice. Many general practitioners, however, prefer to start antimicrobial therapy at the initial visit in most women who present with a single symptomatic episode. This is acceptable practice provided that a urine specimen has been taken for culture before treatment has commenced.

The prescribing of an alkalinizing agent does not eradicate bacteriuria, although it may alleviate the lower urinary tract symptoms, at least temporarily. The traditional advice to 'drink plenty of water' is a useful adjunct to antimicrobial therapy. Urinary tract hydrodynamics appear to be the most important protective effect in man and have been well demonstrated in elegant kinetic studies (O'Grady and Cattell 1966). Although urinary concentrations of the administrated drugs will be reduced in the presence of a diuresis, this is of no practical importance.

Ideally, women with uncomplicated UTI should be treated with the shortest course of the safest and cheapest antimicrobial agent that will eradicate the causal organism. The potential side-effects of the chosen drug should be weighed against the severity of the illness. Antimicrobial treatment regimens for UTI can be classified as:

- Curative
- Prophylactic or preventive
- Suppressive (not a consideration in women with uncomplicated infections)

Duration of treatment

It has been well documented that many patients with symptomatic UTI will stop their prescribed treatment when their symptoms resolve, often after the first few doses. This no doubt explains why women with recurrent infections nearly always have a supply of antimicrobial agents available at home.

There is a strong ecological argument for a patient to be treated in a manner most likely to discourage the development of bacterial resistance. Most recurrent infections are re-infections from the faecal flora and most antimicrobial agents act on these commensal gut organisms to select resistant strains, which may compromise further treatment. Single-dose treatment could be most beneficial if the drug had no appreciable effect on the development of resistant gut organisms. It has been shown that one week of treatment with amoxycillin in a dose of 250 mg taken 8 hourly rendered faecal Enterobacteriaceae resistant to that drug, whereas a single 1 g dose did not (Anderson 1983). In addition, there was a parallel increase in resistance to co-trimoxazole, suggesting both antibiotic-induced resistance transfer and selection, rather than selection alone.

There is now increasing interest in the use of antimicrobial agents that eradicate potential uropathogens from the vaginal reservoir, and perhaps the bowel, that are the sources for vaginal colonization (Stamey and Condy 1975; Kunin 1987; Rubin *et al.* 1992*b*).

A single dose of an antimicrobial drug is associated with fewer side-effects, such as rashes, gastrointestinal upsets, and vaginal candidiasis, and a lower risk of toxicity than a prolonged course of treatment (Stamm 1983; Tolkoff-Rubin and Rubin 1987).

Bacterial cystitis is, pathologically, a superficial mucosal infection of the bladder and successful treatment is dependent on the concentration of antimicrobial drug achieved in the urine. Most of these drugs are primarily excreted in the urine and extremely high concentrations are achieved adjacent to the bladder mucosa. Some guidance as to the likely efficacy of a single dose of an antimicrobial agent is provided by a mechanical model that simulates aspects of the dynamic conditions of bacterial growth in the bladder (O'Grady *et al.* 1973; O'Grady 1983).

Not only does a large single dose of an antimicrobial drug produce high urinary concentrations for a prolonged period (Neu 1983; Slack and Greenwood 1987), but many of these drugs have an additional post-antibiotic effect (Craig and Vogelman 1987). The latter is the phenomenon of continuing suppression of bacterial growth after a short exposure of a pathogen to an antimicrobial agent. This effect appears to be a feature of most antimicrobial drugs and has been observed with the common bacterial pathogens when they are exposed to drug concentrations that approach or exceed the minimum inhibitory concentration. Increasing the concentration of the drug and lengthening the exposure time of the pathogen prolong the post-antibiotic effect to a point of maximum effect (Craig and Vogelman 1987). Those antimicrobial drugs that work by inhibiting protein or nucleic acid synthesis induce prolonged post-antibiotic effects against Gram-negative bacilli, while the cell wall active agents and trimethoprim induce very short or no effects against Gram-negative bacilli. Although the mechanisms by which different antibacterial drugs produce this effect is uncertain, the likely explanations are either limited persistence of the drug at its site of action or drug-induced nonlethal change. The post-antibiotic effect could have a major influence on the frequency of administration of a drug.

Recent studies, however, have thrown some doubt on this phenomenon. When an *in vitro* dynamic model with no host defence factors was used to simulate *in vivo* pharmacokinetics, the post-antibiotic effect observed with gentamicin was minimal and related to the first dose only (Begg *et al.* 1992). A similar phenomenon has been reported with lomefloxacin (Chambers *et al.* 1991). More work is clearly necessary on this interesting phenomenon.

Localization of the site of infection

Over the years, there has been great interest and enthusiasm for developing methods of localizing the site of a UTI. Is the infection simply confined to the bladder, or does it involve the upper urinary tract, and in particular the renal parenchyma? The argument is that infection involving the kidney requires longer treatment than an infection of the bladder alone.

The early methods used to localize the site of infection were invasive, requiring general anaesthesia and bilateral ureteric catheterization (Stamey *et al.* 1965), while Fairley *et al.* (1967) developed the time-consuming bladder washout technique. In the mid 1970s the antibody-coated bacteria test generated considerable interest. (Thomas *et al.* 1974). After much initial enthusiasm, however, it became discredited (Mundt and Polk 1979) and is certainly of no value in the clinical management of an individual patient.

Considerable interest has been generated by the observation that failure to eradicate a UTI with a single dose of an antimicrobial agent (i.e. single-dose failure) is a valuable and simple clinical test for identifying those patients with renal parenchymal infection who require more intensive treatment, investigation, and follow-up (Ronald *et al.* 1976; Bailey and Abbott 1977).

Uncomplicated acute urinary tract infection (bacterial cystitis)

There is now convincing evidence that the antimicrobial treatment for this type of UTI need not be extended beyond three days, and in fact a single dose of an appropriate agent is highly effective.

Choice of antimicrobial drug

Drug regimens for an oral three-day course of treatment for uncomplicated bacterial cystitis are set out in Table 6.1.

The sulphonamides, such as sulphamethizole, have become unfashionable for the treatment of UTI. The proportion of urinary tract pathogens resistant to this group of antimicrobial agents varies considerably from country to country. For sensitive pathogens, however, the sulphonamides remain effective drugs.

One of the most popular choices of antibiotics has been ampicillin or amoxycillin. Unfortunately, in many countries as many as 40 per cent of urinary tract isolates of *E. coli* in the community and 60 per cent in hospital are now resistant to these antibiotics. For this reason they are now a poor choice as a first-line drug for treating most pathogens, except *Streptococcus faecalis*, before the antibacterial sensitivity profile is known. An attempt has been made to overcome the problem of widespread resistance to ampicillin/amoxycillin by the concomitant use of clavulanic acid or sulbactam. These are beta-lactamase inhibitors, which neutralize some of the beta-lactamase enzymes produced by bacteria. A clavulanic acid-potentiated form of amoxycillin (Augmentin) has been widely promoted in some countries, but some of the clinical studies have proved disappointing and

Table 6.1 Drug regimens for an oral 3-day course of treatment for bacterial cystitis

Drug	Dose	Comment
Trimethoprim	300 mg daily	An ideal agent
Co-trimoxazole	960 mg 12 hourly	Should be replaced by trimethoprim alone
Nitrofurantoin	50 mg 8 hourly	Not effective against *Proteus* spp.
Nalidixic acid	500 mg 8 hourly	Not effective against *Staph. saprophyticus*
Norfloxacin	400 mg 12 hourly	Valuable agents
Ciprofloxacin	250 mg 12 hourly	
Pefloxacin	400 mg daily	
Lomefloxacin	400 mg 12 hourly	
Fleroxacin	200–400 mg daily	
Cephalexin	250 mg 8 hourly	Useful if renal insufficiency present
Cephradine	250 mg 8 hourly	
Cefaclor	250 mg 8 hourly	
Sulphamethizole	1g 8 hourly	Unfashionable
Pivmecillinam	200 mg 8 hourly	
Amoxycillin	250 mg 8 hourly	High incidence of resistance: useful for *Strept. faecalis*
Augmentin	500 mg amox/125 mg clavulanic acid 12 hourly	Disappointing

have been associated with a high incidence of gastrointestinal side-effects (Bailey *et al.* 1983). In addition, resistance of *E. coli* to Augmentin has already become a problem. Similarly, an oral formulation of sulbactam/ampicillin (sultamicillin) has not fulfilled its early promise in the treatment of UTI.

Co-trimoxazole has been a most effective and widely used oral antibacterial agent. The combination of sulphamethoxazole and trimethoprim, however, remains an important cause of adverse drug reactions and in some countries has been withdrawn from use for the management of UTI. Trimethoprim alone has been used widely with comparable efficacy but with a reduced incidence of side-effects compared to co-trimoxazole. Trimethoprim is more active than sulphamethoxazole against most bacterial species and, in the treatment of UTI, the activity of trimethoprim is so dominant as to be almost entirely responsible for the action of co-trimoxazole. In addition, there is no convincing evidence that combining trimethoprim with a sulphonamide will reduce the likelihood of resistance developing to the former drug.

Nitrofurantoin remains a valuable drug, except that it is ineffective against *Proteus mirabilis*. Many clinicians continue to prescribe nitrofurantoin in a dose of 100 mg, 6 hourly. This high dose frequently causes nausea or vomiting which is reduced if the macrocrystalline formulation is used. Extensive clinical experience has shown equal effectiveness with a dose of 50 mg, 8 hourly.

Nalidixic acid is effective for treating UTI with Gram-negative organisms. It is inactive against *Staph. saprophyticus*. Unfortunately, this drug is still recommended for use in a dose of 1 g, 6 to 8 hourly. This large dose has an unacceptably high incidence of unpleasant side-effects. A dose of 0.5 g is just as effective and has a more acceptable incidence of side-effects (Little *et al.* 1979). In fact, nalidixic acid is most bactericidal at a concentration similar to that obtained in urine after an 0.5 g dose. Oxolinic acid has similar drawbacks to nalidixic acid and is effective in a dose of 375 mg, 12 hourly. Both nalidixic acid and oxolinic acid have now been superseded by the new 4-quinolones such as norfloxacin, enoxacin, pefloxacin, ofloxacin, ciprofloxacin, lomefloxacin, and fleroxacin. To date, norfloxacin and ciprofloxacin have been the most extensively investigated of these nalidixic acid analogues, with results comparable to co-trimoxazole (Bailey 1992). These broad-spectrum synthetic compounds are highly effective against a wide range of organisms, including hospital-acquired urinary tract pathogens. The quinolones have already become competitors of both the aminoglycosides and the newer beta-lactam antibiotics for the treatment of severe or complicated UTI. Their role in the treatment of simple, uncomplicated infections is less certain. Some investigators still believe that the quinolones should be reserved for the treatment of the more resistant pathogens, or for use in complicated clinical situations.

Mecillinam (6-β-amidinopenicillanic acid) belongs to a group of penicillanic acid derivatives with high *in vitro* activity against the Enterobacteriaceae. Mecillinam itself is poorly absorbed by the oral route, but the hydrochloride of its pivaloyloxymethyl ester, pivmecillinam, is well absorbed and rapidly hydrolysed with the liberation of mecillinam. Clinical studies have shown pivmecillinam to be particularly effective against UTI with *E. coli*.

Orally absorbed cephalosporins, such as cephalexin, cephradine, cefaclor and cefuroxime axetil, are also effective for the treatment of UTI. These compounds, like amoxycillin, act as bacterial cell-wall toxins. In the urinary tract this may result in the production of persisting forms that regain their former structure when the antibiotic has been discontinued. This probably explains the higher failure rate of these agents compared with drugs that act by interfering with intermediary metabolism or DNA replication in the bacteria (Kunin 1987).

The above discussion applies only to patients with normal renal function. When renal insufficiency is present, any UTI becomes, by definition, complicated. In this context the pharmacology of the agent intended for use must be known. In the presence of renal functional impairment, trimethoprim, amoxycillin, and the cephalosporins are the preferred agents, the sulphonamides are contraindicated, and co-trimoxazole is best avoided or the dose reduced. The use of nitrofurantoin is also contraindicated because of reduced renal excretion with accumulation in the serum increasing the risk of peripheral neuropathy. Nalidixic acid is best avoided because of accumulation of potentially toxic metabolites. The 4-quinolones have a reduced clearance in renal insufficiency making a dose reduction necessary. Their efficacy in renal insufficiency is still uncertain.

Single-dose treatment

The historical development of treating uncomplicated bacterial cystitis or asymptomatic bacteriuria with single-dose antimicrobial therapy goes back to 1967 when Grüneberg and Brumfitt reported cure of 22 of 25 women with a single 2 g dose of sulphormethoxine, a long-acting sulphonamide (Bailey 1990). In a randomized, controlled trial ampicillin in a dose of 500 mg 8 hourly for 7 days cured the same number of patients but produced more side-effects. Williams and Smith (1970) used single-dose combination therapy in four different regimens for treating women with bacteriuria in pregnancy. The most successful of these was a single dose of both streptomycin and sulfametopyrazine, which resulted in a 77 per cent cure rate among the 47 women treated. This cure rate was achieved despite the fact that about one-third of the urinary tract pathogens treated were resistant to sulphonamides. Some would regard the use of streptomycin in pregnancy as potentially hazardous, while sulphonamides should be avoided in the last trimester because of the potential risk to the neonate from bilirubin displaced from binding by sulphonamides.

Brumfitt *et al.* (1970) treated 25 pregnant women with a single 2 g intramuscular dose of cephaloridine curing 13 (52 per cent). The sole criterion for cure was eradication of the original infecting pathogen. Involvement of the renal parenchyma was detected by measuring the antibody titre directed against the 0 antigen of the infecting organism. This test was undertaken in 19 of the 25 pregnant women. Of those with an antibody titre suggesting kidney involvement only one of 10 was cured, compared with eight of the nine in whom the titre indicated infection confined to the bladder. The authors concluded that the response to a single dose of cephaloridine appeared to be a good indicator as to whether or not the infection involved the kidney. The authors suggested that although cephaloridine was known to be bactericidal its effect was not as rapid as that of some other antibiotics, such as the aminoglycosides.

In the late 1960s the author observed the effects of treating pregnant women with asymptomatic bacteriuria with a single 100 mg oral dose of nitrofurantoin (Bailey 1990). One half were cured as defined by a sterile urine specimen one week following treatment. These women cured were subsequently shown to have radiologically normal urinary tracts, but of those women who remained infected, half had a significant urinary tract abnormality. It was suggested that a possible advantage of single-dose treatment in pregnancy could be a reduction in the incidence of side-effects in the mother or in the risk of drug toxicity to the fetus.

After these early studies, which were mainly in pregnant women, there was little interest in this approach to therapy until the mid to late 1970s. Subsequently, Bailey and Abbott (1977) reported that the cure rate following a single 3 g oral dose of amoxycillin was comparable to that of a conventional course of the same antibiotic. They also showed that a single dose of amoxycillin cured 16 of 17 with radiologically normal urinary tracts compared to 10 of 18 with a urinary tract abnormality. These findings suggested that failure to eradicate a UTI with a single dose of amoxycillin might indicate which patients were likely to have a urinary tract abnormality. Ronald *et al.* (1976), using the bladder washout test to localize the site of infection, showed that 36 of 39 women (92 per cent) with organisms localized to the bladder were cured after a single 0.5 g intramuscular dose of kanamycin sulphate, whereas 47 of 65 women (72 per cent) with bacteria coming from the upper urinary tract relapsed almost immediately.

These last two studies stimulated numerous further clinical trials, initially with amoxycillin and later co-trimoxazole and trimethoprim which showed a single dose to be just as efficacious as a course of either drug. Encouraging results were also reported with single oral doses of the sulphonamides, nitrofurantoin 100–200 mg, tetracycline 2 g, doxycycline 300 mg, pivmecillinam 600 mg, cefaclor 2 g, and cephalexin, 2–3 g. Of the drugs administered parenterally the aminoglycosides (e.g. kanamycin 0.5 g; netilmicin 150 mg) are the most effective. A number of cephalosporins or other beta-lactam antibiotics have been used in single-dose parenteral regimens with results generally similar to ampicillin or amoxycillin, but inferior to trimethoprim or co-trimoxazole (Philbrick and Bracikowski 1985; Leibovici and Wysenbeek 1991). Drugs studied in this group included cephaloridine 2 g, cephamandole 1 g, cefuroxime 1.5 g, oral cephalexin 2–3 g, ceftriaxone 0.5–1.0 g, cefotaxime 1 g, cefadroxil 1 g, and aztreonam 1 g.

A compound with a pharmacokinetic profile that makes it particularly attractive for single-dose treatment of uncomplicated UTI is fosfomycin trometamol. A 3 g dose has been shown to be highly effective in both open (Moroni 1987) and randomized, controlled trials (Neu and Williams 1988), and it is now marketed in several countries specifically for the treatment of women with cystitis.

More recently, the 4-quinolones have been the focus of attention for single-dose regimens. Norfloxacin in a dose of 800 mg has been shown to be successful in both non-comparative and comparative studies (Bailey 1992). Bailey *et al.* (1987) undertook a randomized, comparative study comparing enoxacin 400 mg with trimethoprim 600 mg. The two drugs were comparable for the treatment of *E. coli*, but enoxacin was a little less effective against *Staph. saprophyticus.* A range of other quinolones, including pefloxacin 800 mg, lomefloxacin 400 mg, and fleroxacin 400 mg, have also been shown to be just as efficacious in single-dose regimens as a 3- to 13-day course of either a quinolone or co-trimoxazole (Bailey 1992). Some workers remain concerned as to the effectiveness of the quinolones in single dose against *Staph. saprophyticus.* Others believe that the quinolones should be kept for the treatment of more serious UTIs with pathogens that are resistant to the commonly used agents.

Of the orally administered agents, trimethoprim 600 mg, co-trimoxazole 1.92 g, fosfomycin trometamol 3 g, and the 4-quinolones (e.g. norfloxacin 800 mg), have been shown to be the most effective when administered as a single dose (Table 6.2).

In 1983, Neu discussed the ideal pharmacological properties of an antimicrobial agent for single-dose administration. Any new agent being assessed for its use in a single-dose regimen should be compared with either trimethoprim or co-trimoxazole in randomized, controlled trials of sufficient size to eliminate a type II statistical error (Philbrick and Bracikowski 1985).

The many advantages of single-dose therapy of women with cystitis or asymtomatic bacteriuria have been well documented (Bailey 1983), and are summarized in Table 6.3. There is now impressive evidence that single-dose antimicrobial therapy should be considered as the treatment of choice for uncomplicated UTI presenting in general practice.

Table 6.2 Single-dose orally administered drug regimens for the treatment of bacterial cystitis

Trimethoprim	600 mg*
Co-trimoxazole	1.92 g*
Fosfomycin trometamol	3 g*
Norfloxacin	800 mg*
Enoxacin	400 mg*
Ciprofloxacin	500 mg*
Pefloxacin	800 mg*
Fleroxacin	400 mg*
Sulphafurazole	1–2 g
Sulphamethizole	3 g
Amoxycillin	3 g
Pivmecillinam	600 mg
Doxycycline	300 mg
Cephalexin	3g
Cefaclor	2g

*Recommended.

Table 6.3 Advantages of single-dose antimicrobial therapy for bacterial cystitis

1. Simple
2. Effective
3. Cheap
4. Well tolerated
5. Preferred by patients
6. Assured compliance
7. Fewer side-effects
8. Less hazard to fetus
9. Less risk of resistant organisms developing
10. Simple method of localizing the site of infection
11. Indicator of the need for urinary tract investigation

A suggested algorithm for the management of simple UTI is shown in Fig. 6.1.

Questions posed by single-dose therapy

Is single-dose therapy effective for the treatment of infections with pathogens other than E. coli? Although single-dose therapy is highly effective for the treatment of UTI due to *E. coli* it has been questioned as to whether this approach to treatment is equally effective for women infected with *Staph. saprophyticus.* The latter organism has a seasonal variation and during the spring and summer

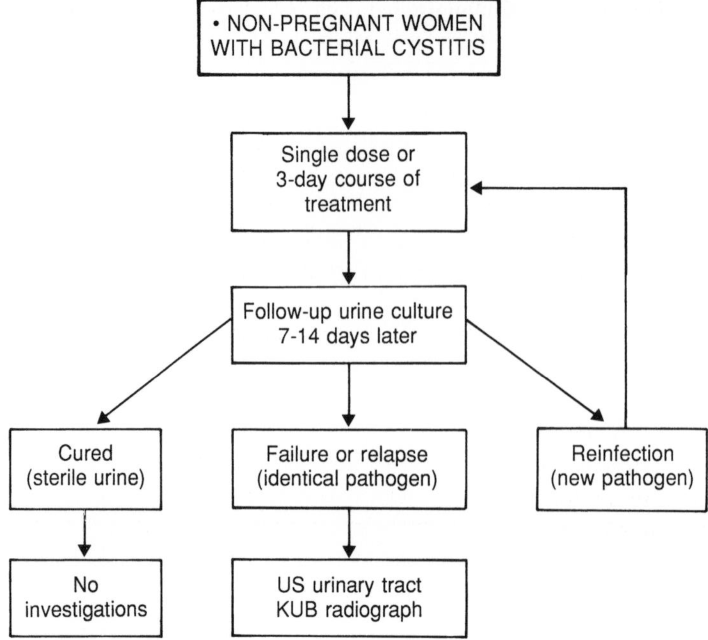

Fig. 6.1 A suggested algorithm for the management of non-pregnant women with bacterial cystitis (US, ultrasonography; KUB, plain abdominal radiograph, including kidney, ureter, and bladder areas). (Reproduced with permission of the Editor, *Clinical Drug Investigations* (1995), **9** (Suppl. 1), 8–13.

months is the second most common urinary tract pathogen causing bacterial cystitis in most communities.

This question was analysed by Bailey (1989) from several of his studies. Of 44 women infected with *Staph. saprophyticus* and treated with a single dose of either amoxycillin, trimethoprim, co-trimoxazole, or doxycycline, 39 (89 per cent) were cured. The drug that was found to be disappointing for eradicating this organism was a single dose of enoxacin (Bailey *et al.* 1987). Some other workers have reported this observation with other quinolones. With the possible exception of the quinolones these findings would suggest that single-dose therapy is effective for the treatment of bacterial cystitis due to *Staph. saprophyticus*.

Of the pathogens other than *E. coli* and *Staph. saprophyticus* that cause uncomplicated UTI in general practice, the most common is *Proteus mirabilis*. In 10 single-dose studies undertaken by Bailey (1989) there were a total of 43 pathogens other than *E. coli* and *Staph. saprophyticus*; 22 were strains of *P. mirabilis* and only 11 were cured. Some of these studies were randomized, controlled trials which also had five-day treatment arms. The latter included a total of 16 women infected with *P. mirabilis* of whom 14 were cured. Single-dose therapy was therefore less successful for the treatment of infections with *P. mirabilis* and the same applied to *Strep. faecalis*. The former organism is frequently localized to the upper urinary tract, whereas the latter is usually present in an abnormal host or urinary tract. Women infected with these two pathogens should have their urinary tract investigated.

Does duration of therapy affect the time for the urinary tract symptoms to resolve? The question has been asked as to whether urinary tract symptoms take longer to resolve in patients treated with single-dose therapy compared to those who receive a course of treatment. In one of the few studies where this question was addressed, women treated with a single 600 mg dose of trimethoprim lost their symptoms in a mean time of 1.5 days, compared with 2.2 days for a single 1.92 g dose of co-trimoxazole, and 3.4 days for those women receiving a 5-day course of trimethoprim (Bailey *et al.* 1985). The only statistically significant difference in this study was that women treated with a single dose of amoxycillin took a significantly longer time for their symptoms to settle than those treated with a single dose of trimethoprim.

As many women continue to have urinary tract symptoms for 24 hours or more after a single dose they may be concerned that the treatment regimen may have been inadequate. The patients should be reassured that a single dose of a drug such as trimethoprim, co-trimoxazole, or a quinolone will sterilize the urine very rapidly, but the symptoms will take a little longer to settle.

Does single-dose therapy predispose to earlier or more severe recurrences? There has been some concern that single-dose therapy may predispose to earlier recurrence of infection. Bailey (1983) followed 104 women included in two trials which compared a single dose with a five-day course of co-trimoxazole. During follow-up, the number of recurrences was similar, and of those treated with a single dose the mean number of days to recurrence was 203 compared with 193 for those that received a course of co-trimoxazole. These findings suggest that a single-dose therapy does not predispose to earlier or more frequent recurrences. Unfortunately, most comparative studies have only a short period of follow-up.

Tolkoff-Rubin and Rubin (1987) reviewed more than 200 women or children who had had a suspected relapse following single-dose antimicrobial therapy. No relapse was associated with clinical symptoms or signs that were worse than in the initial illness and there was no associated long-term morbidity.

Asymptomatic bacteriuria

The presence of asymptomatic bacteriuria indicates that the urine is colonized with bacteria. However, unless there is invasion and an associated inflammatory response, many workers believe it cannot be considered as an infection. Asymptomatic bacteriuria, however, has great predictive value in epidemiological studies, particularly in pregnancy, and should be considered as an abnormal finding. Its significance can only be interpreted in the clinical context.

The balance of evidence now suggests that asymptomatic bacteriuria is well tolerated and should be left untreated, except in settings, such as pregnancy,

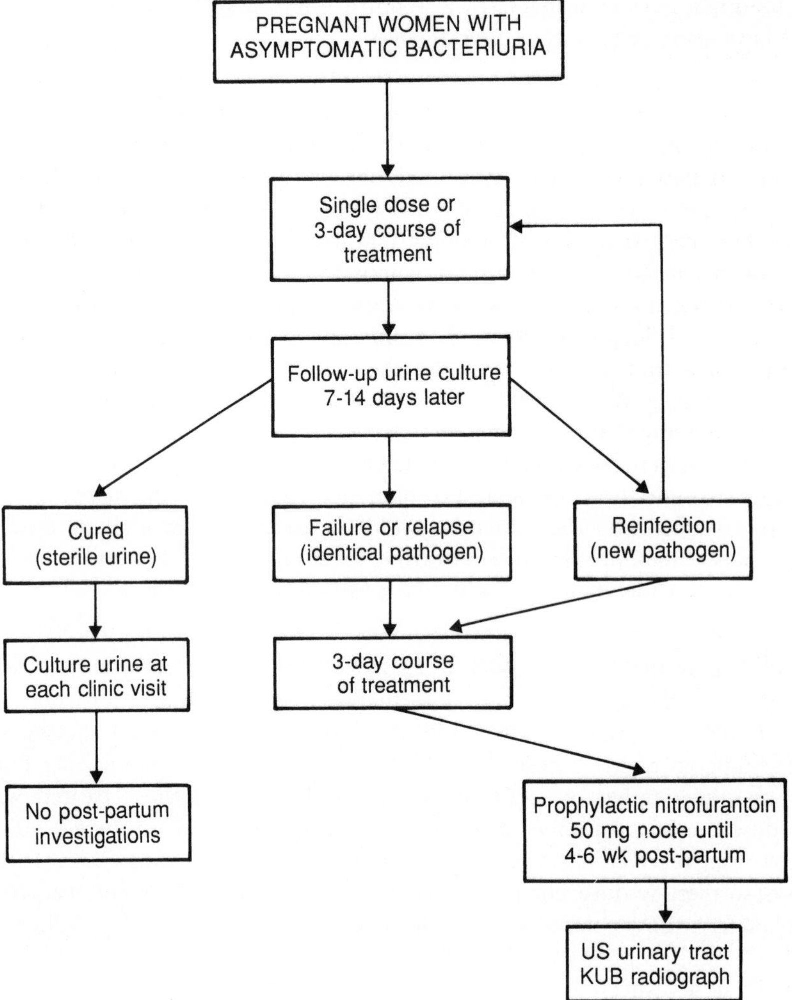

Fig. 6.2 A suggested algorithm for the management of pregnant women with asymptomatic bacteriuria (US, ultrasonography; KUB, plain abdominal radiograph, including kidney, ureter, and bladder areas).

prior to joint prosthetic or urological surgery, or after urinary catheter removal (see Fig. 6.2). The important topics of asymptomatic bacteriuria in pregnancy and the high prevalence in the elderly, especially in those who are institutionalized, will be dealt with elsewhere in this monograph.

The area of concern is that many patients who have asymptomatic bacteriuria eradicated are at risk of having their urinary tract infected with a more virulent organism which is associated with a clinical episode (Asscher *et al.* 1969).

Abacterial cystitis (urethral syndrome)

Up to one-half of women presenting with dysuria and frequency will have a bacterial colony count in voided urine of < 100 000/ml of a potential pathogen. Many of these women will be infected with a potential pathogen if urine is taken by suprapubic aspiration (Stamm *et al.* 1981; Fihn *et al.* 1988). Clearly, these women simply have bacterial cystitis. A small proportion, however, have a sterile urine specimen or one with a low count (< 1000/ml) of contaminating organisms and are diagnosed as having the urethral syndrome or abacterial cystitis. Many of these women have accompanying pyuria, indicating an associated inflammatory reaction (Stamm *et al.* 1981; Bailey 1983). The aetiology of the urethral syndrome is unclear, but is almost certainly multifactorial (Tait *et al.* 1985). A study of female university students with the urethral syndrome showed that this was often due to urethritis caused by *Chlamydia trachomatis* (Stamm *et al.* 1980). In one study (Stamm *et al.* 1981), 11 of 19 symptomatic women with sterile pyuria on suprapubic aspirates or catheter urine samples had proven infection with this organism. If *C. trachomatis* infection is confirmed the patient and her partner should be treated with a 7- to 14-day course of doxycycline or a sulphonamide.

For those women with the urethral syndrome and no identifiable pathogenic cause there is some debate as to whether they respond to antimicrobial therapy or resolve spontaneously whether or not a drug is given. Some have suggested that those without pyuria do not respond to antibacterial treatment (Stamm *et al.* 1981). In clinical practice, however, these women are usually treated with antimicrobial drugs before the result of the urine culture is available.

Bailey (1983) assessed the response to treatment of 70 women with dysuria and frequency who had a voided urine specimen that was sterile or had a bacterial count of < 10 000/ml. They were enrolled in three controlled trials comparing a single-dose regimen of either doxycycline, cefuroxime, or pivmecillinam with a five-day course of co-trimoxazole, but were excluded when the urine culture results became available. When assessed one week after completing treatment, the only women whose symptoms had not completely resolved, or at least improved, were two women treated with a single dose of pivmecillinam. Four women had a bacterial count of > 100 000/ml one week after treatment; two of these had pyuria at the initial presentation. Of the 27 women (39 per cent) with pyuria, 26 had their symptoms completely alleviated. It appeared that single-dose therapy was associated with a rapid resolution of the urinary tract symptoms.

If a woman with abacterial cystitis does not respond to a single dose or a three-day course of therapy, and does not have *C. trachomatis* urethritis, then other approaches to management should be considered. These include the use of analgesics or antispasmodics, a search for a gynaecological disorder, such as atrophic vaginitis or bacterial vaginosis, an alteration to personal hygiene, or consideration for a urodynamic assessment. It is also important to remember that sexually active women with frequency and dysuria, but sterile urine, may have a sexually transmitted disease.

Uncomplicated acute pyelonephritis

Many patients with acute pyelonephritis (APN) are sufficiently ill to warrant hospitalization for rehydration, pain relief, parenteral antibiotic treatment, and urinary tract investigation. Only the last can indicate to the clinician whether the APN is uncomplicated or associated with a urinary tract abnormality which may or may not require urgent attention (see Fig. 6.3).

Parenteral therapy is usually indicated in patients with high fever and especially those with vomiting. For those who need parenteral treatment the choice of antimicrobial agent will be between an aminoglycoside, a quinolone or a beta-lactam (Table 6.4).

The aminoglycosides are extremely effective and in the ill patient remain the preferred agents until the sensitivity profile of the infecting pathogen is known.

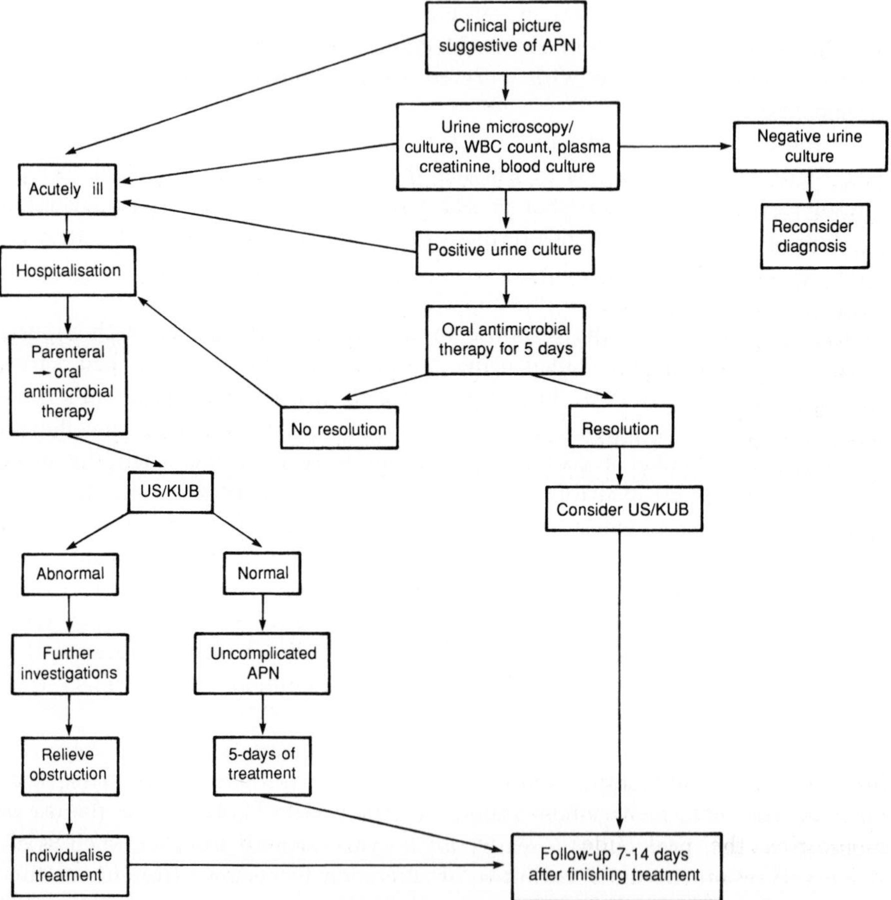

Fig. 6.3 A suggested algorithm for the management of women with suspected acute pyelonephritis (APN).

Table 6.4 Drug regimens for a parenteral 5-day course of treatment for uncomplicated acute pyelonephritis

Gentamicin* Tobramycin* Netilmicin*	Loading dose 2–3 mg/kg body weight; maintenance doses according to drug levels and renal function
Ciprofloxacin	100 mg 12 hourly
Lomefloxacin	400 mg daily
Cephradine	1 g 8 hourly
Cefazolin	1 g 8 hourly
Ceftriaxone	2 g daily
Ceftazidime	0.5–1.0 g 12 hourly
Aztreonam	1 g 12 hourly
Ipipenem/cilastin	500 mg/500 mg 8 hourly
Amoxycillin	1 g 8 hourly
Clavulanic acid/amoxycillin	200 mg/1 g 8 hourly

*4–7 mg/kg as a single daily dose is just as effective and is less toxic.

Some clinicians prefer netilmicin or tobramycin to gentamicin, because of their reduced risk of nephrotoxicity and ototoxicity. Others believe the cheapness of gentamicin is more attractive than the possible benefits of reduced toxicity. Amikacin should be retained for the treatment of resistant organisms. Some of these very ill patients may have disturbed renal function necessitating careful monitoring of both renal function and the serum peak and trough concentrations of the drug. All patients, irrespective of their renal function, require a full loading dose (2.5–3.0 mg/kg gentamicin, tobramycin, or netilmicin). The maintenance dose of 1.0–1.5 mg/kg should then be adjusted according to the measured or estimated creatinine clearance, and given at an increased interval. For the treatment of UTI this method is preferred to giving a smaller dose every eight hours. For a rapid guide to dosage the creatinine clearance can be easily estimated at the bedside by using the variables of age, weight, sex, and plasma creatinine in the Cockcroft and Gault (1976) formula:

$$\text{Creatinine clearance (ml/min)} = \frac{140 - \text{Age (yr)} \times \text{Weight (kg)}}{815 \times \text{Plasma creatinine (mmol/l)}}$$

Females: × 0.85

Some clinicians now use computer modelling to predict more accurately the maintenance dose of the aminoglycosides. There is no substitute, however, for monitoring the peak (ideally > 10 mg/l) and trough or pre-dose (ideally < 2 mg/l) serum concentrations of the aminoglycosides every second or third day and daily if treatment is extended beyond five days or renal function is changing.

There is increasing evidence that patients with serious UTI are just as effectively managed with a once-daily dose of an aminoglycoside (Barclay *et al.* 1994).

In animal models of UTI and in clinical studies, dosage regimens that provide the same total dose of aminoglycoside given once or twice daily have been shown to be equally or more effective than divided dosing regimens. In addition, aminoglycoside toxicity is reduced when these drugs are administered as a large single daily dose (Parker and Davey 1993; Prins *et al.* 1993).

There is now considerable interest in the use of the 4-quinolones for treating APN. The availability of some of the new quinolones (e.g. ciprofloxacin, lomefloxacin) for parenteral administration has enabled these drugs to be administered to patients who are vomiting. As soon as the patient feels better, often after 24–48 hours, she can be switched to the oral formulation of the quinolone, and sent home earlier. This practice has enormous potential for cost savings.

There is a steadily expanding list of beta-lactam antibiotics including the third- and fourth- generation cephalosporins, the semi-synthetic or ureido penicillins, the penems, and the monobactams (e.g. aztreonam). The place of these new antibiotics is not yet clear, but some are associated with the risk of side-effects including skin rashes, hypersensitivity reactions, vitamin-K-dependent coagulation disorders, neutropenia, thrombocytopenia, diarrhoea, pseudomembranous colitis, and disturbance of renal function. Ampicillin/amoxycillin should be avoided in initial treatment of an ill patient because of the high risk that the pathogen will be resistant.

The duration of treatment for uncomplicated APN remains the subject of much debate (Kunin 1981; Pinson *et al.* 1992; Bailey 1994*a*). Without any scientific basis, it is not an uncommon practice for some patients with uncomplicated APN to be given a 4- to 6-week period of treatment. This is now widely regarded as excessive. Stamm *et al.* (1987) showed that a 2-week course of treatment with co-trimoxazole or ampicillin proved as efficacious as a 6-week treatment with either drug.

Some authors consider that even a treatment period of 14 days is excessive. Over the past 25 years in this unit we have shortened the duration of antimicrobial therapy progressively from 14 days to 5 days. We reviewed (Bailey and Peddie 1987) 91 consecutive women who were admitted to our unit with uncomplicated APN and enrolled in prospective clinical studies of 5-day treatment. All women were sufficiently ill to warrant hospitalization and were subsequently shown to have a structurally normal urinary tract and normal renal function. Of the total of 91 women, 79 (87 per cent) were cured. This group included 35 patients treated with an aminoglycoside antibiotic (tobramycin, sisomicin, netilmicin) of whom 33 (94 per cent) were cured. A further 38 women were treated with a beta-lactam antibiotic (cefoxitin, cefotiam, cefoperazone, cefamandole, ceftriaxone, aztreonam) and 32 (84 per cent) were cured. Finally, 14 of 18 (78 per cent) treated with an oral quinolone (norfloxacin, enoxacin) were cured. In a recent study, 15 of 17 patients treated with netilmicin (intravenously) and 15 of 17 with ciprofloxacin (intravenously initially and later orally) were cured. The women treated with ciprofloxacin required a significantly shorter period of hospitalization as they were able to go home on oral therapy (Bailey *et al.* 1992). These results using a 5-day course of antimicrobial therapy for the treatment of hospitalized women with severe APN were most impressive and comparable to cure rates expected when treating women with acute cystitis or asymptomatic bacteriuria.

Patients with uncomplicated APN nearly always respond rapidly to treatment and after one to three days in hospital are well enough to go home. It is our current practice to either switch the parenteral agent to an orally absorbed drug or, alternatively, to have the patient return each day as an outpatient for a parenteral dose. In the latter instance, drugs that have a long action are especially attractive. This early discharge policy has found favour with the health economists.

There is no justification to use more than a single drug for the treatment of uncomplicated APN. A suggested protocol for the management of patients with suspected APN is set out in Fig. 6.4.

Recurrent urinary tract infections

Urinary tract investigations

It would be impossible, and not cost-effective, to investigate all those women in the sexually active age group who suffer isolated episodes of bacterial cystitis or asymptomatic bacteriuria. In such a group, less than 10 per cent of women have a urinary tract abnormality and only a small proportion of these abnormalities are significant or correctable (Kunin 1987).

It is therefore a matter of considerable importance to determine which of these women require investigation of the urinary tract such as organ imaging and cystoscopy. A factor that has rarely been addressed is that the major expense in the management of UTI is the cost of the urinary tract investigations. When should these women be investigated? All women with acute pyelonephritis require investigation. In this department, 24 per cent of a series of women hospitalized with acute pyelonephritis had a urinary tract abnormality. We believe that women with atypical symptomatology, an unusual pathogen, a systemic disorder, such as diabetes mellitus, and persistent pyuria, or persistent microscopic haematuria require investigation. Investigation should be carried out before commencing a period of long-term, low-dose antimicrobial prophylaxis. Many women who have had recurrent proven infections are anxious and concerned about possible renal damage and also warrant investigations (see Fig. 6.4).

Any simple diagnostic aid that could minimize the need for expensive investigations must be advantageous. In the mid 1970s it was suggested that failure of single-dose therapy might be a simple guide to the need for further urinary tract investigation. Since then there has been increasing support for this approach. It is our current practice that women with bacterial cystitis or asymptomatic bacteriuria who are not cured with single-dose therapy (i.e. single-dose failures) are referred for imaging of the urinary tract (urinary tract ultrasonography; plain abdominal, KUB, radiograph; and/or renal area tomography).

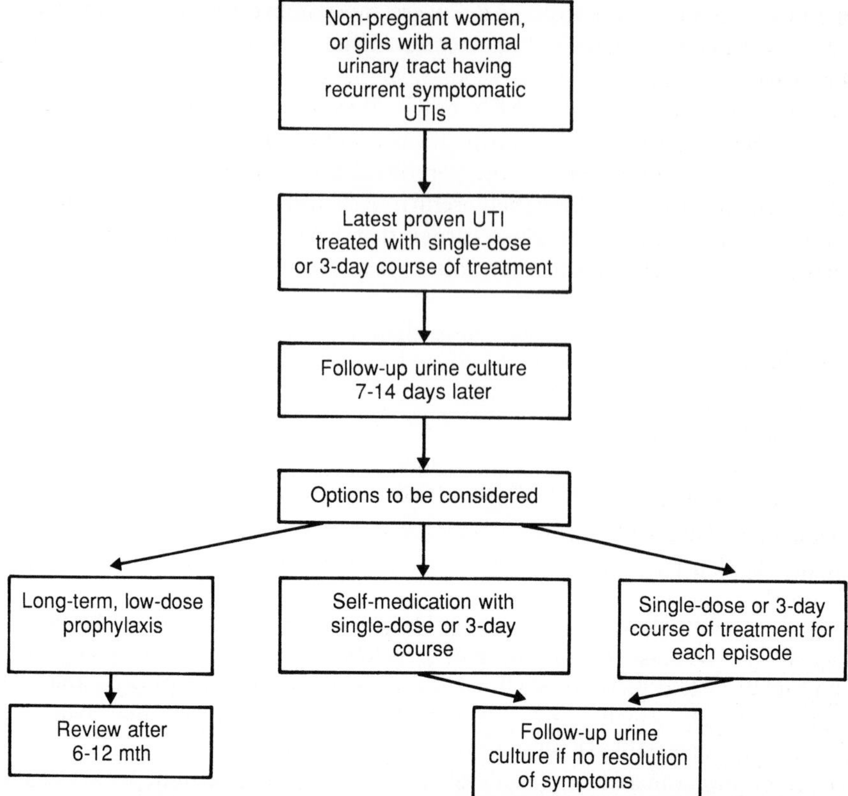

Fig. 6.4 A suggested algorithm for the management of either non-pregnant women or girls with a normal urinary tract who are having recurrent symptomatic urinary tract infection.

Thus, single-dose therapy has not only become a simple way of managing these patients, but has also become a reliable and inexpensive diagnostic indicator.

Some urologists still include cystoscopy as an essential investigation for women with UTI. This is a very expensive procedure and rarely alters the management of these women. Experience in this unit over 25 years has led us to believe that there is no indication for cystocopy in women suffering occasional UTI whose follow-up urine culture is sterile and free of pyuria or microscopic haematuria. Some clinicians recommend cystoscopy for women with well-documented abacterial cystitis which recurs.

Follow-up

Ideally, a patient who has had a UTI should be reviewed 10–14 days after treatment and a urine specimen obtained for culture. Up until recently it has been recommended practice that seven days was an ideal time to assess cure, but some of the new antimicrobial agents (e.g. long-acting quinolones) may be excreted in the urine for up to a week.

The early reappearance of the same bacterial species or the same biotype or serotype of *E. coli* suggests that the original pathogen has not been eradicated and that the patient may require a longer period of treatment and further investigation. A genuine relapse will rarely occur if the urine is sterile 10 days after treatment. Most recurrences are re-infections with a different bacterial species. This is no reflection on the previous treatment but merely indicates the recurrent nature of this problem.

Prophylactic or preventive treatment

Some women have recurrent or closely spaced symptomatic infections which cause considerable anxiety and much morbidity. This is especially a problem in young, sexually active females. All patients should be warned that recurrences may occur and that invariably these are with new organisms and are not due to inadequacy or failure of the last course of treatment. Women with uncomplicated UTI should also be reassured that although clinical episodes of infection are unpleasant they will not lead to any damage to renal function.

The number of books written by lay authors and the endless lists of alternative therapies for UTI attests to the lack of knowledge and the unsatisfactory manner in which the medical profession has managed this recurrent problem. Personal hygiene, perineal toilet, bowel habit, cold or humid weather, nylon underwear, tight knickers or pantyhose, deodorants, bubble baths, allergies, stress, and psychological factors have all been incriminated as possible predisposing factors, but their precise role, if any, is unproven.

What is now clear is that women who use diaphragms, with or without spermicides, for contraception are at an increased risk of both symptomatic (Fihn *et al.* 1985) and asymptomatic UTI (Peddie *et al.* 1986), compared with women using oral contraceptives, intra-uterine contraceptive devices, condoms or no contraception.

Many women with recurrent infections are helped by ensuring that they have an intake of at least 2 litres of water daily and always empty their bladder completely, particularly before going to bed and after intercourse. Some benefit may be obtained by applying an antiseptic cream (e.g. 0.5 per cent cetrimide w/w) to the periurethral area before intercourse.

If these simple measures have been employed, but have failed, the use of low-dose antimicrobial prophylaxis should be discussed with the patient (see Fig. 6.4). The pattern of recurrences can be interrupted by instituting prophylactic therapy after the urine has been sterilized. Nitrofurantoin in a dose of 50 mg taken last thing at night after the patient has emptied the bladder is highly effective, as is 100 mg of trimethoprim, 0.24 g of co-trimoxazole or 200 mg of norfloxacin (Ohkoshi and Naber 1992; Bailey 1994*b*). There have also been satisfactory results with a 1 g oral dose of hexamine hippurate and, in patients with renal insufficiency, 125 mg of cephalexin. Trials have shown that it is just as effective to give a dose on alternate nights or even three nights a week (Harding *et al.* 1979). In women whose bacteriuria is clearly related to sexual activity, a dose after intercourse is highly effective and has become a widely accepted approach to treatment (Stapleton *et al.* 1990).

The excellent results with nitrofurantoin may reflect the fact that the drug causes no alteration to the faecal flora. Trimethroprim may have advantages as a prophylactic agent because it is secreted partly through the vagina and thus may eliminate a potential source of infecting pathogens from the periurethral area. (See Table 6.5)

Table 6.5 Drug regimens for long-term, low-dose prophylaxis of recurrent urinary tract infection

Drug	Dose*
Nitrofurantoin	50 mg
Trimethoprim	100 mg
Co-trimoxazole	0.24 g
Norfloxacin	200 mg
Ciprofloxacin	125 mg
Cephalexin	125 mg (useful if renal insufficiency)
Hexamine hippurate	1 g

*Treatment is effective if taken each night, alternate nights, three times a week, or just after intercourse.

The treatment of atrophic vaginitis should be given early consideration in post-menopausal women with recurrent symptomatic UTI. It is correctable with the use of oral or topical oestrogen therapy (Privette *et al.* 1988; Raz and Stamm 1993). This promotes accumulation of glycogen by vaginal epithelial cells thus allowing the growth of *Lactobacillus* spp. and the production of lactic acid. This causes a marked acidification of vaginal secretions with suppression of vaginal growth of potential urinary pathogens.

Economics of treating urinary tract infection

Shortening the duration of therapy

With the increasing cost of health care delivery a number of approaches for managing UTI have been suggested which require further evaluation as possible cost-saving manoeuvres. If any current management practice could be changed without a detrimental effect this could be beneficial. Shortening the duration of therapy is one such approach.

The cost of the recommended single doses of trimethoprim (600 mg), co-trimoxazole (1.92 g), or norfloxacin (800 mg) is less than the cost of a three-day course of these agents.

In the United States, the cost of the medication accounted for only 12.6 per cent of the total cost (excluding the costs of urinary tract investigations) of managing a UTI in the conventional manner. The other expenses were accounted for by the doctor's fees, the cost of pre-treatment, and follow-up urine examination (Schultz *et al.* 1984). When a single 1.92 g dose of co-trimoxazole was used instead of a 10-day course the cost of the drug fell to only 1 per cent of the total costs.

Patients in many countries pay for their medicines or have a fixed prescription charge. In those countries with the latter a woman will expect more tablets for her money than just a single dose. This is something local drug regulatory authorities should address if they are sincere in their intention of reducing the cost of health care. Should a woman prescribed a single dose of an antibiotic for the treatment of bacterial cystitis have to pay the same amount as another receiving a one-month course of the same drug for a chronic chest infection?

Not surprisingly, single-dose treatment of UTI has generated relatively little interest from the pharmaceutical industry until quite recently. The savings on a nation's annual drug bill, however, would be substantial. The manufacturers of antimicrobial agents are always fearful that their product will not be effective, and therefore advise its use in large doses for long periods of time, and rationalize this over-kill and the high number of side-effects which accompanies it, by expressing concern about the potential risks of developing resistant bacterial strains. Some pharmaceutical companies, however, are now actively promoting single-dose treatment of simple bacterial cystitis.

Fair *et al.* (1980) calculated that the use of a 3-day instead of a 10- to 14-day antimicrobial regimen for urinary infections would result in a saving of US$62 million annually in the United States. Källenius *et al.* (1983) indicated that the cost of antimicrobial agents used for UTI in Sweden was about Skr40 million. This corresponded to US$1.2–1.4/ inhabitant/year, or about 3.4 per cent of Sweden's annual drug bill. These authors concluded that if treatment periods could be shortened without a loss of efficacy then costs could be considerably reduced. Moreover, if the ecological effects of treatment were reduced, this would probably reduce the need for pharmaceutical companies to develop more potent and more expensive drugs.

In lesser developed countries, where urine culture or organ imaging facilities may be unavailable or too expensive, the cost of treating a UTI is almost completely confined to the cost of the antimicrobial agents used. In this context the advantages of single-dose therapy are compelling. The cost of the drugs, however, is only minor when compared with the expenses of pre-treatment and follow-up urine cultures, doctors' fees, and the expenses involved in investigating the urinary tract of some of these patients.

Any approach to the management of UTI that could avoid these expensive investigations, without missing the diagnosis of a lesion that is correctable, must be cost-saving.

Pre-treatment urine cultures

Another suggestion for reducing the costs of treating an uncomplicated episode of bacterial cystitis has been to forego a pre-treatment urine culture. In clinical practice, women presenting with acute lower urinary tract symptoms usually will demand, and be given, treatment before the culture result is available. It could be argued that as most women respond rapidly to treatment and remain free of further symptoms indefinitely or for long periods, there is little to be gained from laboratory investigations if the result is not available prior to treatment and merely confirms clinical suspicion after the patient has recovered. It would, of course, never be known whether the patient had bacterial cystitis or abacterial cystitis (urethral syndrome). This practice would upset the purist who correctly appreciates that a UTI is a bacteriological entity. Many doctors, however, only examine the urine after treatment, or if the symptoms either fail to settle or recur.

This approach to management is considered acceptable by many clinicians for those women with an isolated clinical episode, whereas those with recurrent symptoms justify a pre-treatment urine culture.

A decision–analysis model has been developed (Carlson and Mulley 1985) to estimate the effects and costs of alternative initial management strategies for the treatment of women with bacterial cystitis. Obtaining an initial culture in all patients reduced the expected symptom days by about 10 per cent, but increased the expected cost by about 40 per cent. Schultz *et al.* (1984) carried out a study to assess the cost-effectiveness of routine urinalysis and culture, and the efficacy of single dose co-trimoxazole, in a prospective, randomized trial of 200 women who presented with acute lower urinary tract symptoms. Considerable savings could be achieved by reserving urinalysis and urine culture for women with persistent or recurrent symptoms. The authors also concluded that empirical therapy with co-trimoxazole for selected women with lower urinary tract symptoms was practical, safe, and cost-effective.

General practitioners frequently complain (and usually with justification) of large time delays in the reporting of urine cultures. Many laboratories are now able to provide the results of the urine culture, together with the likely pathogen and sensitivity profile by 10.00 a.m. the following morning.

Notwithstanding the above, only pre-treatment cultures will provide information on infection with unusual or resistant pathogens, or permit the monitoring of antimicrobial resistance in a community, and therefore the formulation of prescribing policies.

Is antibacterial sensitivity testing worthwhile?

The clinical value of routine antibacterial sensitivity testing has been questioned (Fair and Fair 1982). In a study on 2413 urological patients simple identification of the pathogen provided the authors with sufficient information to make a choice of an 'effective' drug. For example, if *E. coli* was isolated then there was more than an 80 per cent chance that the organism would be sensitive to trimethoprim, nitrofurantoin, nalidixic acid, and cephalexin. It was concluded that in a high percentage of patients, the clinical response could be predicted without the need for antimicrobial sensitivity testing.

Elimination of routine sensitivity testing would significantly reduce the costs of treatment. Perhaps only organisms other than *E. coli* should have their antibacterial sensitivity profile studied? An alternative approach would be to ask the laboratory to store the cultures for subsequent sensitivity testing if necessary.

Routine follow-up urine cultures

Another consideration in the management of uncomplicated UTI is the benefit of a routine follow-up culture in those women who have lost their symptoms. There is little published information on the yield and clinical usefulness of such cultures. Clinical practice varies markedly. Winickoff *et al.* (1981) in a retrospective study, concluded that a routine follow-up culture in asymptomatic women may be unjustified. However, Savard-Fenton *et al.* (1982) considered a follow-up urine culture was mandatory, as it reliably identified the minority of patients who needed more intensive treatment and investigation. Obviously, the cost of a routine follow-up culture would be the same whether the patient was treated with a single dose or a course of an antimicrobial agent. Clearly if single-dose therapy was inferior to a course of treatment then there would be a stronger case for obtaining follow-up cultures from those treated with single-dose regimens. This is not the case. The authors also showed that a single dip-slide culture was just as efficient and much cheaper than a urine specimen sent to the laboratory for processing. Patients could be asked to deliver or post one to the laboratory one week after treatment. This cheap method of urine culture has not found favour in most countries, while clinical experience has brought to attention a number of technical problems.

It is the practice of most clinicians to culture routinely the urine one to two weeks after the completion of treatment to document cure. This is ideal clinical practice, as there is no other way of proving cure. The value, however, of a follow-up culture for those women who have lost their symptoms remains unclear. If the patient was asked to return only if her symptoms persisted, or recurred, then there would be a saving on the doctor's time and fee.

Self-medication

Another approach to cost cutting has been the use of self-therapy for selected patients. Wong *et al.* (1985) compared the effect of low-dose prophylaxis with co-trimoxazole (0.24 g at bedtime) for six months, with a regimen in which the patient gave herself a single 1.92 g dose of co-trimoxazole when she suspected that she had an infection. The prophylactic regimen reduced the number of infections from 2.2 to 0.2 per patient year. There was no significant cost difference between the prophylactic and intermittent self-therapy groups for those women having two or more infections each year. More specifically, 30 of 35 symptomatic infections that occurred during self-therapy responded to a single dose of co-trimoxazole. None of the five women who did not respond, or had a relapse, after single-dose therapy developed acute pyelonephritis or a bacteraemia and all were cured with a course of treatment. The authors (Wong *et al.* 1985) concluded that in selected patients, single-dose self-therapy was efficacious and economical when compared with conventional therapy or prophylaxis. As pointed out in the *Lancet* (1985), the financial arguments in this study were complex and the drug costs were only a small part of the reckoning.

It seems a reasonable practice to encourage selected patients with closely spaced episodes of bacterial cystitis, who are not willing to take long-term, low-dose prophylaxis, to take a single dose of an appropriate antimicrobial agents (e.g. trimethoprim 600 mg) when symptomatic, and provide a urine specimen for culture 10–14 days later, or earlier if the symptoms do not resolve within 3 days.

Possible approaches to cost-cutting that warrant further evaluation

As the majority of UTI occur in healthy, sexually active women who have a normal urinary tract and normal renal function a number of cost-saving approaches have been suggested (Bailey 1987), but require further assessment. It is important that such approaches do not increase morbidity or prevent identification of the small proportion of women who have a correctable urinary tract abnormality. The biggest savings would be made in avoiding expensive and often inappropriate urinary tract investigations. My suggestions are:

1. Instruct the woman with acute lower urinary tract symptoms to increase her oral fluid intake, or to take an alkalinizing agent, and only contact her doctor if the symptoms persist. This approach may improve or even eradicate her symptoms, but will usually not eradicate the bacteriuria.

2. Have the patient seen by a practice nurse, rather than a doctor, who will take a urine specimen and either await the result of the culture or prescribe a single dose of an antimicrobial agent.

3. Alternatively, the woman could be seen by her general practitioner who would follow a similar approach to (2).

4. A doctor, nurse, or technician skilled in urine microscopy could obtain information rapidly. Only those women with pyuria ($\geqslant$10 white blood cells per cubic millimetre of uncentrifuged urine), or obvious organisms would then receive immediate antimicrobial treatment.

5. A more convenient and economical way of culturing the urine is by the use of the commercially available dip inoculum methods (dip-slides) in the doctor's office and in the home. This practice would be cheaper than sending the urine, or the patient, to a private or hospital laboratory. These simple and cheap methods of culturing urine should be more widely promoted.

6. If the pre-treatment urine culture was infected with *E. coli* a routine antibacterial sensitivity profile should be eliminated.

7. If a doctor is actually going to treat a symptomatic patient before the urine is examined or cultured, is it really worthwhile obtaining a pre-treatment specimen?

8. Is it necessary to see the woman for a routine follow-up clinical assessment and urine examination if she has lost her symptoms? Perhaps she should be instructed to return only if the symptoms fail to settle or recur? A cheap alternative would be to give the woman a dip-slide and ask her to inoculate it and post it to the laboratory.

9. Should a woman with an occasional symptomatic infection have a supply of medication available at home with instructions to take a single dose if she develops symptoms, and to then visit her doctor only if the symptoms do not resolve? Alternatively, a woman self-medicating in this way should have a routine urine culture 10–14 days after treatment.

10. How can a reduction be made in the need for expensive urinary tract investigations? It is suggested that the latter be withheld on women with bacterial cystitis or asymptomatic bacteriuria who are cured with single-dose therapy.

Conclusions

Urinary tract infections are the most common bacterial infections treated in general practice. The majority of these occur in women in the sexually active age group and present as bacterial cystitis. Although these episodes are unpleasant they are infrequently associated with a systemic illness and there is no danger of renal damage occurring if the patient has a normal urinary tract. It is now widely considered that traditional regimens for simple, uncomplicated UTI are extravagant. There is convincing evidence that a three-day course, a single-day, or single-dose treatment is just as effective as a more prolonged course of treatment. Similarly, the duration of treatment can be safely reduced to five days for patients with uncomplicated APN. The many advantages of this simple approach to a common problem have been discussed in this chapter. Several suggestions have also been made for reducing the costs of managing uncomplicated UTI. Although the search should continue for more effective antimicrobial drugs and the ideal dosage regimens in which they should be used, more investigations are required on alternative approaches to treatment and prevention. In recent years there have been several working parties, symposia, and reviews which have addressed these issues (Kunin 1987; Neu and Williams 1988; Cass and Svanborg-Edén 1989; Ohkoshi and Yawada 1990; Kaye 1991; Ward and Jones 1991; Cattell 1992; Ohkoshi and Naber 1992; Rubin *et al.* 1992*a*,*b*; Forland 1993; Roland and Nicolle 1993; Bailey 1994*c*; Ohkoshi *et al.* 1994).

References

Anderson, J. D. (1983). Single dose studies with special reference to the emergence of antibiotic resistance. In *Single dose therapy of urinary tract infection*, (ed. R. R. Bailey), pp. 33–9. ADIS Health Science Press, Sydney.

Asscher, A. W., *et al.* (1969). Asymptomatic significant bacteriuria in the non-pregnant woman. II. Response to treatment and follow-up. *British Medical Journal*, **1**, 804–6.

Bailey, R. R. (1983). *Single dose therapy of urinary tract infection*, pp. 1–125. ADIS Health Science Press, Sydney.

Bailey, R. R. (1987). Cost–benefit considerations in the management of uncomplicated urinary tract infections in sexually active women. *New Zealand Medical Journal*, **100**, 680–3.

Bailey, R. R. (1989). Single-dose therapy for uncomplicated urinary tract infections: an overview. In *Host-parasite interactions in urinary tract infections*, (ed. E. H. Kass and C. Svanborg Edén), pp. 405–10. University of Chicago Press.

Bailey, R. R. (1990). Review of published studies on single dose therapy of urinary tract infections. *Infection*, **18**(Suppl. 2), S53–6.

Bailey, R. R. (1992). Quinolones in the treatment of uncomplicated urinary tract infections. *International Journal of Antimicrobial Agents*, **2**, 19–28.

Bailey, R. R. (1994*a*). Duration of antimicrobial treatment and the use of drug combinations for the treatment of uncomplicated acute pyelonephritis. *Infection*, **22**(Suppl. 1), S550–2.

Bailey, R. R. (1994*b*). Management of uncomplicated urinary tract infections *International Journal of Antimicrobial Agents*, **4**, 95–100.

Bailey, R. R. (1994*c*). Urinary tract infection. In *Textbook of renal disease*, (2nd edn), (ed. J. Whitworth and J. R. Lawrence), pp. 249–63. Blackwells, Edinburgh.

Bailey, R. R. and Abbott, G. D. (1977). Treatment of urinary tract infection with a single dose of amoxycillin. *Nephron*, **18**, 316–20.

Bailey, R. R. and Peddie, B. A. (1987). Acute renal infection in women: duration of antimicrobial therapy. *Annals of Internal Medicine*, **107**, 30.

Bailey, R. R., Bishop, V., Peddie, B., Chambers, P. F. M., Davies, P. R., and Crofts, H. G. (1983). Comparison of augmentin and co-trimoxazole for treatment of uncomplicated urinary tract infections. *New Zealand Medical Journal*, **96**, 970–2.

Bailey, R. R., Gorrie, S. I., Peddie, B. A., and Davies, P. R. (1987). Double blind, randomised trial comparing single dose enoxacin and trimethoprim for treatment of bacterial cystitis. *New Zealand Medical Journal*, **100**, 618–9.

Bailey, R. R., Keenan, T. D., Eliott, J. C., Peddie, B. A., and Bishop, V. (1985). Treatment of bacterial cystitis with a single dose of trimethoprim, co-trimoxazole or amoxycillin compared with a course of trimethoprim. *New Zealand Medical Journal*, **98**, 387–9.

Bailey, R. R., Lynn, K. L., Robson, R. A., Peddie, Catt, B. A., and Smith A. (1992). Comparison of ciprofloxacin with netilmicin for the treatment of pyelonephritis. *New Zealand Medical Journal*, **105**, 102–3.

Barclay, M. L., Begg, E. J., and Hickling, K. G. (1994). What is the evidence for once daily aminoglycoside therapy? *Clinical Pharmacokinetics*, **27**, 32–48.

Begg, E. J., Peddie, B. A., Chambers, S. T., and Boswell, D. R. (1992). Comparison of gentamicin dosing regimens using an in vitro model. *Journal of Antimicrobial Chemotherapy*, **29**, 427–33.

Brumfitt, W., Faiers, M. C., and Franklin, I. N. S. (1970). The treatment of urinary infection by means of a single dose of cephaloridine. *Postgraduate Medical Journal*, **46**(Suppl.), 65–9.

Carlson, K. J. and Mulley, A. G. (1985). Management of acute dysuria: decision-analysis model of alternative strategies. *Annals of Internal Medicine*, **102**, 244–9.

Cattell, W. R. (1992). Lower and upper urinary tract infection in adults. In *Oxford textbook of clinical nephrology* (ed. S. Cameron, A. M. Davison, J-P Grunfeld, D. Kerr, and E. Ritz), pp. 1676–99 Oxford University Press, Oxford.

Chambers, S. T., Peddie, B. A., Begg, E. J., and Boswell, D. R. (1991). Antibacterial effects of lomefloxacin in vitro. *Journal of Antimicrobial Chemotherapy*, **27**, 481–9.

Cockcroft, D. W. and Gault, M. H. (1976). Prediction of creatinine clearance from serum creatinine. *Nephron*, **16**, 31–41.

Craig, W. A. and Vogelman, B. (1987). The postantibiotic effect. *Annals of the Internal Medicine*, **106**, 900–2.

Fair, W. R. and Fair, W. R.III (1982). Clinical value of sensitivity determinations in treating urinary tract infections. *Urology*, **19**, 565–9.

Fair, W. R., Crane, D. B., Peterson, L. J., Dahmer, C., Taque, B., and Amos, W. (1980). Three-day treatment of urinary tract infections. *Journal of Urology*, **123**, 717–21.

Fairley, K. F., Bond, A. G., Brown, R. B., and Habersberger, P. (1967). Simple test to determine the site of urinary tract infection. *Lancet*, **2**, 427–31.

Fihn, S. D., Latham, R. H., Roberts, P., Running, K., and Stamm, W. E. (1985). Association between diaphragm use and urinary tract infection. *Journal of American Medical Association*, **254**, 240–5.

Fihn, S. D., Johnson, C., Roberts, P. L., Running, K., and Stamm, W. E. (1988). Trimethoprim-sulfamethoxazole for acute dysuria in women: a single dose or 10-day course: a double-blind, randomized trial. *Annals of Internal Medicine*, **108**, 350–7.

Forland, M. (1993). Urinary tract infection: how has its management changed? *Postgraduate Medicine*, **93**, 71–86.

Grüneberg, R. N. and Brumfitt, W. (1967). Single dose treatment of acute urinary tract infection: a controlled trial. *British Medical Journal*, **3**, 649–51.

Harding, G. K. M., Buckwold, F. J., Marrie, T. J., Thompson, L., Light, R. B., and Ronald, A. R. (1979). Prophylaxis of recurrent urinary tract infection in female patients: efficacy of low-dose, thrice-weekly therapy with trimethoprim-sulfamethoxazole. *Journal of the American Medical Association*, **242**, 1975–7.

Källenius, G., Kallings, L. O., and Winberg, J. (1983). Single dose treatment of children using sulphafurazole. In *Single dose therapy of urinary tract infection*, (ed. R. R. Bailey), pp. 63–72. ADIS Health Science Press, Sydney.

Kass, E. H. and Svanborg-Edén, C. (1989). *Host-parasite interactions in urinary tract infections: Proceedings of the Fourth International Symposium on Pyelonephritis*, pp. 1–473. University of Chicago Press.

Kaye, D. (1991). Urinary tract infections. *Medical Clinics of North America*, **75**, 241–520.

Kunin, C. M. (1981). Duration of treatment of urinary tract infections. *American Journal of Medicine*, **71**, 849–54.

Kunin, C. M. (1987). *Detection, prevention and management of urinary tract infections*, pp. 1–447. Lea & Febiger, Philadelphia.

Lancet (1985) Editorial. Self-medication for recurrent urinary infection? *Lancet*, **1**, 1199–200.

Leibovici, L. and Wysenbeek, A. J. (1991). Single-dose antibiotic treatment for symptomatic urinary tract infections in women: a meta-analysis of randomized trials. *Quarterly Journal of Medicine*, **78**, 43–57.

Little, P. J., Peddie, B. A., and Sincock, A. (1979). The treatment of symptomatic urinary tract infections. *Australian Family Physician*, **8**, 985–7.

Moroni, M. (1987). Monuril in lower uncomplicated urinary tract infections in adults. *European Urology*, **13**(Suppl. 1), 101–4.

Mundt, K. A. and Polk, B. F. (1979). Identification of site of urinary-tract infections by antibody-coated bacteria assay. *Lancet*, **2**, 1172–5.

Neu, H. C. (1983). Single dose treatment of urinary tract infections: a pharmacologist's view. In *Single dose therapy of urinary tract infection*, (ed. R. R. Bailey), pp. 92–7. ADIS Health Science Press, Sydney.

Neu, H. C. and Williams, J. D. (1988). *New trends in urinary tract infections: the single-dose therapy*, pp. 1–357. Karger, Basel.

O'Grady, F. (1983). Single dose treatment of urinary tract infection: a microbiologist's view. In *Single dose therapy of urinary tract infection*, (ed. R. R. Bailey), pp. 79–91. ADIS Health Science Press, Sydney.

O'Grady, F. and Cattell, W. R. (1966). Kinetics of urinary tract infection. II. The bladder. *British Journal of Urology*, **38**, 156–62.

O'Grady, F., Mackintosh, I. P., Greenwood, D., and Watson, B. W. (1973). Treatment of 'bacterial cystitis' in fully automatic mechanical models simulating conditions of bacterial growth in the urinary bladder. *British Journal of Experimental Pathology*, 283–90.

Ohkoshi, M. and Kawada, Y. (1990). *Clinical evaluation of drug efficacy in UTI*, pp. 1–233. Excerpta Medica, International Congress Series No. 938, Amsterdam.

Ohkoshi, M. and Naber, K. G. (1992). International consensus discussion on clinical evaluation of drug efficacy in urinary tract infection. *Infection*, **20**(Suppl. 3), S135–42.

Ohkoshi, M., Naber, K. G., and Kawada, Y. (1994). International consensus discussion on clinical evaluation of drug efficacy in urinary tract infection. *Infection*, **22** (Suppl 1), 53–66.

Parker, S. E. and Davey, P. G. (1993). Editorial. Antimicrobial therapy: once-daily aminoglycoside dosing. *Lancet*, **341**, 346–7.

Peddie, B. A., Bishop, V. A., Blake, E. A., Gorrie, S. I., Bailey, R. R., and Edwards, D. (1986). Association between diaphragm use and asymptomatic bacteriuria. *Australia and New Zealand Journal of Obstetrics and Gynaecology*, **26**, 225–7.

Philbrick, J. T. and Bracikowski, J. P. (1985). Single-dose antibiotic treatment for uncomplicated urinary tract infections. Less for less? *Archives of Internal Medicine*, **145**, 1672–8.

Pinson, A. G., Philbrick, J. J., Lindbeck, G. M., and Schorling, J. B. (1992). Oral antibiotic therapy for acute pyelonephritis: a methodologic review of the literature. *Journal of General Internal Medicine*, **7**, 544–53.

Prins, J. M., Büller, H. R., Kuipjer, E. J., Tange, R. A., and Speelman, P. (1993). Once versus thrice daily gentamicin in patients with serious infections. *Lancet*, **341**, 335–9.

Privette, M., Cade, R., Peterson, J., and Mars, D (1988). Prevention of recurrent urinary tract infections in postmenopausal women. *Nephron*, **50**, 24–7.

Raz, R. and Stamm, W. E. (1993). A controlled trial of intravaginal oestriol in postmenopausal women with recurrent urinary tract infections. *New England Journal of Medicine*, **329**, 753–6.

Ronald, A. R., Boutros, P., and Mourtada, H. (1976). The correlation between localization of bacteriuria and response to single dose therapy in adult females. *Journal of American Medical Association*, **253**, 1854–6.

Ronald, A. R. and Nicolle, L. E. (1993). Infections of the upper urinary tract. In *Diseases of the kidney*, (5th edn), (ed. R. W. Schrier and C. W. Gottschalk), pp. 973–1006, Little Brown, Boston.

Rubin, R. H., Beam, T. R. jun., and Stamm, W. E. (1992*a*). An approach to evaluating antibacterial agents in the treatment of urinary tract infection. *Clinical Infectious Diseases*, **14**(Suppl. 2), S246–51.

Rubin, R. H., Shapiro, E. D., Andriole, V. T., Davis, R. J., and Stamm, W. E. (1992*b*). Evaluation of new anti-infective drugs for the treatment of urinary tract infection. *Clinical Infectious Diseases*, **15**(Suppl. 1), S216–27.

Savard-Fenton, M., Fenton, B. W., Reller, L. B., Lauer, B. A., and Byyny, R. L. (1982). Single-dose amoxicillin therapy with follow-up urine culture. Effective initial management for acute uncomplicated urinary tract infections. *American Medical Journal*, **73**, 808–13.

Schultz, H. J., McCaffery, L. A., Keys, T. F., and Nobrega, F. T. (1984). Acute cystitis: a prospective study of laboratory tests and duration of therapy. *Mayo Clinic Proceedings*, **59**, 391–7.

Slack, R. and Greenwood, D. (1987). The microbiological and pharmacokinetic profile of an antibacterial agent useful for the single-dose therapy of urinary tract infection. *European Urology*, **13**(Suppl. 1), 32–6.

Stamey, T. A. and Condy, M. (1975). The diffusion and concentration of trimethoprim in human vaginal fluid. *Journal of Infectious Diseases*, **121**, 261–6.

Stamey, T. A., Govan, D. E., and Palmer, J. M. (1965). The localization and treatment of urinary tract infections: the role of bactericidal urine levels as opposed to serum levels. *Medicine*, **44**, 1–36.

Stamm, W. E. (1983). Single dose treatment of urinary tract infections: an overview. In *Single dose therapy of urinary tract infection*, (ed. R. R. Bailey), pp. 98–106. ADIS Health Science Press, Sydney.

Stamm, W. E., *et al.* (1980). Causes of the acute urethral syndrome in women. *New England Journal of Medicine*, **303**, 409–15.

Stamm, W. E., Running, K., McKevitt, M., Counts, G. W., Turck, M., and Holmes, K. K. (1981). Treatment of acute urethral syndrome. *New England Journal of Medicine*, **304**, 956–8.

Stamm, W. E., McKevitt, M., and Counts, G. W. (1987). Acute renal infection in women: treatment with trimethoprim-sulfamethoxazole or ampilicin for two or six weeks: a randomized trial. *Annals of Internal Medicine*, **106**, 341–5.

Stapleton, A., Latham, R. H., Johnson, C., and Stamm, W. E. (1990). Postcoital antimicrobial prophylaxis for recurrent urinary tract infection: a randomized, double-blind, placebo controlled trial. *Journal of American Medical Association*, **264**, 703–6.

Tait, J., *et al.* (1985). Urethral syndrome (abacterial cystitis)—search for a pathogen. *British Journal of Urology*, **57**, 552–6.

Thomas, V., Shelokov, A., and Forland, M. (1974). Antibody-coated bacteria in the urine and the site of urinary tract infection. *New England Journal of Medicine*, **290**, 588–90.

Tolkoff-Rubin, N. E. and Rubin, R. H. (1987). New approaches to the treatment of urinary tract infection. *American Journal of Medicine*, **82**(Suppl. 4A), 270–7.

Ward, T. T. and Jones, S. R. (1991). Genitourinary tract infections. In *A practical approach to infectious diseases*, (3rd edn), (ed. R. F. Reese and R. F. Betts), pp. 357–89, Little Brown, Boston.

Williams, J. D. and Smith, E. K. (1970). Single dose therapy with streptomycin and sulfamethopyrazine for bacteriuria during pregnancy. *British Medical Journal*, **4**, 651–3.

Winickoff, R. N., Wilner, S. I., Gall, G., Laage, T., and Barnett, G. O. (1981). Urine culture after treatment of uncomplicated cystitis in women. *Southern Medical Journal*, **74**, 165–9.

Wong, E. S., McKevitt, M., Running, K., Counts, G. W., Turck, M., and Stamm, W. E. (1985). Management of recurrent urinary tract infections with patient-administered single-dose therapy. *Annals of Internal Medicine*, **102**, 302–7.

7
Urinary tract infection in children

G. D. Abbott

Introduction

Urinary tract infection (UTI) in infancy and childhood is among the most common infections caused by bacteria, probably second only to otitis media. UTI causes significant morbidity, particularly where children experience repeated attacks which can affect their well-being and schooling. Mortality from the acute disease is fortunately infrequent but can arise, particularly in infancy, from associated bacteraemia and sepsis. Long-term morbidity and mortality are engendered by renal scarring causing hypertension and chronic renal failure. Children who develop renal scars very commonly have vesicoureteric reflux (VUR) or obstructive uropathy and urinary infection. Early and accurate diagnosis is essential and this must be followed by prompt and adequate treatment leading to sterilization of the urinary tract. Appropriate imaging investigations and follow-up of patients with defined abnormalities, such as VUR, obstruction, or repeated infections, are required. This chapter will deal with these various aspects of diagnosis and management.

Epidemiology

Infants

A number of epidemiological studies have been carried out in infants and children of different age groups. There are inherent difficulties in interpreting many of these studies as diagnostic criteria vary and methods of urine collection are not standard. In many studies in infancy, the diagnosis of UTI has been based on examination of bag urine samples on some, through to suprapubic urine aspirates in others. Many of the studies include only infants who have been symptomatic, but others have assessed unselected newborn populations. Prevalence rates of infection differ among the populations tested, but, in general, urinary infections in this age group are much more common in boys than girls. Lincoln and Winberg (1964) studied 584 infants, the urine being collected by the clean-catch method. The incidence of bacteriuria in males was 2.7 per cent and females 0 per cent. In the same year Randolph and Greenfield (1964), using a strap-on device for urine collection, reported the results of the study of 400 newborn infants in which the incidence of bacteriuria in males was 2 per cent and 0 per cent in females. Littlewood *et al.* (1969) reported their findings from 600 asymptomatic infants. Urine was collected by clean catch or bag, and bladder puncture was used to confirm some cases. The incidence of bacteriuria was 2.3 per cent in males and 0.3 per cent in females. Abbott (1972) reported the findings of a large prospective study involving 1460 infants. These infants were studied between the third and sixth day of life. Diagnosis was established by bladder puncture if the initial clean-catch urine was suggestive of infection. The incidence of bacteriuria was 1.5 per cent in males and 0.4 per cent in females. Five of the 14 infants with UTI had symptoms suggestive of infection, one had bacteraemia, and six out of the 14 cases had moderate VUR. Edelmann *et al.* (1973) reported their findings from a population of 836 full-term infants and 206 premature infants. The overall incidence of bacteriuria was 0.7 per cent in the term infants and 2.9 per cent in the premature infants. Urine was obtained initially by the clean-catch method and bladder puncture used to confirm cases. Maherzi *et al.* (1978) reported a large study of 1762 infants of whom 1014 were full-term and 634 were premature. Voided urines were tested with dip-slides and confirmed by bladder puncture. The overall incidence of UTI was 2.9 per cent in full-term infants and 1.6 per cent in premature infants.

It has been suggested that there may be an increase in the incidence of UTI in infants born to mothers who have had UTI during pregnancy. Patrick (1967) reported that some women with asymptomatic bacteriuria during pregnancy had infected amniotic fluid at term. In addition, positive cultures were obtained from the umbilical vein, blood, placenta, and the urine of infants born to mothers with UTI. However, Ives *et al.* (1971) found no evidence that maternal urinary infection was associated with either urinary infection or bacteraemia in the newborn infant.

The increased incidence of UTI in males seems to only be apparent in the first 3 months of life. After that there is a sharp increase in the incidence in females. Ginsburg and McCracken (1982) reported a clinical study of 100 infants hospitalized in the first year of life because of UTI. Male infants accounted for 75 per cent of patients in the first 3 months and thereafter females predominated. Similarly, Bourchier *et al.* (1984), in a study of 100 hospitalized infants under the age of 1 year, observed that males accounted for 46 of the 59 patients less than 3 months of age.

Children aged 1–5 years

Studies of bacteriuria in this age group have reported a prevalence of infection ranging between 1 and 3 per cent in girls but few cases among boys. Saxena *et al.* (1974) surveyed 1000 children and found the prevalence in males was 0.4 per cent and females 0.7 per cent. Mair (1973) in a survey of 2165 new entrants to school found a prevalence of bacteriuria in boys of 0.2 per cent and 2.6 per cent in girls. Similarly in studies of girls only, Savage *et al.* (1969) found a prevalence of bacteriuria of 2.1 per cent and Kunin *et al.* (1976), a prevalence of 1.1 per cent.

Schoolchildren aged 5–15 years

Many surveys of schoolchildren have been carried out to establish the incidence of UTI. In a very large study, Kunin *et al.* (1964) surveyed a population of 19 335 children, finding a prevalence of bacteriuria in girls of 1.2 per cent, compared to 0.04 per cent among boys: a ratio of 30:1. Kunin estimated the actual risk of a girl acquiring bacteriuria during the school years is much greater than the prevalence of 1.2 per cent, since this prevalence rate only relates to those found to have bacteriuria at one point in time. He estimated that 5–6 per cent of girls will have had at least one episode of bacteriuria during their time at school. Many groups, including the Newcastle Asymptomatic Bacteriuria Research Group (1975), have confirmed a prevalence rate of bacteriuria of 1–2 per cent in schoolgirls, with a much lower prevalence in boys. (See Table 7.1 for the prevalence of bacteriuria in infants and children.)

Table 7.1 Prevalence of bacteriuria in infants and children

Age		Prevalence (%)
Newborns	Term	1
	Pre-term	2–3
Pre-school (< 5 yrs)	Males	0.2
	Females	0.8
School (5–15) yrs)	Males	0.03
	Females	1–2

*Published with permission from G. H. McCracken (1989).

Urinary tract infection and circumcision

There now seems to be overwhelming evidence that infant boys with symptomatic or asymptomatic UTI are usually uncircumcised. In the study by Ginsberg and McCracken (1982) of 100 hospitalized infants with UTI, 95 per cent of the male infants were uncircumcised. Wiswell and Roscelli (1986) corroborated these findings in their survey of infants hospitalized with UTI during a 10-year period. Uncircumcised boys had the highest rate of infection at 1.12 per cent compared to 0.57 per cent of girls, and 0.11 per cent of circumcised boys. In a retrospective analysis of 427 698 infants born during a 10-year period, Wiswell *et al.* (1985) found that although only 21 per cent of the boys were uncircumcised, 72 per cent of male UTI occurred among these infants. Herzog (1989) made similar observations. Overall, these studies suggest that uncircumcised boys have a 10–30 times increase likelihood, compared to those circumcised, of having a UTI in the first year of life. There is now a tendency in some countries to advocate the return to routine circumcision in all males. The risks and benefits of this procedure have to be weighed up carefully. There may be a place for circumcision in boys with a history of recurrent infection and with serious underlying anatomical abnormalities. This would particularly apply if UTI could not be controlled by chemoprophylaxis.

Recurrent urinary tract infection

Feld *et al.* (1989) reported a risk of a 25 per cent recurrence rate in neonates with UTI, the risk being 30 per cent after an initial infection in older children. The risk increased substantially to 60–75 per cent after the second and third infections. The recurrence risk is highest among girls during the first 12 months after the initial infection. Many of these recurrent infections are asymptomatic.

Clinical features

The clinical features of UTI vary considerably with the age at presentation. In general, the younger the infant the more non-specific the symptoms. It is very difficult in infants to identify one symptom that specifically directs attention to the genitourinary tract. Neonates and infants under the age of one year may be only mildly unwell, have feeding problems, irritability, vomiting, and loose stools. Unexplained jaundice in the first month of life, along with these more general symptoms, should lead to a search for UTI. The neonate may, however, present extremely unwell and dehydrated, with tachycardia, peripheral circulatory failure, and hypotension. Older infants are usually febrile but neonates may have hypothermia.

In the pre-school age group, symptoms are, again, often non-specific, the child presenting with fever only. Roberts *et al.* (1983) demonstrated that among 193 febrile children less than 2 months of age with no obvious cause for fever on physical examination, the incidence of UTI was 4.1 per cent. The rate of UTI in an age-matched control group of 312 asymptomatic infants was only 0.3 per cent. More recently, Bauchner *et al.* (1987) evaluated the frequency of UTI in 664 febrile children who had no symptoms referable to the genitourinary tract. The overall rate of UTI in this group was only 1.7 per cent, but in infants less than 6 months of age, the incidence was 7.5 per cent.

The usual symptoms of cystitis or acute pyelonephritis are much more variable or even absent in children, particularly in the pre-school child. Symptoms of bladder inflammation, such as frequency, dysuria and urgency, may be present in some children over the age of 2 years. Loss of urinary control in a previously continent child and recurrence of nocturnal enuresis are suggestive of UTI. Children with cystitis may have some degree of fever but this is usually less than 38 °C. Some mild associated systemic upset and lower abdominal pain may be present. Older children may present with symptoms suggestive of classical acute pyelonephritis with high fever, rigors, and loin tenderness. They usually have temperatures greater than 39 °C, vomit frequently, and are often delirious.

Parents often report foul-smelling and cloudy urine in children with urinary infection. Abbott and Allen (1984) in a prospective study found that offensive smell alone was predictive of UTI in 50 per cent of cases. Cloudiness of urine is often due to urates in urine. After heating and acidification the cloudiness due to urates disappears, and persistent cloudiness appears to be due to white cells and bacteria. It was found in this study that when persisting cloudiness and foul smell were combined this finding was predictive of UTI infection in 75 per cent of cases. Haematuria is not uncommon but invariably accompanies symptoms of cystitis and is often found in association with pyuria (Kunin 1987).

Physical examination is usually unrewarding, particularly in infants. The physical findings that can be detected usually relate to associated urinary tract anatomical abnormalities, genital inflammation, and abnormalities in the central nervous system. Genital inflammation in girls is a common cause of dysuria and the symptoms caused by this are often indistinguishable from symptoms of lower UTI. Urge incontinence, frequency, and dysuria are often associated with vulvitis and constipation. An uncircumcised boy with symptoms of frequency and dysuria may have balanitis. Careful abdominal examination may reveal loin or suprapubic tenderness. Associated constipation is indicated by palpable faecal masses in the left colon. Enlarged kidneys may be noted in babies with pyelonephritis or there may be obvious enlargement due to hydronephrosis or cystic lesions. In children with recurrent UTI and symptoms of poor urinary control, careful examination of the central nervous system in the perineal region and lower extremity is important. The back should be examined for evidence of spina bifida occulta or spinal dysrhaphia. The blood pressure should always be taken as children with UTI may have significant hypertension associated with underlying obstruction or reflux nephropathy.

Diagnosis of urinary tract infection

The diagnosis of UTI in childhood is fraught with difficulties relating to obtaining an uncontaminated specimen of urine for microscopy and culture. The younger the child the greater the risk of contamination, particularly in the female. Midstream specimens of urine can be adequately collected from older continent and co-operative children using similar techniques to adults. The major problem of urine collection lies in the neonatal period, infancy, and the incontinent toddler.

Urine collection

Neonates, infants, and incontinent toddlers

The usual techniques for urine collection in this age group are:

- Bag collection
- Clean-catch urine collection
- Suprapubic aspiration (bladder puncture)
- Catheterization

Bag and clean-catch specimens Obtaining urine from neonates, infants and incontinent toddlers is usually by bag collection or by a clean-catch technique.

With both of these methods, careful soap and water preparation of the perineal region is required. Where possible, the infant or young child should be given a feed and preparations made for urine collection while feeding is proceeding. The soiled diaper should be removed and the perineal area and genitals washed clean. A clean diaper should be placed under the buttocks; in the female, the labia should be separated with thumb and index finger, and the labial meatus cleansed with sponges. In the male, the foreskin and glans should be similarly cleaned. The adhesive plastic bag is then applied to the area and the infant observed until urine is passed. The baby should preferably be held upright during this time. The bag should be removed immediately the child voids. The lower corner of the bag is then cut with scissors and the urine collected into a sterile container placed immediately below the bag.

In the clean-catch method, similar preparation is carried out. The parent, nurse, or doctor then waits for the child to void and immediately catches a stream of urine in a sterile container during voiding.

Studies in the late 1960s by Braude *et al.* (1967) and Cruickshank and Edmond (1967) showed that properly collected clean-catch specimens could yield a high number of urines that were either sterile or contained less than 10^4 organisms per ml (10^4 org/ml). In a study of 1460 infants, Abbott (1978) demonstrated that in 76 per cent of infants a sterile urine or less than 10^4 org/ml could be obtained using a clean-catch or bag specimen. However, in this study if the colony count was greater than 10^5 org/ml a bladder puncture performed within 24 hours confirmed the diagnosis of bacteriuria in only 19 per cent if there was a pure growth on culture on the voided specimen. If the colony count lay between 10^4 and 10^5 org/ml there was only a 2 per cent chance of the bladder puncture being positive in this group. Thus, if neonates have less than 10^4 org/ml in a bag collected or clean-catch specimen then UTI can be reliably excluded. If the colony count is greater than 10^4 org/ml and particularly if greater than 10^5 org/ml suprapubic aspiration is required to confirm or exclude UTI.

Older infants and incontinent toddlers Shannon *et al.* (1969) carried out a study on 230 infants and children in this age group and compared the results of bag specimens with suprapubic aspirates obtained within 24 hours. When the colony count was greater than 10^5 org/ml the bladder puncture was positive in 50 per cent of children in whom there was a single organism on culture of the voided specimen. If there was a mixed growth of organisms with a colony count in this range, bladder puncture was positive in 22 per cent of children. If the colony count lay between 10^4 and 10^6 org/ml, the bladder puncture was positive in only 15 per cent of children. Thus, although the reliability of voided specimens in diagnosing UTI is greater than in the neonate, suprapubic aspiration should be performed to confirm or exclude urinary infection.

Older continent children In this age group a midstream specimen can be obtained using similar techniques to those in adults and the significance of bacterial counts is similar. In adult women with a bacterial count on a single midstream specimen of greater than 10^5 org/ml the confidence limit of certain infection is

80 per cent, increasing to 95 per cent if there are two consecutive urine specimens obtained. If there are intermediate levels of bacteriuria between 10^4 and 10^5 org/ml, suprapubic aspiration is positive in approximately 50 per cent of patients (Bailey and Little 1970).

Suprapubic aspiration (bladder puncture) This technique is valuable, widely used, and generally safe and reliable for obtaining urine in children. As urine is aspirated directly from the bladder, any growth of a single organism is significant. The presence of multiple organisms usually indicates that accidental penetration of adjacent bowel may have occurred. Although this is uncommon, it is more likely to occur if urine is aspirated as the needle is being withdrawn. It appears to be a more frequent problem in neonatal intensive care units where there are many infants of extremely low birthweight and prematurity. The indications and contraindications for suprapubic aspiration are set out in Tables 7.2 and 7.3, respectively.

Technique for suprapubic aspiration Bladder puncture should be obtained 10–15 minutes after the baby has been fed and the diaper is dry. The bladder should be palpable or percussable. Older children should be given copious fluids to drink and asked to refrain from voiding (Abbott and Shannon 1970).

The child needs to be securely restrained during the procedure. The suprapubic skin should be disinfected. A 22-gauge $\frac{1}{2}$-inch needle is attached to a 10 ml

Table 7.2 Indications for suprapubic aspiration

1. Colony counts exceeding 10^5 org/ml on bag urines
2. Repeated low or intermediate colony counts of 10^4–10^5 org/ml with a single organism on voided urine, particularly if there are persisting symptoms of infection or pyuria
3. Repeated heavy mixed growths of organisms on voided specimens exceeding 10^5 org/ml with one organism predominating, particularly if there are symptoms of infections or pyuria
4. Acutely ill infants or children in whom a rapidly obtained reliable specimen can allow an urgent presumptive diagnosis to be made

From G. D. Abbott (1978).

Table 7.3 Contraindications to suprapubic aspiration

1. Unexplained abdominal distension
2. Abdominal masses
3. A known bleeding disorder

Note: The contraindications in (1) and (2) may be resolved by guided fine-needle aspiration under ultrasonography (US). From G. D. Abbott (1991).

syringe which is then inserted 1–2 cm suprapubically in the midline. The needle is pushed downwards and caudally at an angle of 80–90 degrees. A definite sensation of entering the bladder can usually be felt following which urine is aspirated. The urine is then either left in the syringe sealed with a sterile cork or transferred to a sterile container.

Catheterization Catherization of the bladder is usually not required for the diagnosis of UTI but can prove preferable to a series of unsuccessful attempts to obtain urine by suprapubic aspiration in a distressed child. Kunin (1987) has clearly defined the role and techniques of catheterization and catheter care. He states that, in general, single catheterizations are associated with a much lower frequency of infection than with indwelling catheters. The prevalence of induced infection by single catheterization appears to range between about 1 per cent and 22 per cent in adult patients. The prevalence of infection induced by single catheterization has not yet been established in children.

Pyuria

White cells in the urine indicate inflammation of the genitourinary tract. Although these cells may originate from the bladder or kidney, they may also enter urine from adjacent structures such as the vagina. Stamm (1983) reported that more than 96 per cent of symptomatic adults with significant bacteriuria and urinary infection had greater than 10 white blood corpuscles per cubic mm. In contrast, fewer than 1 per cent of asymptomatic non-bacteriuric individuals had evidence of pyuria. In the neonatal period the presence of pyuria can be confusing as renal tubular cells can resemble white cells in the urine unless special stains are used. Houston (1963) and Braude *et al.* (1967) suggested that counts of greater than 50–75 wbc/mm^3 in female neonates, and greater than 150 wbc/mm^3 for girls is significant in clean-catch specimens. In large screening surveys Kunin *et al.* (1964, 1976) showed that pyuria was absent in 50 per cent of children with significant bacteriuria. The finding of pyuria is suggestive but not diagnostic of UTI.

Proteinuria

The presence of proteinuria is an unreliable indicator of UTI in screening surveys. Kunin *et al.* (1964) showed that only 30 per cent of children had proteinuria in the presence of significant bacteriuria.

Chemical tests for bacteriuria

There are a number of chemical tests that have been used for the detection of bacteriuria. No test is ideal, and in children the problem of contamination of the urine by bacteria arising from outside the genitourinary tract tends to negate a high proportion of these tests. Kunin (1987) stated that the nitrite method is the chemical test with the greatest potential for use in mass screening and for the follow-up of patients.

Microorganisms in UTI in children

In the majority of cases of UTI in children the infecting organism is a member of the Enterobacteriaceae, Pseudomonas, and Enterococci species, and much less commonly Staphylococci. *Staphylococcus saprophyticus*, an organism commonly found in young women, appears to be rare in childhood urinary infection (Kunin 1987).

Escherichia coli accounts for about 80 per cent of all cases in children. *Proteus mirabilis* is more common in uncircumcised boys. Uncomplicated UTI is usually caused by single organisms. In some patients with complex urological abnormalities more than one organism may be cultured (Zelikovic *et al.* 1992).

Localization of urinary infection

There is a wide range of direct and indirect methods for localizing UTI. No one test, short of culturing kidney tissue, is entirely reliable or correlates well with symptomatology. In general, the sick child with a high fever, a polymorph leucocytosis, and an elevated C-reactive protein or sedimentation rate is likely to have acute pyelonephritis. Kunin (1987) has reviewed the various methods of localizing infection in considerable detail. In the infant and young child it is virtually impossible, because of the non-specific nature of symptoms, to have any certainty as to whether the child may have pyelonephritis or a lower urinary tract infection.

Recently, there has been increasing interest in the role of dimercaptosuccinic acid (DMSA) labelled with technetium (^{99m}Tc) in the detection and localization of parenchymal inflammatory changes associated with acute pyelonephritis. The studies of Rushton and Majd (1992) have clearly shown the accuracy of DMSA scintigraphy in the diagnosis of experimentally induced acute pyelonephritis in piglets using strict histopathological criteria as the standard of reference. The sensitivity and specificity of the DMSA scan for the diagnosis of acute pyelonephritis was 91 per cent and 99 per cent, respectively. Rushton and Majd then went on to conduct a prospective clinical study in 94 hospitalized children with a diagnosis of acute febrile UTI. These studies demonstrated that the DMSA scan is highly sensitive and reliable for the diagnosis of acute pyelonephritis, and confirmed that the diagnosis of acute pyelonephritis in children based on clinical and other laboratory observations is unreliable. They found that the decreased uptake of DMSA in acute pyelonephritis is due to both ischaemia and tubular cell dysfunction, and concluded that the DMSA scan probably becomes positive in the early phase of the inflammatory response as a result of ischaemia, and before significant tubular damage has occurred. They also noted that acute pyelonephritic changes were common in the absence of vesicoureteric reflux (VUR). The acute parenchymal inflammatory changes appeared to be reversible and did not lead to renal scarring in the majority of cases. They also found that renal scarring only occurred at sites corresponding to previous areas of acute pyelonephritis. However, in contrast, Roseburg *et al.* (1992) found that an abnormal DMSA scan at the time of infection identified most children with significant VUR on subsequent voiding cystourethrograms.

Currently, in acute hospital practice the most useful way of identifying whether a child has acute pyelonephritis is to perform a DMSA scan as a relatively urgent procedure.

Other investigations

Infants and children with acute urinary infection may have bacteraemia. Up to 30 per cent of neonates and infants are said to have a positive blood culture (McCracken 1989). Documented bacteraemia in older infants and children appears to be much less common.

Polymorph leucocytosis, a sedimentation rate greater than 20 mm/h, or a C-reactive protein greater than 0.001 mg/ml along with a fever greater than 38.5 °C have been found in some studies to correlate with upper tract infection. These findings are, however, relatively non-specific and correlate poorly with the findings on DMSA scan performed during the acute phase of urinary infection (Rushton and Majd 1992).

In more seriously ill hospitalized children significant renal dysfunction may occur during urinary infection. Berg (1989) demonstrated that there were significant changes in glomerular filtration rate and PAH clearance during acute infection. In addition, the fractional excretion of sodium, maximum urine concentrating capacity, free water clearance, and distal tubular sodium excretion were all reduced compared with controls. The reduction in urinary concentrating capacity has been documented previously by Winberg (1959).

Management of urinary tract infection

The management of a child with UTI involves a number of steps. In general, febrile, vomiting, and unwell children, and all infants with suspected or proven urinary infection should be admitted to hospital. Older children who are less unwell can usually be safely managed in the community. Management consists of:

1. An accurate diagnosis of UTI.
2. Appropriate antimicrobial therapy.
3. Follow-up urine cultures.
4. Treatment of recurrent infections.
5. Appropriate imaging of the genitourinary tract to detect underlying congenital and anatomical abnormalities.
6. Long-term follow-up of children with renal scarring to detect the development of hypertension and deterioration of renal function.

Antimicrobial therapy

Treatment should not be delayed pending full culture and sensitivity results, particularly if the child is unwell; or in any infant. Urine obtained by suprapubic aspiration, catheterization, or midstream collection that shows bacteria on Gram stain, should allow the prompt introduction of an antimicrobial agent. Older children who are less unwell and have symptoms highly suggestive of lower UTI can usually await the results of urine culture before commencing therapy.

Parenteral antimicrobials are indicated for all infants and for sick febrile older children suspected of having acute pyelonephritis (McCracken 1989).

Neonates and infants less than 3 months old Ginsberg and McCracken (1982) and Israeli *et al.* (1987) reported that one-third of neonates and one-fifth of infants under the age of 3–4 months with UTI have positive blood cultures. In this age group, initial therapy is provided with parenterally administered gentamicin and amoxycillin (Table 7.4). Parenteral therapy is continued until the infant is clinically improved, and blood and urine culture are sterile, usually 24–48 hours after the commencement of therapy. At that time change to a suitable oral agent can be made. Treatment should be continued for 7–10 days.

Older infants and children Bacteraemia in older infants and children appears to be uncommon. However, febrile, unwell children with symptoms and signs suggestive of acute pyelonephritis should be hospitalized and receive parenteral antimicrobial agents (Table 7.5). Once there is evidence of clinical improvement and blood cultures are found to be sterile, these children can be changed to an oral agent. Treatment should continue for 7–10 days. Older children who are less unwell and have symptoms suggestive of cystitis can receive oral therapy from the beginning and can be treated in the community.

Table 7.4 Antimicrobial therapy of urinary infections in infants younger than 1 month

Initial therapy

Amoxycillin 75–100 mg/kg daily in 3 or 4 divided doses, intravenously (IV), and gentamicin 7.5 mg/kg daily in 3 doses, IV.

Parenteral therapy is continued until there is evidence of clinical improvement and blood and urine cultures are sterile.

Subsequent therapy

Oral therapy with either amoxycillin 50 mg/kg daily in 2 or 3 doses, Augmentin[a] 50 mg/kg daily in 2 or 3 doses, cephalexin 50 mg/kg daily in 2 or 3 doses, or cotrimoxazole[b] (trimethoprim 4 mg, sulphamethoxazole 20 mg) daily in 2 doses.

Duration of therapy

Therapy should be given for 7–10 days. In those with bacteraemia, parenteral antimicrobial therapy should be given for the entire 10 days.

[a] Amoxycillin plus clavulanate potassium.

[b] Sulphonamides should be avoided in infants who are jaundiced or those who are premature.

Table 7.5 Antimicrobial therapy of urinary infections in infants over 1 month and children

Pyelonephritis
Amoxycillin 100 mg/kg daily intravenously (IV) in 3 doses, and gentamicin 7.5 mg/kg daily in 3 IV doses.
Amoxycillin (as above) and cefotaxime 100–150 mg/kg daily IV in 3 doses, or ceftriaxone 100 mg/kg daily IV in 2 doses and amoxycillin 100 mg/kg daily IV in 3 doses.
For oral therapy, co-trimoxazole in a dosage of 6–8 mg of trimethoprim and 30–40 mg of sulphamethoxazole per kg daily in 2 doses or trimethoprim 4 mg/kg daily in 2 doses.

Cystitis
Amoxycillin 50 mg/kg daily in 2 or 3 oral doses, co-trimoxazole or trimethoprim as above, cephalexin 50 mg/kg daily in 2 or 3 doses, or Augmentin 50 mg/kg daily in 2 or 3 doses.

Duration of therapy
Therapy is conventionally provided for 7–10 days.

Duration of antimicrobial therapy

In general, terms neonates and young infants should receive standard duration of therapy of 7–10 days. In older infants and children there has been considerable interest in recent years in shorter treatment. In adults, there is widespread use of short-course therapy in the treatment of UTI. The first report of single-dose treatment in children was by Bailey and Abbott (1976). Since then there have been a number of papers reporting the use of single-dose or short-term therapy. Moffatt *et al.* (1988) carried out a methodological review of 14 published studies on short-term antimicrobial therapy for urinary infection. Overall, there was no significant difference in cure rates of UTI with short-term versus conventional regimes of 7–10 days treatment. However, there were a number of differences in study design producing a number of methodological flaws, principally those of small sample size, patient heterogeneity, and a lack of double-blinds. These studies involved a total of less than 300 patients. None addressed patient compliance, adverse reactions, nor effects of treatment on gastrointestinal or genito-urinary flora. Moreover, the groups studied generally included patients of widely differing ages. Subsequently, Madrigal *et al.* (1988) reported their study of short-course therapy for childhood UTI involving 132 Costa Rican children aged 3 months to 12 years. They compared co-trimoxazole given as a single dose or for 3 or 7 days. Cure rates were similar for all dosage regimes but there was a significantly higher incidence of recurrent infections in the single-dose group. A further study by Grimwood *et al.* (1988) reported the results of a randomized controlled study in Christchurch, New Zealand, comparing the cure rates of single-dose gentamicin and conventional therapy with an appropriate oral anti-microbial agent, such as co-trimoxazole or amoxycillin, given for 7 days. Cure was defined as sterile urine 7 days after completing therapy. Sixty-nine children ranging from 1 month to 12 years of age were studied and included patients with suspected acute pyelonephritis and also those with a history of recurrent UTI. In this study, the overall cure rates were equal. However, children with a history of recurrent UTI and those with radiological abnormalities had higher failure rates with both treatments. Children who relapsed or failed treatment were mostly in the single-dose treatment group, while those who were re-infected with a different organism were mostly from the conventional treatment group. Rectal and periurethral swabs showed greater bacterial suppression in children on conventional therapy compared to those who received single-dose gentamicin.

Overall, from the reported studies it appears clear that single-dose or very short-course therapy of less than 3 days is contraindicated in infants and in children who have clinical acute pyelonephritis. It may be reasonable to treat older children who have cystitis but no anatomical abnormalities with single-dose or short-course therapy. However, because of the uncertainty of knowing whether there is upper tract infection present, conventional therapy is generally recommended for all children.

Follow-up urine cultures

As UTI has a likelihood of relapsing or recurring, follow-up urine culture should be done 48 hours, 7 days, and 6 weeks after stopping antimicrobial agents, and then monthly for several months following the initial episode. In those patients with recurrent urinary infections, dip-slides can be used at home.

Chemoprophylaxis pending imaging investigations

Pending further radiological and imaging investigations, infants and younger children should be placed on chemoprophylaxis following the therapeutic course. Recommended drugs for chemoprophylaxis are co-trimoxazole or trimethoprim in half the therapeutic dosage, or nitrofurantoin 1–2 mg/kg/day. These agents should be continued until the radiological and imaging investigations have been reviewed and VUR has been excluded (Smellie and Normand 1985).

Treatment of recurrent urinary tract infections

Urinary infections frequently recur. These re-infections are most likely to occur in the first few months after treatment is discontinued. Children who suffer recurrent infections experience a good deal of morbidity from recurrent symptoms, and are at risk from renal scarring, particularly if they have underlying VUR. Smellie *et al.*, in a series of papers (1967, 1978, 1982), reported their results using co-trimoxazole and trimethoprim in the prophylaxis of UTI in children. Smellie and Normand (1985) stated that the aim of prophylaxis was to prevent re-infection in a susceptible urinary tract after infection has been eradicated, and not just to suppress inadequately treated infection. The ideal prophylactic drugs should be effective against the usual urinary tract pathogens, and should preferably be absorbed from the proximal part of the alimentary tract to minimize the effect on bowel flora and hence the emergence of resistant organisms. The drug should have a high excretion rate in the urine. The agents most effectively fulfilling these criteria are co-trimoxazole, trimethoprim, and nitrofurantoin. Co-trimoxazole and trimethoprim are usually given in half the therapeutic dosage and nitrofurantoin 1–2 mg/kg/day. Other less-frequently used agents are nalidixic acid and cephalexin. These drugs are administered once or twice a day. A single daily dose seems to be effective, and is best given at bedtime when urine is in the bladder for the longest period of time. Regular monthly urine cultures or dip-side cultures are useful while on chemoprophylaxis. Frequent emphasis on the importance of taking the medication is required as Smyth and Judd (1993) have reported that compliance in their treated children was only 60 per cent.

Indications for low-dose antimicrobial prophylaxis

1. If there is frequent recurrence of symptomatic infections (three within a 6-month period).
2. Following the successful treatment of an infection in infants and young children until radiological assessment has been carried out and VUR has been excluded.
3. If VUR is present and thus the kidneys are potentially at risk from infection in the infant and child under the age of 5 years.

Prophylaxis is usually continued for a period of several months. If given for symptomatic recurrences alone, a trial off chemoprophylaxis is indicated after 6 months treatment. If the child has VUR, chemoprophylaxis is usually continued until the reflux has resolved spontaneously or has been surgically corrected. Frequent recurrences of UTI with a resistant organism during low-dose chemoprophylaxis are reported to be uncommon. Smellie and Normand (1985) reported that no significant side-effects had been observed or reported in children receiving co-trimoxazole, trimethoprim, nitrofurantoin, or nalidixic acid in the low dosages recommended for chemoprophylaxis, even when given for periods of up to 10 years. They also reported that although an increase in the proportion of trimethoprim-resistant Gram-negative organisms had been observed between 1970 and 1980, there had been no apparent corresponding decrease in efficacy of trimethoprim or co-trimoxazole in that period.

General measures in the prevention of recurrent infections

Apart from chemoprophylaxis, a number of general measures are often recommended (Smellie and Normand 1985). Many of the recommendations are based on clinical experience rather than documented efficacy.

1. Complete bladder emptying: children with recurrent infections should be encouraged to void every two or three hours and to practise double micturition. This helps to ensure that the bladder is emptied. Many children, particularly girls, are inclined to delay voiding for long periods and to void incompletely.

2. Children should be encouraged to drink, particularly during pre-school and school years, when fluid intake may be minimal. Drinking with meals and at regular intervals at school, such as playtime, is to be encouraged.
3. Children with constipation need this problem corrected using high-fibre diets and agents such as lactulose. Constipation, dysfunctional voiding, and recurrent infections frequently occur together.
4. Other measures. Other simple measures, such as the treatment of threadworm infestation, is frequently advocated. Threadworm infestation of the perineum and vulval region frequently leads to symptoms of frequency and dysuria, dysfunctional voiding, and incomplete emptying (Kunin 1987). Children should be encouraged to wear looser clothing and to use cotton pants instead of nylon. Vaginal irritants such as bubble baths and chlorinated water are best avoided. Children should shower instead of having baths.

At each attendance at the outpatient clinic or general practitioner's surgery, reinforcement of these general measures, and particularly encouragement to maintain compliance with chemoprophylaxis, is important.

Imaging of the genitourinary tract

Following an accurate diagnosis and sterilization of the urine by adequate treatment, the next step in management is imaging of the urinary tract. An underlying urinary tract abnormality cannot be predicted with any certainty by either the clinical presentation or response to treatment. All children, regardless of age or sex, should undergo appropriate investigations (Abbott 1991). Investigations are directed at identifying obstruction, calculi, neurogenic bladder, and VUR (Whittaker and Sherwood 1984). These are the major anomalies that are amenable to intervention.

Exclusion of obstruction, calculi, and neurogenic bladder

In the acutely ill infant and child, renal ultrasonography (US) should be carried out urgently to exclude obstruction in the genitourinary tract. If upper tract dilatation is seen on ultrasound, further investigations will be necessary to distinguish between obstruction, VUR, non-obstructive megaureter, and neurogenic bladder. A neurogenic bladder is suggested by abnormalities of bladder shape or thickening of the bladder wall, incomplete emptying on micturition, and accompanying dilatation of the upper tracts. Plain radiographs of the abdomen will demonstrate radiopaque calculi, spina bifida occulta, and constipation.

If reliable US is not available, the intravenous urogram (IVU) remains an effective method for demonstrating renal size, structure, function, and calyceal pattern. The calibre of the ureters and bladder morphology including filling defects such as ureterocoeles, diverticula, or trabeculation, can be seen. In addition, spinal defects and overloaded bowel are visualized on the plain film (Smellie and Normand 1985).

Vesicoureteric reflux (VUR)

It is now clearly established that VUR is the most commonly demonstrated abnormality found in infants and children undergoing radiological investigation following UTI—being found in 30–50 per cent. Over the last 30–40 years a wealth of literature has evolved on the nature of the defect, natural history, genetics, mechanisms of renal damage, and management. Key observations were made by Hutch (1952), Hodson and Edwards (1960), and Rolleston *et al.* (1970) concerning the relationship between VUR and renal scarring. In the intervening years an enormous amount of both experimental and clinical information has emerged. While considerable controversy remains regarding the actual mechanisms of renal damage, a good deal of consensus has been achieved. Woodward and Rushton (1987) clearly summarized some of the general agreements and assumptions that could be made from this wealth of clinical, experimental, and radiological data, and Bailey (1992) carried out an extensive review of the literature. The following can generally be concluded from these reviews:

1. Most primary reflux is due to a congenital anatomical abnormality of the bladder trigone.
2. In many instances this anomaly improves with growth and development of the child so that the reflux may cease spontaneously. In low-grade (I–II) reflux with undilated ureters, approximately 75–85 per cent will stop refluxing. In higher grades (III–V) with dilated ureters reflux ceases in 25–30 per cent.
3. Although radiological grading is helpful in predicting the likelihood of spontaneous cessation, it is possible to improve that predictability by cystoscopic evaluation of the size, configuration, and position of the ureteric orifice plus the length of the submucosal tunnel.
4. VUR in combination with urinary infection can and does lead to renal scarring.
5. Renal scarring infrequently occurs in patients with primary reflux and normal voiding pressures in the absence of urinary infection.
6. Renal growth may proceed normally despite continuing sterile reflux.
7. In severely refluxing patients, approximately 10 per cent will have bacteriuria despite continuous antimicrobial chemoprophylaxis and these ‘breakthrough’ infections may cause renal scars.
8. Some patients prove either unwilling or unable to comply with continuous medications and are vulnerable to scar formation.
9. A successful anti-reflux operation may not change the recurrence rate of urinary infection, but it appears to significantly reduce the likelihood of pyelonephritis and the necessity for continued chemoprophylaxis.

Debate continues on the mechanisms of renal scarring, and although previous information and reviews have closely linked the necessity to have both VUR and urinary infection for the development of renal scarring, some recent studies have tended, at least in part, to refute this. The studies of Roberts (1991) concerning the aetiology and pathophysiology of pyelonephritis, and those of Rushton and Majd (1992), showed that not all patients with pyelonephritis have demonstrable reflux, and that the likelihood of renal scars developing as a consequence of pyelonephritis is the same regardless of whether reflux is documented or not. Rosenburg *et al.* (1992) however found a close associaton between initial DMSA changes and significant VUR. There is no doubt that bacterial pyelonephritis produces renal scars experimentally and clinically. This has been shown by the studies of Rushton and Majd (1992) and those of Winberg *et al.* (1982). It is uncertain why only a proportion of patients with acute inflammatory changes during acute pyelonephritis progress to subsequent renal scarring. The studies of Rushton and Majd (1992) would suggest that only half of the patients with acute pyelonephritis will have permanent scarring. It is, however, of considerable interest that some of the most marked examples of renal scarring associated with reflux are detected soon after birth. Presumably, such injury is of developmental origin and has occurred *in utero*. The studies of Yeung *et al.* (1991) suggested the possibility of transient bladder outflow tract obstruction with elevated intraluminal pressure that might damage kidneys during development.

Recently, the use of antenatal ultrasound examination has identified infants with pre-natal hydronephrosis. Many have subsequently been shown to have VUR post-natally. Infants found to have VUR have been predominantly male and have had high-grade reflux which spontaneously resolves in the first few months of life (Rosenberg 1991; Elder 1992). In clinical practice, however, VUR and renal scarring are found predominantly in girls. Therefore, the usefulness of antenatal ultrasound screening for VUR has been questioned. In a recent study, however, Anderson *et al.* (1992) have reported a much higher incidence in females. In this study, 38 infants were found to have VUR and of this number, 10 (25 per cent) had changes on the initial DMSA scan performed within 3 months of birth. Only three of these children had urinary infection post-natally prior to the DMSA scan being performed.

The long-term studies of Smellie (1991) and Bailey *et al.* (1992), have shown that reflux tends to resolve spontaneously with time, but there is a decided difference in the rate of resolution depending on the initial grade of reflux. In lower grades of reflux (I–II) it is as high as 85 per cent but this rate may be less than half for those with dilating reflux, as shown by Edwards *et al.* (1977). Overall, it would appear that approximately 50 percent of reflux resolves within five years. Recurrent UTI and new scar formation appear to become much less frequent as the child grows older.

Genetics of vesicoureteric reflux

Stevens *et al.* (1972) observed VUR in identical twins and Hayden and Koff (1984) reported the incidence of VUR in triplets. The mechanism of inheritance has since been debated. Some authors have suggested a multifactorial trait (Jenkins and Noe 1982), or alternatively an autosomal dominant gene with reduced penetrance (Miller and Kaspari 1972). Others have suggested an X-linked inheritance (Middleton *et al.* 1975; Tobenkin 1964). Chapman *et al.* (1985) studied 88 affected families who were subjected to segregation analysis using a mixed model (Lalouel and Morton 1981) and a computer program (Pointer). Eighteen families were identified through a proband with end-stage reflux nephropathy, two through a proband with severe renal failure, and 68 through a proband with reflux and normal renal function. In 30 of the 88 families, additional affected members were found. Of the 242 relatives investigated, 48 were affected. Three generations were affected in six families and two generation in a further 15 families. In a few cases, apparently non-affected relatives were probable asymptomatic carriers of the gene because they had both an affected offspring and an affected parent. In one family both parents were affected but the only child was unaffected. This was consistent with a dominant but not recessive mode of inheritance. The model indicated that the gene frequency was 1 in 600 and that mutation was uncommon. According to the model and using information on the prevalence of end-stage reflux nephropathy it was calculated that 45 per cent of gene carriers will have VUR or reflux nephropathy as adults and 15 per cent will develop end-stage renal failure. Of the non-carriers of the gene, 0.05 per cent will have VUR or reflux nephropathy and 0.001 per cent will go on to renal failure from this cause. Thus, this trait for reflux is one of the commonest Mendelian dominant traits described in humans. Noe (1992), in a large prospective study of siblings of the index patient with VUR, found 34 per cent of siblings had reflux. These authors therefore concluded that there was a necessity for family studies. All children born to parents with known VUR or reflux nephropathy or who have siblings with these abnormalities should have their urinary tract investigated within a few weeks of birth. A voiding cystourethrogram or radioisotope cystourethrogram should be performed in infants and young children and in older age groups, the kidneys should have an imaging procedure to detect renal scarring and if scars are found, a voiding cystourethrogram should be performed.

Vesicoureteric reflux and renal scarring

The precise mechanism of renal scarring in the presence of VUR remains controversial. Several explanations have been forthcoming, including the following outlined by Woodward and Rushton (1987).

1. The embryonic ureteral bud may develop from an abnormal site, therefore inducing abnormal renal development with subsequent dysplasia.
2. Sterile reflux and its concomitant 'water hammer' effect may produce renal damage, perhaps mediated through an immunological response.
3. Intra-renal reflux of infected urine with or without symptoms may occur in susceptible renal papillae and damage the parenchyma.

Many clinical studies have confirmed the frequent association between VUR, urinary infection, and renal scarring, particularly those of Smellie and Normand

(1975) and Scott and Stansfield (1968). Rolleston *et al.* (1970), in a hallmark paper, described the relationship of infantile VUR to renal damage. Scarring is already present at the time of initial investigation in many patients with VUR and urinary infection. Development of new scars in previously normal kidneys has been documented but is considered uncommon, particularly in children over the age of 5 years (Cardiff–Oxford Bacteriuria Study Group 1978). When it does occur it appears almost always to be associated with previous UTI and more severe grades of reflux (Smellie *et al.* 1981). In some cases, the progression of scarring may represent a continuing evolution of the scarring process with growth and hypertrophy of adjacent normal renal parenchyma. The delineation of scarring in earlier studies has been on the basis of intravenous urograms. It is thought that renal scarring can be modified by the early adequate treatment of acute pyelonephritis as demonstrated by Winter *et al.* (1983).

Detection of vesicoureteric reflux

Optimal methods for detection of VUR have recently been reviewed by Lebowitz (1992). The two major methods are the voiding cystourethrogram (VCU) and radionuclide cystography. Lebowitz summarizes the situation by stating that VCU is more accurate in quantifying and grading reflux but monitoring is intermittent. Conversely radionuclide cystography has a lower radiation dose and its continuous monitoring leads to fewer false negative results but its ability to grade reflux is inferior to VCU.

A variety of methods for grading reflux have evolved, and a uniform radiological classification is essential. Recently, a grading classification of VUR has been agreed by the 26 units participating in the International Reflux Study in Children (IRSC 1981). This classification is as follows:

Grade 1: Ureter only.

Grade 2: Ureter, pelvis, and calyces with no dilatation and normal calyceal fornices.

Grade 3: Mild or moderate dilatation and/or tortuosity of the ureter and mild or moderate dilatation of the pelvis. No or only slight blunting of the fornices.

Grade 4: Moderate dilatation and/or tortuosity of the ureter and moderate dilatation of the pelvis and calyces. Complete obliteration of sharp angles of the fornices but maintenance of papillary impression in the majority of calyces.

Grade 5: Gross dilatation and tortuosity of the ureter, pelvis, and calyces. The papillary impressions are no longer visible in the majority of calyces.

Mild to severe reflux is a continuum and therefore any grading system is inherently arbitrary. If reflux is found to be present, Lebowitz (1992) states that the rate and completeness of drainage must be determined before the examination in complete. Only then can coexistent obstruction of the ureter, pelvis, or vesicoureteric junction be identified. The importance of this is that if co-existing obstruction is not recognized, the grade of reflux will be falsely high.

Neilson (1989) and Seruca (1989) consider that the identification of voiding dysfuction in a child with reflux is also important. Radiographic signs of an unstable bladder include trabeculation, incomplete emptying, and uninhibited contractions during filling. Bladder sphincter dyssynergia may also be noted.

Generally, voiding cystourethrography is used to detect and grade reflux. Radionuclide cystourethrography is usually reserved for screening family members, the follow-up of patients with previously defined and graded VUR, and in the post-operative assessment after ureteric re-implantation for reflux. Once VUR has been found then assessment of the kidneys is required to detect renal scarring.

Reflux nephropathy was originally defined by intravenous urography (IVU), which demonstrated two distinct types of radiographic damage (Bailey 1992).

1. The first type comprises full thickness focal scars, with calyceal clubbling, atrophy, and retraction of the overlying cortex involving one or more renal lobes. This is found most frequently in the polar regions of the kidney and is considered pathognomonic of reflux nephropathy. There is always preservation of at least one normal renal lobe. This is considered the most common form of reflux nephropathy.
2. Occasionally, with the most severe degrees of VUR, the damage is diffuse with involvement of all lobes of the kidney, resulting in a generalized reduction in parenchymal thickness and uniform papillary change. This type of damage resembles that seen in obstructive atrophy.

Whyte *et al.* (1988) demonstrated that as well as defining the changes of reflux nephropathy in children, a carefully performed intravenous urogam could also show non-obstructive dilatation of the ureter and striation of the renal pelvis suggesting previous over-distension. In this study it was therefore considered that the IVU was a useful screening procedure for reflux in children over the age of 2 years.

Ultrasonography (US), although extremely useful in detecting obstruction, multicystic kidneys and kidneys that do not function on IVU, it is not reliable in excluding the presence of significant reflux or for detecting renal scars (Teele and Share 1991).

More recently, in a review of a number of studies Kennedy *et al.* (1991) considered that DMSA scan is the most sensitive detector of renal scarring. In addition to showing anatomical details of the kidney, it also gives valuable functional information (Goldraich 1991).

Radiological investigations for vesicoureteric reflux

A variety of approaches is recommended and no one group of authors appears to achieve absolute agreement.

The practical issue is whether VUR needs to be detected in children of all ages or whether voiding cystourethrography should be confined only to infants and younger children. It seems clear the process starts very early in life, and scarring develops usually in association with UTI. Subsequent damage, particularly after the age of 5 years, is less likely, and continuing reflux, which has not already caused renal scarring, is probably of much less consequence. On this basis many would restrict voiding cystourethrography to the younger age group. Some restrict it to children under the age of 5 years, and others recommend it only in children up to the age of 1 or 2 years (Maling 1991). A scheme for investigation of children presenting with their first UTI, as carried out in Christchurch, New Zealand, is *included* in Table 7.6. It is important to emphasize that the scheme outlined by Maling is used for the *initial* investigation of UTI. If the child continues to have recurrent infections, voiding dysfunction, or has a family history of VUR, then further investigations to exclude VUR should be undertaken. The other key issue is the availability of the different imaging techniques and the confidence and experience of the person performing the investigation.

Although the detection of VUR is considered essential, it is also extremely important to detect obstruction and renal scarring. Once renal scarring has been defined then investigation to find any possible underlying associated mechanism, such as VUR, must be pursued vigorously.

Treatment of vesicoureteric reflux

The optimal management for VUR has been controversial for several years. The main aim of treatment must be to try to prevent renal scarring with consequent

Table 7.6 Radiological investigations for urinary infections in children

1. *Under 2 years* (Maling 1991)
   (a) Voiding cystourethrogram (VCU).
   (b) Ultrasound (US)..
   (c) Dimercaptosuccinic acid (DMSA) scan and/or intravenous urography (IVU), only if one of the above is abnormal.
2. *2–5 years*
   US and DMSA scan, or IVU. VCU need only be performed if an abnormality is seen in one of these examinations or if recurrent urinary infections continue to be a major problem. By pursuing this policy the number of VCUs in this difficult age group will be restricted and it is unlikely that many cases of significant VUR will be missed.
3. *Over 5 years*
   US examination and only further imaging if this is abnormal. Further imaging when necessary will be chosen from:
   (a) IVU
   (b) DMSA scan
   (c) VCU
   The choice of imaging will depend upon the US findings.

development of hypertension and chronic renal failure. Fortunately, two recent studies have gone a long way to evaluating the relative merits of surgical re-implantation of refluxing ureters, or chemoprophylaxis to prevent UTI while reflux persists.

In 1975, the Birmingham Reflux Study Group (BRSG) establish a controlled prospective trial in which children with severe VUR were randomly allocated to operative or non-operative management, and were reassessed functionally and structurally five years after entry. The results reported from the BRSG (1987) after five years confirmed and extended observations made after two years. The study failed to demonstrate significant differences between the two treatment groups in either the incidence of 'breakthrough' UTI, glomerular filtration rate, renal concentrating ability, renal growth, progression of existing scars, or new scar formation.

Recently, results of the International Reflux Study in children (IRC 1981) were summarized by Smellie (1992). In this study the outcome of medical and surgical management of children with severe VUR (international Grades III or IV) was compared after a five-year observation period. As children with this severity of reflux are not common, a multi-centre study was necessary to recruit sufficient numbers to achieve a statistically valid result. A total of 434 children was entered: 128 were from centres in America and 306 from Europe. They were randomly allocated and stratified to a medical or surgical regimen. Of the children, 50 per cent had scarred kidneys at entry, evenly distributed between the groups. After five years there was no difference in outcome between the two treatment groups in terms of renal size and growth, development of new, or of progression of established radiological scarring. In the European sector, infection recurred in equal numbers of children but pyelonephritic symptoms were more common in the medical treatment group. New scars developed in 19 of the 155 children treated medically and 20 of the 151 children treated surgically, including 5 and 7, respectively, with previously normal kidneys.

It was concluded that factors influencing the choice of treatment include patient age, availability of expert surgical care and experienced medical supervision, parental choice, and compliance. Follow-up studies indicate that renal scarring rather than the persistence of reflux determines the prognosis and, therefore, emphasis should be place on the prevention of scarring.

Medical management of vesicoureteric reflux in infants and young children

1. Children should be placed on low-dose chemoprophylaxis. As discussed previously, the three most effective agents appear to be co-trimoxazole, trimethoprim, or nitrofurantoin. These agents should be given once or twice a day and, if in a single dose, preferably at bedtime to keep the urine sterile while it is in the bladder for the longest period.

2. Urine cultures on a monthly basis should be carried out on chemoprophylaxis. If 'breakthrough' infections occur these should be treated with

another agent, either parenterally or orally for a standard course of 7–10 days. Once the child's urine is sterile chemoprophylaxis is recommenced.

3. Chemoprophylaxis should be continued until the reflux has been demonstrated to have ceased. For lesser degrees of reflux this will usually occur within two years, but less frequently and over a longer period of time for those with Grades III–IV reflux. Either the voiding cystourethrogram or the radioisotope cystogram should be repeated every one to two years until the reflux has been shown to have resolved.

4. As has been discussed earlier, it is important to establish whether there is any renal scarring present and this is best defined by a DMSA scan or, if unavailable, an intravenous urogram (IVU). A DMSA scan is usually done early in the investigation of UTI and should be repeated at the time of the cystogram a year later to see whether any scarring defined earlier has persisted or new scars have developed. A renal ultrasound (US) performed at the time of annual review is also useful to show whether there has been satisfactory renal growth but is much less reliable in defining whether there are scars present.

5. If, after a period of chemoprophylaxis and appropriate radiological follow-up, it has been shown that the reflux has resolved then chemoprophylaxis can be stopped. If the child has renal scarring then long-term follow-up is required, particularly if the scarring is extensive and bilateral. These children are at risk of developing hypertension and some will develop deterioration of renal function and chronic renal failure. The development of persistent proteinuria is an ominous sign, and appears to be due to the development of a glomerular lesion of focal and segmental sclerosis with hyalinosis, involving unscarred segments of kidney or the structurally normal contralateral kidney in patients with unilateral reflux nephropathy (Bailey 1992). Children with renal scarring should be seen at least annually to check their blood pressure and to assess for proteinuria. Reflux nephropathy is the commonest cause of severe sustained hypertension in children (Dillon 1985).

Surgical correction of VUR

Currently, it appears that the only absolute indication for surgical intervention remains failure of medical therapy to prevent UTI and pyelonephritis. However, parental preference, problems with compliance, the expense of long-term follow-up, and the availability of an appropriately experienced paediatric urologist or paediatric surgeon, are important considerations.

Grade V VUR is generally considered a surgical condition requiring re-implantation of the ureters. Montford *et al.* (1992) reported their 20-year experience on 68 patients with Grade V reflux. Those with very early diagnosis or detected antenatally appeared to have a better prognosis from the point of view of the development of chronic renal failure. If renal failure was already established, surgery did not appear to change the rate of chronic renal failure in these patients.

The place of endoscopic correction of VUR is evolving. Dewan (1991), when reviewing the topic, concluded that although this was an easier method of definitive management of all grades of reflux, the role of the technique and the ideal injection material had not yet been clearly defined. He also pointed out that while it is a simpler technique, it does not resolved the dilemma of the place of anti-reflux surgery versus medical management.

Following surgical reimplantation of ureters an US or IVU is usually performed some weeks post-operatively. Antimicrobial chemoprophylaxis is usually continued until either a voiding cystourethrogram or radioisotope cystogram has demonstrated that reflux has stopped. Following successful surgery the duration of follow-up is dependent on the presence or absence of renal scarring. If renal scarring is present then long-term follow-up of these patients to detect hypertension, proteinuria, or deterioration of renal function is required.

References

Abbott, G. D. (1972). Neonatal bacteriuria: a prospective study in 1,460 infants. *British Medical Journal*, **1**, 267–9.

Abbott, G. D. (1978). Neonatal bacteriuria—the value of bladder puncture in resolving problems of interpretation arising from voided urine specimens. *Australian Paediatric Journal*, **14**, 83–6.

Abbott, G. D. (1991). Urinary tract infection in children: Diagnosis, investigation and management. *New Ethicals*, **12**, 117–27.

Abbott, G. D. and Allan, J. (1984). *Diagnosis of UTI by sight and smell.* Paper presented at The Paediatric Society of New Zealand Annual Conference, Abstract 21. Wellington, New Zealand.

Abbott, G. D. and Shannon, F. T. (1970). How to aspirate urine suprapubically in infants and children, *Clinical Pediatrics*, **9**, 277–8.

Anderson, N., Abbott, G. D., and Mogridge, N. (1992). *Prenatal screening for vesico-ureteric reflux: preliminary results.* Paper presented at Proceedings, Christchurch Medical Research Society, 15 April 1992. *New Zealand Medical Journal*, **105**, 385–6.

Bailey, R. R. (1992). Vesico-ureteric reflux and reflux nephropathy. In *Oxford textbook of clinical nephrology*, (ed. S. Cameron, A. Davison, J. Grunfeld, D. Kerr, and E. Ritz), Vol. 3, pp. 1983–2002. Oxford University Press.

Bailey, R. R. and Abbott, G. D. (1976). Treatment of urinary tract infections with a single dose of amoxycillin. *New Zealand Medical Journal*, **84**, 324–5.

Bailey, R. R. and Little, P. J. (1970). *Suprapubic bladder aspiration in renal infection and renal scarring.* Paper presented at Proceedings of an International Symposium on Pyelonephritis, Vesico-ureteric Reflux and Renal Papillary Necrosis, pp. 81–4. Melbourne, Australia.

Bailey, R. R. Lynn, K. L., and Smith A. H. (1992). Long-term follow-up of infants with gross vesico-uretic reflux. Part 2. *Journal of Urology*, **148**, 1709–11.

Bauchner, H., *et al.* (1987). Prevalence of bacteriuria in febrile children. *Pediatric Infectious Disease Journal*, **6**, 239–42

BRSG (Birmingham Reflux Study Group) (1987). A prospective trial of operative versus non-operative treatment of severe vesico-uretic reflux, five years observation. *British Medical Journal*, **295**, 237–41.

Berg, U. B. (1989). Renal dysfunction in recurrent urinary tract infection in childhood. *Paediatric Nephrology*, **3**, 9–15.

Bourchier, D., Abbott, G. D., and Maling, T. (1984). Radiological abnormalities in infants with urinary tract infections. *Archives of Disease in Childhood*, **59**, 620–4.

Braude, H., *et al.* (1967). Cell and bacterial counts in the urine of normal infants and children. *British Medical Journal*, **4**, 697–700.

Cardiff–Oxford Bacteriuria Study Group (1978). Sequelae of covert bacteriuria in schoolgirls: A four year follow-up study. *Lancet*, **i**, 1889–96.

Chapman, C. A., Bailey, R. R., Janus, E. D., and Abbott, G. D. (1985). Vesico-ureteric reflux: segregation analysis. *American Journal of Medical Genetics*, **20**, 577–85.

Cruickshank, G. and Edmond, E. (1967). Clean catch urines in the newborn: Bacteriology and cell excretion patterns in the first week of life. *British Medical Journal*, **4**, 705–9.

Dewan, P. A. (1991). Endoscopic management of vesico-ureteric reflux. In *Second C. J. Hodson Symposium on Reflux Nephropathy*, pp. 65–8. Design Printing Services, Christchurch, New Zealand.

Dillon, M. J. (1985). Hypertension. In *Clinical paediatric nephrology*, (ed. R. T. Postlethwaite Wright), pp. 1–25. John Wright, Bristol.

Edelman, C. M., *et al.* (1973). The prevalence of bacteriuria in full term and premature newborn infants. *Journal of Pediatrics*, **82**, 125–32.

Edwards, D., Normand, I. C. S., and Smellie. J. M. (1977). The disappearance of vesico-ureteric reflux during long-term prophylaxis of urinary tract infection in children. *British Medical Journal*, **2**, 285–8.

Elder, J. S. (1992). Importance of antenatal diagnosis of vesico-ureteric reflux. *Journal of Urology*, **148**, 1750–4.

Feld, L., Greenfield, S., and Ogra, P. (1989). Urinary tract infections in infants and children. *Pediatric Review*, **11**, 71–7.

Ginsberg, C. M. and McCracken, G. H. (1982). Urinary tract infections in young infants. *Pediatrics*, **69**, 409–12.

Goldraich, N. P. (1991). Reflux nephropathy: the place of the DMSA scan. In *Second C. J. Hodson Symposium on Reflux Nephropathy*, pp. 9–13. Design Printing Services, Christchurch, New Zealand.

Grimwood, K., Abbott, G. D., and Fergusson, D. M. (1988). Single dose gentamicin treatment of urinary infections in children. *New Zealand Medical Journal*, **101**, 539–41.

Hayden, L. J. and Koff, S. A. (1984). Vesico-ureteric reflux in triplets. *Journal of Urology*, **132**, 516–18.

Herzog, L. (1989). Urinary tract infections in circumcision. *American Journal of Disease in Children*, **143**, 348–50.

Hodson, C. J. and Edwards, D. (1960). Chronic pyelonephritis and vesico-ureteric reflux. *Clinical Radiology*, **11**, 219–25.

Houston, I. B. (1963). Pus cell and bacterial counts in the diagnosis of urinary tract infection in childhood. *Archives of Disease in Children*, **38**, 600–4.

Hutch, A. A. (1952). Vesico-ureteric reflux in the paraplegic: cause and correction. *Journal of Urology*, **68**, 457–61.

IRSC (International Reflux Study Committee) (1981). Medical versus surgical treatment of primary vesico-ureteric reflux. A prospective reflux study in children. *Journal of Urology*, **125**, 277–85.

Israeli, V., Darabi, A., and McCracken, G.H. (1987). The role of bacterial virilance factors and Tam Horsfall protein in the pathogenesis of *E. coli* urinary tract infection in infants. *American Journal of Disease in Children*, **141**, 1230–4.

Ives, J. A., Abbott, G. D., and Bailey R. R. (1971). Bacteriuria of pregnancy and infection in amniotic fluid and infant. *Archives of Disease in Childhood*, **46**, 82–4.

Jenkins, G. R. and Noe, H. N. (1982). Familial vesico-ureteric reflux: a prospective study. *Journal of Urology*, **128** 774–6.

Kennedy, J. D., Abbott, G. D., McRae, C. U., and Maling, T. M. J. (1991). A protocol for the investigation of infants and children presenting with urinary tract infection. *Second C. J. Hodson Symposium on Reflux Nephropathy*, pp. 15–17. Design Printing Services, Christchurch, New Zealand.

Kunin, C. M. (1987). In *Detection, prevention and management of urinary tract infections*, (4th edn), pp. 60–3; 76–81; 125–39; 224–30; 245–6. Lea & Febiger, Philadelphia.

Kunin, C. M., Dutscher, R., and Paquin, A. J. (1964). Urinary tract infection in school children: Epidemiologic, clinical and laboratory study. *Medicine*, **43**, 91–130.

Kunin, C. M., deGroot, J. E., Uehling, D., and Ramgopal, V. (1976). Detection of urinary tract infection in 3–5 year old girls by mothers using a nitrite indicator strip. *Pediatrics*, **57**, 829–35.

Lalouel, J. M. and Morton, N. E. (1981). Complex segregation analysis with pointers. *Human Hereditary*, **31**, 312–20.

Lebowitz, R. L. (1992). The detection and characterisation of vesico-ureteral reflux in the child. *Journal of Urology*, **148**, 1640–2.

Lincoln, K. and Winberg, J. (1964). Studies of urinary tract infection in infancy and childhood. 2. Quantitative estimation of bacteriuria in unselected neonates with special reference to the recurrence of asymptomatic infections. *Acta Paediatrica Scandinavica*, **53**, 307–16.

Littlewood, J. M., Kyte, P., and Kyte, B. A. (1969). Incidence of neonatal urinary tract infection. *Archives of Disease in Childhood*, **44**, 617–20.

Madrigal, G., Odio, C. M., Mohs, E., Guevara, J., and McCracken, G. H. (1988). Single dose antibiotic therapy is not as effective as conventional regimens for management of acute urinary tract infection in children. *Pediatric Infectious Diseases Journal*, **7**, 316–9.

Maherzi, M., Gougnard, J. P., and Torrado, A. (1978). Urinary tract infection in high risk newborn infants. *Pediatrics*, **62**, 521–3.

Mair, M. I. (1973). High incidence of asymptomatic urinary tract infection in infant schoolgirls. *Scottish Medical Journal*, **18**, 51–5.

Maling, T. M. J. (1991). The appropriate organ imaging investigation to detect vesico-ureteric reflux. In *Second C. J. Hodson Symposium on Reflux Nephropathy*, p. 76. Design Printing Services, Christchurch, New Zealand.

McCracken, G. H. (1989). Options in antimicrobial management of urinary tract infection in infants and children. *Pediatric Infectious Diseases Journal*, **8**, 552–5.

Middleton, G. W., Howards, S. S., and Gillenwater, J. Y. (1975). Sex linked familial reflux. *Journal of Urology*; **114**, 36-40.

Miller, H. C. and Kaspari, E. W. (1972). Ureteral reflux as a genetic trait. *Journal of the American Medical Association*, **220**, 842–8.

Moffatt, M., Embree, J., Grimm, P., and Law. B. (1988). Short course antibiotic therapy for urinary tract infection in children. *American Journal of Diseases of Childhood*, **142**, 57–61.

Montford, G., Beseghi, W., and Riccipetoni, G. (1992). *Surgical treatment and follow-up of primary Grade V bilateral vesico-ureteric reflux*. Paper presented at The Ninth Congress of the International Paediatric Nephrology Congress, Jerusalem.

Nielsen, J. B. (1989). Lower urinary tract function in vesico-ureteral reflux. *Scandinavian Journal of Urology*, **125**(Suppl.), 15–7.

Newcastle Asymtomatic Bacteriuria Research Group (1975). Asymptomatic bacteriuria in schoolchildren in Newcastle-upon-Tyne. *Archives of Disease in Childhood*, **50**, 90–102.

Noe, H. N. (1992). The long term results of prospective sibling reflux screening. Part 2. *Journal of Urology*, **148**, 1739–41.

Patrick, M. J. (1967). Influence of maternal renal infection on the fetus and infant. *Archives of Disease in Childhood*, **42**, 208–11.

Randolph, M. F. and Greenfield, M. (1964). The incidence of asymptomatic bacteriuria and pyuria in infancy. *Journal of Pediatrics*, **65**, 57–66.

Roberts, J. A. (1991). Aetiology and pathophysiology of pyelonephriris. *American Journal of Kidney Disease*, **17**, 1–6.

Roberts, K., Charney, E., and Sweren, R. (1983). Urinary tract infections in infants with unexplained fever. A collaborative study. *Journal of Pediatrics*, **103**, 864–7.

Rolleston, G. L., Shannon, F. T., and Utley, W. L. F. (1970). Relationship of infantile vesico-ureteric reflux to renal damage. *British Medical Journal*, **1**, 460–5.

Rosenberg, A. R. (191). Vesico-ureteric reflux and antenatal ultrasonography. In *Second C. J. Hodson Symposium on Reflux Nephropathy*, pp. 1–3. Design Printing Services, Christchurch, New Zealand.

Rosenburg, A., Rossleigh, M., Brydon, M., Bass, S., Leighton, D., and Farnsworth, R. (1992). Evaluation of acute urinary tract infection in children by dimercaptosuccinic acid cintography: a prospective study. *Journal of Urology*, **148**, 1746–9.

Rushton, H. G. and Majd, M. (1992). Dimercaptosuccinic acid renal scintigrophy for evaluation of pyelonephritis and scarring: Review of experimental and clinical studies. *Journal of Urology*, **148**, 1726–32.

Savage, D. C., Wilson, M. I., and Ross, E. M. (1969). Asymptomatic bacteriuria in girl entrants to Dundee primary schools. *British Medical Journal*, **3**, 75–80.

Saxena, S. R., Collis, A., and Laurance, B. M. (1974). Bacteriuria in pre-schoolchildren. *Lancet*, **2**, 517–8.

Scott, J. E. S. and Stansfield, J. M. (1968). Ureteric reflux and kidney scarring in children. *Archives of Disease in Childhood*, **43**, 468.

Seruca. H. (1989). Vesico-ureteral reflux and voiding dysfunction. A prospective study. *Journal of Urology*, **142**, 499–502.

Shannon, F. T., Sepp, E., and Rose, G. R. (1969). The diagnosis of bacteriuria by bladder puncture in infancy and childhood. *Australian Paediatric Journal*, **5**, 97–9.

Smellie, J. M. (1991). Reflections on 30 years of treating children with urinary tract infection. Part 2. *Journal of Urology*, **146**, 665–709.

Smellie, J. M. (1992). Management of children with severe vesico-ureteric reflux. Commentary on the international reflux study in children. *Journal of Urology*, **148**, 1676–8.

Smellie, J. M. and Normand, I. C. S. (1975). Bacteriuria, reflux and renal scarring. *Archives of Disease in Childhood*, **50**, 581–5.

Smellie, J. M. and Normand, I. C. S. (1985). Management of urinary tract infection. In *Clinical paediatric nephrology*, (ed. R. J. Postlethwaite), pp. 372–93. John Wright, Bristol.

Smellie, J. M., Gruneberg, R. N., Leakey, A., and Aitken, W. S. (1976). Long term low dosage co-trimoxazole in the management of urinary tract infection in children. *Journal of Antimicrobial Chemotherapy*, **2**, 287–91.

Smellie, J. M., Katz, G., and Gruneberg, R. N. (1978). Controlled trial of prophylactic treatment in childhood urinary tract infection. *Lancet*, **2**, 175–8.

Smellie, J. M., Normand, I. C. S. and Katz, G. (1981). Children with urinary infection: a comparison of those with and those without vesico-ureteral reflux. *Kidney International*, **20**, 717–20.

Smellie, J. M., Gruneberg, R. N., Normand, I. C. S., and Bantock, H. (1982). Trimethoprim sulfamethoxazole and trimethoprim alone in the prophylaxis of childhood urinary tract infection. *Review of Infectious Diseases*, **4**, 461–6.

Smyth, A. R. and Judd, B. A. (1993). Compliance with antibiotic prophylaxis in urinary tract infection. *Archives of Disease in Childhood*, **68**, 235–6.

Stamm, W. E. (1983). Measurement of pyuria and its relationship to bacteriuria. *American Journal of Medicine*, **75**, 53–6.

Stevens, F. D., Joske, R. A., and Simmons, R. T. (1972). Megaureter with vesicoureteric reflux in twins. *Journal of Urology*, **108**, 635–8.

Teele, R. and Share, L. (1991). *Ultrasonography of infants and children*, pp. 193–213. W. B. Saunders, Philadelphia.

Tobenkin, M. I. (1964). Hereditary vesico-ureteral reflux. *Southern Medical Journal*, **57**, 139–41.

Whittaker, R. H. and Sherwood, T. (1984). For debate: Another look at diagnostic pathways in children with urinary tract infection. *British Medical Journal*, **288**, 839–41.

Whyte, K. M., Abbott, G. D., Kennedy, J. C. and Maling, T. M. J. (1988). Protocol for the investigation of infants and children with urinary tract infection. *Clinical Radiology*, **39**, 278–80.

Winberg, J. (1959). Renal function studies in infants and children with acute non-obstructive urinary tract infections. *Acta Paediatrica Scandinavica*, **48**, 577–89.

Winberg, J., Bollgren, I., Kallenius, G., Mollby, R., and Svenson, S. B. (1982). Clinical pyelonephritis and focal renal scarring: a selected review of pathogenesis prevention and prognosis. *Pediatric Clinics of North America*, **29**, 801–8.

Winter, A. L., Hardy, B. E., and Elton D. J. (1983). Acquired renal scars in children. *Journal of Urology*, **129**, 1190–5.

Wiswell, T. and Roscelli, J. (1986). Collaborative evidence for the decreased incidence of urinary tract infections in circumcised male infants. *Pediatrics*, **78**, 96–9.

Wiswell, T., Smith, F., and Bass, J. (1985). Decreased incidence of urinary tract infections in circumcised male infants. *Pediatric*, **75**, 901–3

Woodward, J. R. and Rushton, G. (1978). Reflux uropathy. *Pediatric Clinics of North America*, **34**, 1349–64.

Yeung, C. K., Dhillon, H. K., Duffy, P. G., and Ransley, P. G. (1991). *Vesico-ureteric reflux in infants with prenatally diagnosed hydronephrosis*. Paper presented at the Annual Meeting of Section of Urology, American Academy of Pediatrics, New Orleans, Louisiana.

Zelikovic, I., Adelman, T., and Nancarrow, P. (1992). Urinary tract infections in children: an update. *Western Journal of Medicine*, **157**, 554–61.

8

Complicated urinary tract infection in adults

Priscilla Kincaid-Smith and Kenneth F. Fairley

Definition

In this chapter 'complicated urinary tract infection' is defined as acute or chronic parenchymal infection associated with a functional or structural urinary tract abnormality. Among functional abnormalities, infection in the immunocompromised transplant recipient is included. Urinary infection in men, which is usually complicated, and infection in other specific conditions, such as diabetes mellitus, are dealt with in other chapters.

Acute pyelonephritis (APN)

Acute pyelonephritis is included in the chapter as a complicated form of urinary tract infection (UTI) because it may cause permanent abnormalities (scarring) in the kidney. In addition, consideration of APN is critical to the remainder of this chapter as this is the form of UTI which usually occurs in patients with structural and functional abnormalities.

Acute pyelonephritis or acute infection of the renal parenchyma is the most common form of complicated urinary infection seen in adults. Formerly, the term 'acute pyelitis' was used to describe infection thought to be confined to the renal pelvis. Renal infection in pregnancy was for many years called 'pyelitis of pregnancy' and the term 'honeymoon pyelitis' was also in common use. This concept of pelvic rather than renal infection in acute pyelonephritis has been finally proven to be incorrect by the demonstration of lesions in the renal parenchyma in many patients with acute renal infection.

The renal lesions, termed 'acute lobar nephronia' by Hodson (Hodson 1978; Rosenfield *et al.* 1979), are areas of renal parenchyma which are heavily infiltrated by inflammatory cells and in which components of the nephron may be completely destroyed. They can be detected by a number of newer imaging techniques including computed tomography (CT), ultrasound (US), and nuclear scanning. In the acute stages, large areas of renal parenchyma may be involved and there is recent evidence that permanent scars may develop in these regions.

Clinical features

Acute pyelonephritis is defined clinically as an acute febrile illness in which loin pain and tenderness are accompanied by pyuria and bacteriuria. The presence of leucocyte or bacterial casts in the urine are virtually diagnostic of acute renal parenchymal infection. Rigors are frequent and reflect bacteraemia. Shortly after the onset of the pyrexia many patients develop generalized symptoms such as headache, nausea, and vomiting. Dysuria and frequency may or may not accompany these symptoms.

Factors which predispose to the development of renal infection are found on intravenous urograms (IVU) in about a third of women who present with symptoms of APN. Two-thirds of men who present in this way have either a radiographic abnormality or have prostatitis as a predisposing factor. Pregnancy should always be considered as a possible underlying factor in young women (Chapter 9).

In adults with APN, reflux nephropathy and renal calculi are the most frequent lesions found on an IVU together accounting for about half the abnormalities. The prevalence of vesicoureteric reflux (VUR) in adults presenting with APN has not been adequately studied. Williams *et al.* (1968) studied women who had had bacteriuria during pregnancy and persisting *Escherichia coli* infection 4 to 6 months after delivery, and reported VUR in two-thirds of these women. It is of particular interest that over half the women with VUR had no renal parenchymal scars so that many adult patients with APN and normal IVU could nonetheless have underlying VUR or occult reflux nephropathy as a predisposing factor (Becker and Kincaid-Smith 1993). Data which suggests this view were presented at the International Nephrology Congress in Jerusalem in June 1993 (Wankowicz *et al.* 1993). These authors investigated 80 adults with recurrent UTI for the presence of VUR and documented this in 61 (76 per cent). This is a higher figure than was reported by Williams *et al.* (1968), but these two studies, taken in conjunction with the documentation of cortical scarring in adults after APN, suggest that the prevalence and role of VUR needs to be carefully reassessed in adults with urinary infection.

Microbiological findings

Escherichia coli is the infecting organism in most cases of APN. It is frequently stated that *E. coli* is isolated in over 80 per cent of cases. In a recent prospective study of 164 consecutive adults presenting with APN, *E. coli* was found in only 69 per cent (Fraser *et al.* 1995). *Escherichia coli* is probably more common in children with acute pyelonephritis.

There has been considerable recent interest in the influence of bacterial adherence and P-fimbriae on *E. coli* on the site of UTI. Fowler and Stamey (1977) and Svanborg-Edén *et al.* (1976) independently identified the importance of bacterial adherence as a step in the initiation of symptomatic UTI. The property of bacterial adherence has been shown to be due to the presence of fimbriae.

P-fimbriae were found in 91 per cent of children with APN, whereas they were present in only 19 per cent of children with cystitis, and 14 per cent with asymptomatic bacteriuria (Kallenius *et al.* 1981). Studies in adults have confirmed the association of P-fimbriae and APN (Fraser *et al.* 1995). In this study, however, the presence of P-fimbriae did not correlate with parenchymal lesions of acute lobar nephronia nor did the presence of type 1 fimbriae. We found that a new cultural characteristic not previously reported, namely inhibition of *E. coli* growth by EDTA, was highly predictive of the development of acute renal parenchymal lesions.

Renal function in acute pyelonephritis

Perhaps because of the focal nature of the lesions it is unusual to see significant deterioration of renal excretory function in APN but formal studies of alterations in this do not appear to have been done. Occasionally, the septicaemia that accompanies APN is associated with severe acute renal failure and acute tubular necrosis.

Impaired concentrating capacity has been emphasized as a feature of renal infection in children. Although this has been confirmed in adults (Ronald *et al.* 1969), not all studies have demonstrated the abnormality (Fairley 1971).

Imaging in acute pyelonephritis

Following the description by Hodson and his colleagues of the lesions of acute lobar nephronia (Hodson 1978; Rosenfield *et al.* 1979), several studies have confirmed the presence of parenchymal lesions on CT scans in APN. The study of Meyrier *et al.* (1989) using CT scans demonstrated lesions in 80 per cent of adults with this disorder. In a few patients, chronic scarring was demonstrated 6–12 months later.

Gallium and dimercaptosuccinic acid (DMSA) nuclear scans have been used mainly in children to document the lesions in APN (Hurwitz *et al.* 1976; Stoller and Kogan 1986). The latter method has been shown to be highly specific (99 per cent) and sensitive (91 per cent) for the detection of the parenchymal lesions in experimental APN in the pig (Majd and Rushton 1992). In a prospective study of 164 consecutive adults presenting with APN, 55 per cent of those with no pre-existing lesions had acute parenchymal lesions demonstrated on CT or DMSA scans, or, both during the acute illness. Abnormalities persisted as scars 3–6 months after the acute episode in 77 per cent of these patients (Fraser *et al.* 1995).

Ultrasonography (US) has also been used to demonstrate parenchymal lesions in APN (Funston *et al.* 1982) but CT and DMSA scans are probably the most accurate methods for detecting the acute lesions and for studying their persistence as scars.

Treatment of acute pyelonephritis

It has been standard practice to admit patients to hospital for treatment of APN and this is still necessary in many cases where generalized signs and symptoms, such as nausea and vomiting, necessitate parenteral treatment.

Many different antibiotics have been used to eradicate the infection in acute pyelonephritis but treatment with gentamicin and ampicillin, both of which have been available for 30 years, is still the recommended treatment in many centres (Forland 1991). We were unable to document any advantage of the new drugs, aztreonam or imipenim-cilastin, over conventional treatment with gentamicin and ampicillin in a prospective randomized trial of treatment in 164 consecutive adults presenting with APN (Fraser *et al.* 1995).

Stamm *et al.* (1987) have advocated oral administration of antibacterial agents in the treatment of APN. In the current climate of cost constraints in health care this has much to commend it particularly in early cases. Stamm compared oral administration of trimethoprim-sulphamethazole and ampicillin in a prospective study and demonstrated a far higher relapse rate due to resistant organisms following ampicillin treatment. In the same study, he showed that two weeks treatment was as effective as six weeks treatment, confirming an earlier study (Kincaid-Smith and Fairley 1969).

Table 8.1 summarizes the treatment used in APN.

Renal and perinephric abscess

Evolution of renal abscesses

Many patients who develop abscesses within the renal parenchyma have underlying predisposing causes, the most frequent being diabetes and renal calculi

Table 8.1 Treatment of acute pyelonephritis

Common pathogens	Antibacterial treatment
Escherichia coli	*Mild symptoms*
Klebsiella pneumoniae	14-day oral treatment with:
Enterococci	Trimethoprim-sulphamethoxazole
Proteus spp.	Fluoroquinolones
Pseudomonas spp.	Ampicillin-clavulanate
Staphylococci	*Severe symptoms with vomiting*
	5-day parenteral treatment with:
	Gentamicin with ampicillin
Ureaplasma urealyticum	Ceftriaxone
Requires tetracyline treatment	Fluoroquinolones
	Aztreonam
	Imipenem-cilastatin
	Trimethoprim-sulphamethoxazole
	Ticarcillin-clavulanate
	Followed by 14-day oral treatment with:
	Trimethoprim-sulphamethoxazole or fluoroquinolones

(Thorley *et al.* 1974). However, it is likely that the localized parenchymal lesions of acute lobar nephronia which are now known to develop in many cases of APN can evolve into abscesses if they are not adequately treated. These parenchymal lesions were observed in 55 per cent of the study by Fraser *et al.* (1995) but in an even higher percentage of the cases reported by Meyrier *et al.* (1989), which included patients with abscess formation. As the latter series was patients referred to a nephrology unit and the former consecutive patients, most of whom were otherwise healthy young women presenting to an emergency department of a major hospital, Meyrier's series would be expected to include more serious cases. They included nine diabetics and four malnourished alcoholics. They do not make specific mention of the criteria used for the clinical or CT diagnosis of abscess formation but, in two of the diabetics the clinical condition was so serious that a nephrectomy was performed as a life-saving procedure. In the pathological description of the kidneys removed 'several abscesses were noted one of which extended into the perinephric fat'. A further indication that abscess formation and APN may represent stages in the evolution of localized parenchymal lesions is seen in the report of June *et al.* (1985). Their evaluation of 28 patients presenting with APN revealed renal abscesses or focal bacterial nephritis in four. Again, they do not define clearly what they mean by 'renal abscess'. None of the 164 consecutive cases of Fraser *et al.* (1995) showed clinical or CT evidence of renal abscess formation but all were treated within a few days of the onset of symptoms.

There is no doubt that the availability of antibacterial treatment has greatly reduced the incidence of renal abscess formation as a complication of acute pyelonephritis. Such lesions were frequent in autopsies done prior to 1945 but rarely observed between 1950 and 1955 (Kincaid-Smith, unpublished data). The fact that we encountered no abscesses diagnosed on CT scans or clinical grounds among 164 consecutive unselected cases of acute pyelonephritis and that Meyrier identified only a small number among 55 referred cases, a quarter of whom were in a high-risk category, also demonstrates that renal abscess formation has become a rare condition, at least in the Western World.

Clinical features and diagnosis

Presenting features in renal abscess formation are similar to those in patients with APN but the features are more severe and last longer. In addition, a renal mass may be present in about one-third of cases. Blood cultures are positive in up to 50 per cent of cases and features of septicaemia are often present. Resolution is slow with fever lasting 7 days or longer and a loin mass and pyuria persisting beyond 5 days, contrasting with most cases of APN, which show clinical resolution within 3 to 4 days.

There has been a resurgence of interest in renal abscess formation with the advent of newer imaging techniques, particularly CT scanning and US. However, although these techniques permit localization of the lesions much more accurately than was previously possible, the features that distinguish acute lobar nephronia from abscess formation using the newer imaging techniques have not been clearly stated.

Recent studies indicate that haematogenous Gram-positive infections are now rarely encountered as a cause of renal abscess. Almost all cases are associated with Gram-negative urinary tract pathogens (Morgan *et al.* 1985; June *et al.* 1985). Although the clinical features of established abscess formation may be similar whether they occur as a complication of UTI or as a result of haematogenous spread, the clinical context in which the latter cases develop are quite different. Haematogenous spread occurs in association with an infected site most commonly within the bloodstream such as an infected shunt, intravascular catheter, or endocarditis. The renal abscesses may be multiple and bilateral.

Treatment includes elimination of the source of infection as well as treatment aimed at the renal lesions. The choice of antibiotics will be different because of the dissimilar nature of the infecting organism in haematogenous cases.

Perinephric abscess

In the same way as acute lobar nephronia may evolve into abscess formation if untreated or in the presence of some complicating factor, it is likely that perinephric abscess formation represents evolution of a renal parenchymal abscess in which the abscess extends into the perinephric fat. Perinephric abscesses are most commonly reported in diabetes and as a complication of renal calculi. They have a high mortality and require surgical intervention. In a review 20 years ago, Thorley *et al.* (1974) reported results in 52 cases and the mortality rate was 50 per cent. One-third of cases were diagnosed at autopsy. Many cases show predisposing factors to abscess formation, the most frequent of these being diabetes and stag-horn calculi. Calculi were present in 25 per cent of the series reported by Thorley *et al.* (1974).

Treatment of renal and perinephric abscesses

Although the treatment of abscess formation within the kidney involves the use of the same group of antibacterial agents as those used in APN, the patients will always require parenteral treatment in hospital. Treatment with gentamicin and ampicillin will cover most urinary tract pathogens but if the response to treatment is not associated with improvement in clinical features, including resolution of the fever, addition of one of the newer agents, such as imipenem-cilastin, aztreonam, parenteral fluoroquinolones, or cephtriaxone may be indicated. Treatment of 10–14 days is indicated. However, if clinical features are improving it may be possible to give a week of parenteral treatment followed by appropriate oral medication. It is very important to ensure that the urine is sterile during treatment and that it remains sterile a week after ceasing treatment. In the presence of renal calculi it may be impossible to eradicate infection.

Because the mortality is so high with perinephric abscesses, early percutaneous drainage or other surgical intervention is necessary in addition to appropriate intravenous antibiotic therapy.

Reflux nephropathy (RN)

The commonest structural abnormality encountered in adults with UTI is reflux nephropathy. This condition is often clearly recognizable from its characteristic radiological parenchymal scars. These were present in 7.3 per cent of an unselected series of consecutive cases presenting to the emergency department at the Royal Melbourne Hospital (Fraser *et al.* 1995). The question has already been raised as to whether vesicoureteric reflux (VUR) may be a much more frequent underlying lesion in adults with UTI than is acknowledged at this time. Very few studies in adults have looked routinely for the presence of VUR. In the two studies where this has been done, both detected VUR in a high percentage of patients. Williams *et al.* (1968) found VUR in 66 per cent of women who had persisting *E. coli* infection after pregnancy bacteriuria. In addition, a recent study from Poland (Wankowicz *et al.* 1993) demonstrated VUR in 76 per cent of adults with recurrent UTI. In the Williams *et al.* (1968) study, 50 per cent of the women had VUR without parenchymal scars. These data fit very well with our own histological data, which suggest that some 10 per cent of patients presenting with proteinuria but with no radiological scars have histological features of RN on renal biopsy (Kincaid-Smith 1983). We have investigated our patients further and found that displacement of the ureteric orifice was similar to that found in patients with proven RN (Becker and Kincaid-Smith 1993).

Reflux nephropathy is so clearly associated with urinary infection that in the past it was called chronic pyelonephritis. The role of VUR and infection in scar formation is now very well established and the exact sequence of events was elegantly demonstrated in the pig by Hodson *et al.* (1975). Hodson postulated and subsequently proved that intra-renal reflux with infected urine led to scar formation in childhood (Hodson 1971, 1978).

In adults with persisting VUR further focal scar formation has rarely been documented. We have occasionally observed scars after an episode of acute symptomatic pyelonephritis but it did not appear to be a major contributing factor to progressive scar formation in adults.

Recent evidence that cortical scars may form after areas of 'acute lobar nephronia' have been identified on CT scans raises the question as to how many of these adults may have underlying VUR. 'Acute lobar nephronia' and subsequent scarring was originally described in the context of VUR (Hodson, 1971, 1975; Hodson *et al.* 1978). It has, however, been accepted that progressive renal failure in adults with RN is more clearly associated with proteinuria and a progressive glomerular lesion that does not appear to be linked to infection (Kincaid-Smith 1975*a*).

Both symptomatic and asymptomatic urinary infection are common in patients with underlying radiological lesions of RN. Unilateral RN is listed below as a cause of persisting infection but, although this does occur, it is rare. Occasionally, we have seen it in patients with small kidneys, with dilated pelvicalyceal systems, parenchymal thinning, and poor renal function on that side. Perhaps this does not allow adequate concentrations of antibacterial agent to be concentrated in the urine on the side of the small kidney.

When recurrent episodes of APN occur in a patient with RN they do not differ significantly from those in patients without RN and should be promptly treated as they should in any patient with APN (Table 8.1).

Much more difficult questions arise as to the role of asymptomatic bacteriuria as a cause of progressive renal impairment in patients with RN and whether asymptomatic bacteriuria should be treated. We have shown that in both pregnant and non-pregnant women the site of asymptomatic infection is very likely to be renal if there is an underlying radiological abnormality such as RN (Fairley *et al.* 1966; Fairley 1971). In such patients it is difficult to document that progressive deterioration of renal function is associated with persistent or recurrent renal infection (Bullen and Kincaid-Smith 1971).

Where there is pyuria, even with a sterile urine, deterioration of renal function is more frequently observed. Some of the patients who deteriorated had occult infection documented as a cause of the pyuria (Fairley and Butler 1971). Studies aimed at determining if upper tract infection arises within the renal parenchyma or is limited to the renal pelvis have supported the likelihood that the renal parenchyma is infected (Whitworth *et al.* 1974).

We have also noted an association between impaired renal function and infection with *Ureaplasma urealyticum* in patients with RN (Birch *et al.* 1981). Such data as are available for Ureaplasma infection suggest that this can be a chronic renal parenchymal infection and positive cultures can be obtained from aspirates from the renal parenchyma (Birch *et al.* 1981).

Cystic disease of the kidney (ADPK)

Polycystic disease of the kidney

Autosomal-dominant polycystic kidney disease (ADPK) occurs throughout the world and is one of the commonest inherited diseases. It accounts for some 10 per cent of cases of end-stage renal failure.

Urinary tract infection (UTI) is the most frequent complication seen in ADPK. Most cases are symptomatic but sterile pyuria is frequently present in asymptomatic cases and may cause difficulties in confirming the diagnosis of urinary infection. The cause of the sterile pyuria has not been elucidated. It has been reported in some 30–50 per cent of cases in different series and may reflect the stage of the disease. Two groups of cases are most likely to show persistent pyuria: (1) those with impaired renal function, and (2) those with recurrent urinary infection.

Sterile pyuria, like UTI, is more common in women (Sklar *et al.* 1987). Young men and women detected through screening for ADPK usually have no pyuria and in the absence of overt urinary infection the urine may remain relatively normal or perhaps show a cast count which is slightly above the normal of 50 per ml. In males, the urine often remains normal for years but if young women develop recurrent episodes of acute pyelonephritis (APN) the urine may, between episodes, show pyuria which may then become persistent. We have searched carefully in some of these patients for evidence of an underlying infection due to anaerobic, slow-growing, or fastidious organisms, but failed to find this evidence. There is no doubt, however, that the pyuria is more likely to be found when recurrent infection has been present in the past suggesting that there is some link between infection and pyuria. The cells in the urine are predominantly polymorphonuclear leucocytes.

Acute pyelonephritis is the usual form of symptomatic UTI encountered in ADPK. It is far more common in women than in men (Schwab *et al.* 1987). It may be severe and life-threatening. Instrumentation of the urinary tract has been identified as an important factor predisposing to APN (Delaney *et al.* 1985). In this study, 50 per cent of patients who developed APN after instrumentation died.

Following an episode of APN the symptoms and signs may persist and be refractory to antibiotic treatment. This usually indicates that infection has become established in one or more cysts in the kidney. Occasionally, severe symptoms are clearly localized to one cyst and may require either aspiration of the purulent contents of the cyst or surgical drainage of the abscess cavity.

Because it can be difficult to treat infection within one or more cysts in the kidney it is particularly important to treat any infection with a bactericidal drug and one which penetrates cyst fluid, in an attempt to eradicate the organism. Selection of an appropriate antibacterial drug is critical to the success of treatment if an infected cyst is suspected. The two drugs that have been regarded as standard treatment for APN (gentamicin and ampicillin), both penetrate cysts poorly and are therefore not the treatment of choice when APN complicates ADPK. Lipid soluble antibiotics penetrate cysts better and should be used to eradicate the infection. Those that are effective against most urinary tract pathogens and which penetrate cysts well are ciprofloxacin, norfloxacin, trimethoprim-sulphomethoxazole, and chloramphenicol (Bennett 1985).

Renal calculi are a common complication of ADPK. Although it has been suggested that a low urinary citrate excretion may predispose to calculi in ADPK, almost all the renal calculi which we encounter are infection stones associated with urea-splitting organisms. These are managed in the same way as other infection stones. If indicated, lithotripsy can be used safely in ADPK.

Infected cysts in the native kidneys may present a difficult and even dangerous complication after renal transplantation when recurrent infection and septicaemia may necessitate nephrectomy of the infected kidney. Patients may require (full-dose) suppressive treatment to prevent recurrent episodes of infection.

Medullary sponge kidney

In this condition, there is dilatation of collecting ducts in one or more papillae. UTI is one of the most common complications of medullary sponge kidney. It may occur in patients who have cysts alone or when the cysts are accompanied by nephrolithiasis. In the latter, it is more difficult to eradicate infection.

Urinary infection is usually renal and accompanied by the clinical features of APN. The area of cortex involved may be quite small but when such kidneys are examined at autopsy they have streaks of scars radiating out from the medulla to the surface of the kidney, which are from previous episodes of UTI (Kincaid-Smith 1975*b*). Ekstrom *et al.* (1959) in a comprehensive review estimated that 11 per cent of patients developed 'chronic pyelonephritis' but we have seen scars at autopsy in all five kidneys which we have examined.

Other cystic conditions

Infection may occur in association with any cysts in the kidney. They are commonly seen in cysts, such as a calyceal diverticulum that communicates with the pelvis, and rarely seen in simple cysts whether these are single or multiple.

Bacterial persistence

There are certain structural abnormalities which make it impossible to eradicate infection from the urinary tract unless the structural abnormality is first corrected. Whenever infection with the same organism persists after appropriate antibacterial treatment the presence of one of these underlying structural abnormalities should be suspected. Table 8.2 lists the causes of bacterial

Table 8.2 Causes of bacterial persistence

Infected renal calculi
Chronic bacterial prostatitis
Unilateral infected reflux nephropathy
Infected calcyceal diverticula
Infected non-refluxing ureteric stump
Medullary sponge kidneys
Infected necrotic papillae
Infected urachal cysts
Vesicovaginal fistulae
Vesicointestinal fistulae
Ectopic ureter draining dysplastic renal segment
Foreign body

Adapted with permission from T. A. Stamey (1980).

persistence. This list includes all the surgically curable causes of bacterial persistence. Some, such as medullary sponge kidneys, cannot be treated surgically. In the case of infected ureteric stump, infected urachal cyst, vesicovaginal and vesicointestinal fistulae, ectopic ureter draining a dysplastic segment, and foreign body, the treatment lies so clearly in the field of the urologist that they will not be discussed further here but will be covered in Chapter 12. It is important, however, to identity the cause because this will always be found to explain bacterial persistence. Some, like the ectopic ureter draining a poorly functioning dysplastic renal segment, may be missed over many years unless carefully investigated. Newer imaging techniques, such as CT and US scans, facilitate the diagnosis. Some of the cases included in Table 8.2, in which the infection cannot be eradicated, may require continuous (full-dose) suppressive antibiotic treatment in order to prevent troublesome recurrent acute pyelonephritis and to prevent the development and growth of infection calculi.

The two most frequent causes of bacterial persistence are infected renal calculi and chronic bacterial prostatitis. The latter clearly belongs in Chapter 13 but the former is a common and important cause of complicated UTI, which warrants discussion in this chapter as well as in Chapter 12.

Infected renal calculi

Infected renal calculi may present with symptoms related to calculi or with symptoms of complicated UTI. Renal calculi of any chemical composition may be associated with episodes of infection but few present significant management problems unless there is associated obstruction. The importance of recognizing the presence of infection is that obstruction may be present and an infected obstructed kidney is a medical emergency because the patient runs a significant risk of developing septicaemia. Both the infection and the obstruction must be treated or treatment of the infection will fail.

Although renal calculi may be associated with any type of bacterial infection the classic and most troublesome association is that of struvite or magnesium ammonium phosphate calculi with urea-splitting bacteria, most commonly *Proteus mirabilis.* Other organisms which may split urea include Klebsiella, Staphylococci, and *Ureaplasma urealyticum.* All may cause struvite or magnesium ammonium phosphate stone formation. The significance of the presence of urea-splitting organisms is that they produce a highly alkaline urine of pH 7.2 or above in which struvite readily precipitates. By this mechanism large stones may form quite quickly and classically these calculi are of stag-horn type in the renal pelvis or assume the shape of the bladder as they enlarge in the bladder.

The association of struvite stones with *P. mirabilis* has been known for many years and also the very high recurrence rate of these calculi after surgery. A recurrence rate of 50–100 per cent often discouraged surgeons from operating on large stag-horn stones in the renal pelvis. Proteus and other urea-splitting organisms become incorporated within the substance of the calculus which makes them impossible to eradicate. Hellstrom (1938) was able to stain bacteria deep within the substance of the stone and Nemoy and Stamey (1971) demonstrated conclusively that bacteria could be cultured from calculi and from fragments of struvite. Even after complete removal of the calculus, positive cultures persist because the pelvis of the kidney or the bladder may be studded with fragments of struvite from which the bacteria can be cultured. Nemoy and Stamey demonstrated that infusion of renacidin dissolved the calculi and struvite deposits and thus allowed cure of the infection. They also showed that quite large calculi could be dissolved by renacidin. Although newer methods of removing stones by percutaneous techniques or shattering them by extra-corporeal shockwave lithotripsy (ESWL) have removed the need for open surgery in most cases, they have not resolved the all-important question of persistence of infection. On a re-visit to a busy lithotripsy unit I was shown a patient being treated for his fourth recurrent stag-horn struvite stone. No attempt had been made to eradicate infection between the lithotripsy treatments so that the continuing recurrences of calculi could be confidently predicted. Lithotripsy in the presence of infection may cause severe acute pyelonephritis and septicaemia. The use of percutaneous renacidin after lithotripsy to remove small stone fragments and those which invariably coat the pelvic mucosa is strongly advocated in cases of stag-horn struvite calculi to allow the eradication of infection and to prevent stone recurrence.

These newer techniques of removal of calculi percutaneously or by lithotripsy can be carried out in almost any patient except perhaps in a very frail individual or one with a serious coagulation disorder. Because procedures for removal of calculi are rarely contraindicated, continuing medical management of the persistent infection in patients with struvite stones is much less frequent than in the past. In patients who do require continuing full-dose suppressive antibacterial treatment if very large calculi are present, it may prove impossible to sterilize the urine because of the sheer bulk of the calculus. Stamey attributes this to the phenomenon of 'critical density' encountered in antibiotic sensitivity-testing (Stamey 1980). Except in the case of very large calculi, the urine can be maintained sterile using full-dose suppressive antibiotic therapy. It is important to do this, not only to prevent recurrent episodes of acute pyelonephritis, but because if the urine remains infected the calculi will continue to grow due to further struvite deposition. Inevitably, as they grow they cause obstruction initially in individual calyces but eventually of all the calyces and the pelviureteric junction. This is how stag-horn calculi cause end-stage renal failure. When obstruction has been present for months then this potentially preventable cause of renal failure becomes irreversible.

Renal papillary necrosis

There are two distinct types of renal papillary necrosis in which UTI is an important associated feature.

The first is an acute form of renal papillary necrosis which is frequently a terminal event. In this, the kidneys are of normal size and the papillae undergo acute necrosis. Acute renal failure accompanies acute renal papillary necrosis if the lesion is bilateral, as it usually is. This type of renal papillary necrosis is associated with severe acute pyelonephritic lesions which are often widespread in the renal parenchyma. If the lesion is unilateral, recovery may occur but nonetheless this condition has most commonly been identified at autopsy. This acute form of renal papillary necrosis may occur in diabetics and was first described in association with UTI and prostatic obstruction (Mandel 1952).

The second form of renal papillary necrosis is much more relevant from a clinical perspective. This is because it is a chronic lesion in which UTI is present over many years and may be difficult or impossible to eradicate because the bacteria are inaccessible to antibacterial drugs within necrotic papillary tissue.

The commonest clinical context in which this occurs is analgesic nephropathy but chronic renal papillary necrosis is sometimes associated with other conditions such as sickle-cell disease. Persisting infection is frequently present and is a constant threat because at any time one or more necrotic papillae may become detached and cause ureteric obstruction. The infected obstructed kidney may then cause fatal septicaemia. Such septicaemic episodes have been recorded as a frequent cause of death in analgesic nephropathy (Kincaid-Smith *et al.* 1971). With episodes of infection and obstruction, the kidney may develop extensive parenchymal lesions of the type described above in acute pyelonephritis and have the distribution of 'acute lobar nephronia'. This process leads to progressive loss of renal function and parenchymal scarring.

Treatment with parenteral antibiotics is necessary in the acute episodes but, in addition, it is often necessary to use continuous full–dose suppressive treatment to prevent recurrent episodes of acute pyelonephritis and to prevent the formation and growth of struvite infection stones (Stamey 1980).

Neurological disorders and urinary tract infection

Many neurological diseases affect bladder function and may predispose to infection. Function may be abnormal in diseases affecting the brain, spinal cord, or peripheral innervation of the bladder. These diseases may cause incontinence or inability to empty the bladder and the bladder may be flaccid or spastic. They may also be responsible for the generation of very high pressures in the bladder associated with detrusor hyper-reflexia (Arnold *et al.* 1984). This may in turn cause high-pressure vesicoureteric reflux (VUR) and transmission of potentially infected urine to the renal pelvis under high pressure. VUR has been demonstrated in a high percentage of both high- and low-pressure neurogenic bladders. Damanski (1965) found that 28 per cent of reflex bladders showed reflux but also so did 19 per cent of flaccid bladders. Scarring of the renal parenchyma identical to that seen in reflux nephropathy and with infected renal calculi is frequently seen in association with infection and intra-renal reflux in the neurogenic bladder (Arnold *et al.* 1984).

Several factors may redispose to infection in such patients, the most important being failure to empty the bladder, bladder catheterization, and instrumentation. Intermittent catheterization is often necessary and is usually performed at 3-hourly intervals in the acute stage after spinal cord injury. In the latter group, which represents a particular challenge in terms of prevention of infection, even with rigorous attention to an aseptic technique it may not be possible to avoid urinary infection. The work of Pearman and England (1973) must be acknowledged here. Using an instillation of 150 mg of kanamycin and 30 mg of colistin they achieved a remarkably low incidence of infection in patients with paraplegia (0.56 per cent in men and 0.97 per cent in women). Although their methods were published over 20 years ago they seem to have attracted surprisingly little attention. Pearman's method or similar methods of preventing infection in patients with bladder dysfunction resulting from neurological disorders appears to be used infrequently.

UTI is usually renal in patients with neurological lesions, particularly when high bladder pressures or VUR are present. The neurological lesion may be such that renal pain is absent, thus depriving the clinician of loin pain as an important symptom indicating the presence of pyelonephritis. In the presence of fever, heavy pyuria, and bacteriuria it is likely that the patient has acute pyelonephritis. The presence of leucocyte and bacterial casts are useful in confirming the diagnosis.

Progressive deterioration in function in the case of the neurogenic bladder can clearly be attributed to the presence of recurrent UTI whether VUR is present or not. The formation of infection stones in some 12 per cent of cases within three years (Jacobson and Bors 1970) and obstruction by these stones is a further cause of deterioration of renal function. The prevention of infection and renal scarring, which results from infection, presents a great challenge because these patients often have resistant urinary pathogens as well as many other, sometimes bizarre, organisms which are introduced by catheterization and instrumentation. Even when infection is due to organisms that are sensitive to antibacterial drugs long term (full-dose) suppressive treatment is frequently required. It is not surprising, in view of difficulties in treating infection in these patients, that they often require dialysis or die of renal failure.

In children with myelodysplasia, as in other forms of neuropathic bladder, UTI and VUR are common. In cases with a thoracolumbar meningomyelocoele an ileal or other form of conduit is commonly performed.

Urinary tract infection and urinary tract diversion

An ileal conduit or other form of pouch is frequently used in patients with neurological lesions accompanied by high bladder pressures such as myelodysplasia. The aim of this diversion is to prevent progressive renal damage which otherwise occurs in association with detrusor hyper-reflexia.

Unfortunately, patients with an ileal conduit commonly have persistent or recurrent UTI, which may be complicated by episodes of acute pyelonephritis, and are often complicated by infection stone formation. Unless infection is controlled in these patients they develop progressive deterioration of renal function due to a combination of obstruction by renal and ureteric calculi and parenchymal lesions of acute pyelonephritis (Price *et al.* 1975).

The principles of treating recurrent infection in these patients are the same as those for other infections. If they show a relapse with the same organism soon after a course of antibiotics then they will usually require long-term suppressive treatment with full doses of antibacterial drugs. Using long-term treatment in such patients with occasional monitoring of the urinary findings, it is often possible to keep the urine sterile and sometimes even free of pyuria for many years (Pearman 1976). This prevents the recurrent episodes of acute pyelonephritis, which can be so debilitating in this group of patients, and also prevents the formation of renal calculi and progressive deterioration of renal function.

Xanthogranulomatous pyelonephritis (XGPN)

This condition, previously regarded as rare, is being recognized with increasing frequency because of the use of new imaging techniques. It occurs mainly in association with Proteus spp. UTI and infection calculi. It is most frequent in women who are also far more likely than men to develop UTI and infection stones. The clinical presentation is with fever, malaise, loin pain, and a mass. The mass may be mistaken for a renal carcinoma and the affected kidney often shows no function on an intravenous pyelogram (IVP). About 80 per cent of the patients will have an associated infection stone, often a stag-horn calculus. The distinction can be made on CT scanning but previously these kidneys were often removed as suspected tumours.

Pathologically, the kidney frequently shows dilatation of the pelvis and calcyes due to the associated calculi which are commonly obstructive. The xanthogranulomatous tissue is rubbery and yellow in colour and may be haemorrhagic. Microscopically it consists of foam-filled macrophages. Essentially, this condition appears to be a chronic granulomatous infection of the kidney. It is almost always unilateral but, if bilateral, causes renal failure.

Treatment has usually been nephrectomy. No data could be found to suggest that removal of the calculus, thus removing the obstruction, and eradication of the accompanying infection, leads to resolution of the condition with a return of renal function but it is reasonable to anticipate that this might occur.

Malacoplakia

This condition, like xanthogranulomatous pyelonephritis, occurs most frequently in women and particularly those in middle age. It most commonly affects the bladder where it causes raised yellow-brown mucosal plaques. It less frequently involves the kidney and rarely other organs such as the gastrointestinal tract, lung, and skin (McClure 1983).

The lesions of malacoplakia are in some respects similar to those of xanthogranulomatous pyelonephritis and some have suggested that it is a different manifestation of the same chronic granulomatous process.

Clinically, there is usually a history of chronic UTI and both loin pain and urinary tract obstruction are present in both conditions. Malacoplakia is usually associated with *E. coli* UTI. The pathology is in some respects similar to xanthogranulomatous pyelonephritis in that the plaques in the bladder or renal pelvis consist of collections of large foamy macrophages, many of which contain a distinctive inclusion called a Michaelis–Gutmann body. This lamellar structure contains iron, and stains well with periodic acid–Schiff stains.

In the kidney it may be confined to the pelvis or massively involve the renal parenchyma. Treatment has been surgical removal.

Urinary tract infection after renal transplantation

Urinary tract infection is common after renal transplantation and screening studies have shown that bacteriuria is present in 50–60 per cent of cases (Leigh 1969; Ramsey *et al.* 1979). Factors which predispose to UTI soon after transplantation are infection in the donor kidney (McCoy *et al.* 1975), catheterization of the bladder in the early post-operative period, and infection within the native kidneys of the recipient. The last factor may also lead to later infection in transplant kidneys (Douglas *et al.* 1974).

There is potential for reducing the rate of infection from all these sources. If the urine of the donor kidney is routinely cultured most infections, which are transmitted in the donor kidney, can be anticipated and treated before infection becomes established. Catheter-induced infections acquired in the early post-graft period can be considerably reduced by closed-system irrigation of the bladder with a bacteriostatic agent such as chlorhexidine (Clark and Grossley 1973). Pearman and England's (1973) technique of instilling antibacterial drugs after catheterization can also be applied in renal transplant patients to prevent infection.

Infection from lesions in the native kidneys of the recipient is not quite so easily prevented. It occurs mainly in kidneys where the infection is difficult or impossible to eradicate. In our experience, the lesions which have proved most troublesome are renal papillary necrosis, polycystic kidneys with infected cysts, and infected renal calculi. The presence of relapsing infections from these sources in the post-transplant period constitutes a serious threat to the transplant patient. They may cause septicaemia and even death and often necessitate continuous suppressive antibacterial treatment. There may be some justification for bilateral nephrectomy in such cases although this has been abandoned as a routine pre-transplant procedure because of the high associated mortality.

Other factors which predispose to urinary infection after transplantation are the use of immunosuppressive drugs, the presence of vesicoureteric reflux and urological complications of transplantation surgery such as obstruction, fistula formation, and ischaemic necrosis of the ureter. Infection is almost always present in such cases.

After transplantation, urinary infection is often asymptomatic. However, it should be treated because at any time an asymptomatic infection can become a life-threatening acute pyelonephritis accompanied by septicaemia.

Early in our transplantation programme we had a high rate of vesicoureteric reflux into the transplant ureter (Mathew *et al.* 1977). At that time, we frequently encountered severe acute pyelonephritis in the transplanted kidney. We demonstrated, in transplant nephrectomy specimens, that such episodes of acute pyelonephritis were followed by large parenchymal scars with the distribution of 'lobar nephronia' (Kincaid-Smith 1975*b*). Now that an anti-reflux procedure is carried out at the time of the ureteric anastomosis we hardly ever encounter such cases.

There has been a suggestion that urinary infections. particularly with *Streptococcus faecalis*, may lead to graft rejection (Byrd *et al.* 1978). This theory has not been fully substantiated.

The principles of treatment of bacterial urinary infection after renal transplantation do not differ from those in other situations except that it is desirable to treat asymptomatic infection.

Fungal urinary tract infections may occur and are discussed in Chapter 15.

There has been considerable interest in cytomegalovirus (CMV) infection in renal transplant recipients both because it constitutes a major clinical problem and because of its possible impact on rejection of the kidney. Richardson *et al.* (1981) reported a glomerulopathy associated with CMV infection in transplants and there had been prior reports of immune complex glomerulonephritis in CMV infections (Stagno *et al.* 1977). Patients with CMV infection show a continuing decline in renal function (Baldwin *et al.* 1983), which may affect the long-term outcome of the transplant (Luby *et al.* 1983). Baldwin's group have proposed that the immunological abnormalities that they demonstrated during CMV infection (i.e. IgM lymphocytotoxins) may be under genetic control.

CMV infection can be treated with the new antiviral agent, gangcyclovir, and this drug also offers some hope of prevention of infection. The best results in preventing CMV infection after transplantation have been achieved with a solution of human anti-CMV immunoglobulin (Cytotect). This has been used with success in heart, bone marrow, and renal transplants (Fassbinder *et al.* 1986).

References

Arnold, E. P., Fukui, J., Anthony, A., and Utley, W. L. F. (1984). Bladder function following spinal cord injury: A urodynamic analysis of outcome. *British Journal of Urology*, **56**, 172–7.

Baldwin, W. M., Class, F. H., and Van Ess, A. (1983). Renal graft dysfunction during infection with cytomegalovirus: Association with IgM Iymphocytotoxins. *British Medical Journal*, **287**, 1332–4.

Becker, G. J. and Kincaid-Smith, P. (1993). Reflux nephropathy: The glomerular lesion and progression of renal failure. *Paediatric Nephrology*, **7**, 365–9.

Bennett, W. E. (1985). General features of autosomal dominant polycystic disease of the kidney: Evaluation and management of renal infection. In *Problems in the diagnosis*, pp. 98–105. PKR Foundation, New York.

Birch, D., Fairley, K. F., and Pavillard, R. (1981). Unconventional bacteria in the urinary tract: *Ureaplasma urealyticum*. *Kidney International*, **19**, 58–64.

Bullen, M. and Kincaid-Smith, P. (1971). Asymptomatic pregnancy bacteriuria. A follow-up study 4–7 years after delivery. In *Renal infection and renal scarring*, (ed. P. Kincaid-Smith and K. F. Fairley), pp. 33–9. Mercedes, Melbourne.

Byrd, L. H., Cheigh, J. S., Stenzel, K. H., Tapia, L., Aronian, J., and Rubin, A. L. (1978). Association between *Streptococcus faecalis* urinary infections and graft rejection in kidney transplantation. *Lancet*, **2**, 1167–9.

Clark, A. D. and Grossley, J. (1973). Closed system bladder irrigation and drainage after major vaginal surgery. *Journal of Obstetrics and Gynaecology of the British Empire*, **80**, 271–3.

Damanski, M. (1965). Vesico-ureteric reflux in paraplegics. *British Journal of Surgery*, **52**, 168–77.

Delaney, V. B., *et al.* (1985). Autosomal dominant polycystic disease: Presentation, complications and prognosis. *American Journal of Kidney Diseases*, **5**, 104.

Douglas, J. F., Clarke, S., and Kennedy, J. (1974). Late urinary tract infection after renal transplantation. *Lancet*, **2**, 1015.

Ekstrom, T., Engfeld, B., and Lagergren, C. (1959). *Medullary sponge kidney*. Almqvist & Wiksill, Stockholm.

Fairley, K. F. (1971). The routine determination of the site of infection in the investigation of patients with urinary tract infection. In *renal infection and renal scarring*, (ed P. Kincaid-Smith and K. F. Fairley) pp. 107–16. Mercedes, Melbourne.

Fairley, K. F. and Butler, H. (1971). Sterile pyuria as a manifestation of occult bacterial pyelonephritis with special reference to intermittent bacteriuria. In *Renal infection and renal scarring*, (ed. P. Kincaid-Smith and K. F. Fairley), pp. 51–67. Mercedes, Melbourne.

Fairley, K. F., Bond, A. G., and Adey D. (1966). The site of infection in pregnancy bacteriuria. *Lancet*, **1**, 939–41.

Fassbinder, W., Ernst, W., Hanke P., Bechstein, P. B., Scheurmann, E. H., and Schoeppe, W. (1986). Cytomegaloviris infections after renal transplantation. Effect of a prophylactic hyperimmunoglobulin. *Transplantation Proceedings*, **XVIII**, 1393–6.

Forland, M. (1991). *Urinary tract infection in therapy of renal disease*, (ed. W. N. Suki and S. G. Massry), (2nd edn), pp. 349–62. Kluwer, Boston.

Fowler, J. E. and Stamey T. A. (1977). Studies of introital colonisation in women with recurrent urinary infections. *Journal of Urology*, **117**, 472–6.

Fraser, I. R., Birch, D., Fairley, K. F., Lichtenstein, J. S., Tress, B., and Kincaid-Smith, P. (1995). A prospective study of cortical scarring in acute febrile pyelonephritis in adults: clinical and bacteriological characteristics. *Clinical Nephrology*, **43**, (3), pp. 159–64.

Funston, M. R., Fisher, K. S., Van Blerk, J. P., and Bortz, J. H. (1982). Acute focal bacterial nephritis or renal abcess? A sonographic diagnosis. *British Journal of Urology*, **54**, 461–6.

Hellstrom, J. (1938) The significance of staphylococci in the development and treatment of renal and ureteral stones. *British Journal of Urology*, **101**, 348–72.

Hodson, C. J. (1971) The mechanism of scar formation in chronic pyelonephritis. In *Renal infection and renal scarring*, (ed. P. Kincaid-Smith and K. F. Fairley), pp. 327–9. Mercedes Melbourne.

Hodson, C. J., Maling, T. M., and McManamon, P. J. (1975). The pathogenesis of reflux nephropathy. *British Journal of Radiology*, (Suppl. 13), 1–26.

Hodson C. J. (1978). The pathogenesis of reflux nephropathy. In *Diagnostic radiology*, (ed. A. R. Margulis and C. A Gooding), pp. 95–107. University of California, San Francisco.

Hurwitz, S. R., Kessler, W., Alazraki, N., and Ashburn, W. (1976). Gallium-67 imaging to localize urinary tract infections. *British Journal of Radiology*, **49**, 156–60.

Jacobson, S. A. and Bors, E. (1970). Spinal cord injury in Vietnamese combat. *Paraplegia*, 7, 263.

June, C. H., Browning, M. D., Smith, P., Wenzel, D. J., Pyatt, R. S., and Checchio, L. M. (1985). Ultrasonography and computed tomography in severe urinary tract infection. *Archives of Internal Medicine,* **145**, 841–5.

Kallenius, G., Svenson, S., Hultberg, H., Mollby, R., Helin, I., Cedergren, B., and Winberg, J. (1981). Occurrence of P-fimbriated *Escherichia coli* in urinary tract infections. *Lancet*, **2**, 1369–72.

Kincaid-Smith, P. (1983). Diffuse parenchymal lesions in reflux nephropathy and the possibility of making a renal biopsy diagnosis in reflux nephropathy. In *Contributions to nephrology. Reflux nephropathy update*, (ed. C. J. Hodson, R. H. Heptinstall, and J. Winberg), pp. 111–15. Karger, Basel.

Kincaid-Smith, P. (1975*a*). *The Kidney*, p. 359. Blackwell, Oxford.

Kincaid-Smith, P. (1975*b*). Glomerular lesions in atrophic pyelonephritis and reflux nephropathy. *Kidney International*, **8**, S81–3.

Kincaid-Smith, P. and Fairley, K. F. (1969). Controlled trial comparing effect of two and six weeks' treatment in recurrent urinary tract infection. *British Medical Journal*, **2**, 145–6.

Kincaid-Smith, P., Nanra R. S., and Fairley, K. F. (1971). *Analgesic nephropathy: A recoverable form of renal failure*, In *Renal infection and renal scarring*. (ed. P. Kincaid-Smith and K. F. Fairley), pp. 385–400. Mercedes, Melbourne.

Leigh, D. A. (1969). The outcome of urinary tract infection in patients after human cadaveric renal transplantation. *British Journal of Urology*, **41**, 406–13.

Luby, J. P., *et al.* (1983). Disease due to cytomegalovirus and its long-term consequences in renal transplant recipients. *Archives of Internal Medicine*, **143**, 1126–9.

Majd M., and Rushton, H. G. (1992). Renal cortical scintigraphy in the diagnosis of acute pyelonephritis. *Seminars in Nuclear Medicine*, **XXII**, 98–111.

Mandel, E. E. (1952). Renal Medullary necrosis. *American Journal of Medicine*, **13**, 322.

Mathew, T. H., Kincaid-Smith, P., and Vikraman P. (1977). Risks of vesico-ureteric reflux in the transplant kidney. *New England Journal of Medicine*, **297**, 414–18.

McClure, J. (1983). Malakoplakia. *Journal of Pathology*, **140**, 275–333.

McCoy, G. C., Loening, S., and Braun W. E. (1975). The fate of cadaver grafts contaminated before transplantation. *Transplantation*, **20**, 467–72.

Meyrier, A., *et al.* (1989). Frequency of development of early cortical scarring in acute primary pyelonephritis. *Kidney International*, **35**, 696–703.

Morgan, W., Rand, M., and Nyberg L. (1985). Perinephric and intrarenal abcess. *Urology*, **26**, 529–33.

Nemoy, N. J. and Stamey, T. A. (1971). Surgical bacteriological and biochemical management of 'infection stones'. *Journal of the American Medical Association*, **215**, 1470–6.

Pearman, J. W. (1976). Urological follow-up of 99 spinal cord injured patients initially managed by intermitten catheterizations. *British Journal of Urology*, **48**, 297.

Pearman, J. W. and England, E. J. (1973). *The urological management of the patient following spinal cord injury*. Charles C. Thomas, Springfield, IL.

Price, M., Koltke, F. J., and Olson, M. E. (1975). Renal function in patients with spinal cord injury: The eighth year of a ten-year continuing study. *Archives of Physical Medicine Rehabilitations*, **56**, 76.

Ramsey D. E., Finch W. T., and Birtch, A. G. (1979). Urinary tract infections in kidney transplant recipients. *Archives of Surgery*, **114**, 1022–5.

Richardson, W. P., *et al.* (1981). Glomerulopathy associated with cytomegalovirus viraemia in renal allografts. *New England Journal of Medicine*, **305**, 57–63.

Ronald, A. R., Cutler, R. E., and Turck, M. (1969). Effect of bacteriuria on renal concentrating mechanisms. *Annals of Internal Medicine*, **70**, 723–33.

Rosenfield, A. T., Glickman, M. G., Taylor, J. W., Crade, M., and Hodson, J. (1979). Acute focal bacterial nephritis (acute lobar nephronia). *Radiology*, **132**, 553–61.

Schwab, S. J., Bauder, S. J., and Klahr, S. (1987). Renal infection in autosomal dominant polycystic disease. *American Journal of Medicine,* **82**, 714.

Sklar A. A., *et al.* (1987). Renal infections in autosomal polycystic kidney disease. *American Journal of Kidney Disease*, **10**, 81.

Stagno, S., *et al.* (1977) immune complexes in congenital and natal cytomegalovirus infections in Man. *Journal of Clinical Investigation*, **60**, 838–45.

Stamey, T. A. (1980). *Pathogenesis and treatment of urinary tract infections*, Ch. 8, pp. 45–6. Williams & Wilkins, Baltimore.

Stamm, W., McKevitt, M., and Counts G. (1987). Acute renal Infection in women: Treatment with trimethoprim-sulfamethoxazole or ampicillin for two or six weeks. *Annals of Internal Medicine*, 106, **341**–5.

Stoller, M. L., and Kogan, B. (1986). Sensitivity of 99m technitium-dimercaptosuccinic acid for the diagnosis of chronic pyelonephritis: Clinical and theoretical considerations. *Journal of Urology*, **135**, 977–80.

Svanborg-Edén, C., Jodal, U., Hanson, L., Lindberg, U., and Sohl Akerlund, A. (1976). Variable adherence to normal human urinary tract epithelial cells of *Escherichia coli* strains associated with various forms of urinary tract infection. *Lancet*, **2**, 490–2.

Thorley, J. D., Jones, S. R., and Sanford, J. P. (1974). Perinephric abcess. *Medicine*, **53**, 441.

Wankowicz, Z., Sulik, J. and Przedlacki, J. (1993). Retrospective analysis of own diagnostic and therapeutic protocol used in urinary tract infections (UTI) in years 1965–1992. (Abstract), XIIth International Congress of Nephrology, p. 612. Kenes, Jerusalem.

Whitworth, J. A., Fairley, K. F., O'Keefe, C., and Johnson W. (1974). The site of renal infection: pylelitis or pyelonephritis? *Clinical Nephrology*, **2**, 9–12.

Williams, G. L., Davies, D. K. L., Evans, K. T., and Williams, J. E. (1968). Vesicoureteric reflux in patients with bacteriuria of pregnancy. *Lancet*, **2**, 1202–5.

9

Urinary tract infection and pregnancy

A. B. MacLean

Introduction

Urinary tract infection (UTI) during pregnancy has all of the seriousness of infection in young women (Wilkie *et al.* 1992), but in addition has problems in respect of diagnosis, subsequent impact on the pregnancy, and the effect of therapy on the fetus. It may be asymptomatic (asymptomatic bacteriuria) or symptomatic (cystitis or acute pyelonephritis). The most common causal organisms are *Escherichia coli*, but infection with Proteus and Klebsiella spp., Enterobacter, *Enterococcus faecalis*, *Staphylococcus saprophyticus* or *Staph. epidermidis*, and group B streptococcus may occur (Kass 1962*a*; Bailey 1990; Wilkie *et al.* 1992).

Prevalence of asymptomatic bacteriuria

The prevalence of asymptomatic bacteriuria in American, British, and Australian studies varies between 4 and 7 per cent, although Norden and Kass (1968) tabulated results for many series with a range from 2 to 13 per cent. The incidence appears to increase with increasing age and parity (Stuart *et al.* 1965; Savage *et al.* 1967) and decrease with increasing social class. Thus, the rates among women confined at the Boston Lying-In Hospital were 1–2 per cent lower than at the Boston City Hospital (Kass 1962*a*; Norden and Kass 1968). Bailey (1972) reported asymptomatic bacteriuria rates as low as 2 per cent among antenatal patients attending a private clinic, and as high as 18.5 per cent among urbanized New Zealand Maori patients.

Prevalence of acute pyelonephritis

Symptomatic bacteriuria is one of the most common medical complications of pregnancy, occurring in some 1 to 2 per cent of pregnant women. One out of five cases of acute UTI is seen during the puerperium (Gilstrap *et al.* 1981*a*). It is a cause of post-operative infection following delivery by Caesarean section, due to indwelling catheterization, disturbance of the bladder in approaching the lower segment, and post-section voiding difficulty, and occurring in one-third of women in the first five days after section (Leigh *et al.* 1990). It may follow catheterization in association with epidural anaesthesia or instrumental vaginal delivery (Stray-Pedersen *et al.* 1990).

Factors predisposing to bacteriuria

Earlier writers (Kass 1962*a*; Beard and Roberts 1968) noted that the prevalence of bacteriuria increased with gestational age and was more likely to recur during pregnancy than in non-pregnant women, and suggested that its presence was due to the pregnancy.

However, other studies showed that bacteriuria pre-dated the pregnancy and had a link with coitus. Turner (1961) suggested marriage was a factor, as only 1 per cent of unmarried women had bacteriuria. Sleigh *et al.* (1964) found no cases among pupil midwives, but a prevalence of 8 per cent among women attending an infertility clinic. Similarly, Bailey (1972) described a rate of 1 per cent among girls leaving school but a rise to 10 per cent when they returned later to Student Health for contraceptive advice. Kunin and McCormack (1968) reported that the incidence of bacteriuria was much lower in nuns than in working class women; the rate in this latter group was not affected by the use of the oral contraceptive pill or the form of menstrual protection used. Thus, it would appear that bacteriuria is a consequence of sexual activity and not a result of pregnancy itself.

The implications of asymptomatic and symptomatic bacteriuria during pregnancy will be considered under the headings of diagnostic difficulty, impact on the pregnancy, and therapy.

Diagnostic difficulty

A diagnosis of symptomatic UTI or acute pyelonephritis in pregnancy is suggested by complaints of being unwell, with nausea, vomiting, dysuria, urinary frequency, abdominal pain radiating into the loin, plus fever and rigors. There is usually pyrexia and tenderness in the costovertebral angle. It must be noted that symptoms of cystitis, such as frequency and lower abdominal pain, occur frequently during pregnancy, and may be overlooked until upper tract symptoms develop. Investigation show leucocytosis, with organisms in the urine and often in blood cultures. The diagnosis is confirmed by the demonstration of significant bacteriuria.

Significant bacteriuria in pregnancy

Although most definitions of UTI require more than 100 000 organisms or colony-forming units per ml of urine, approximately 30 per cent of women with symptoms and a true infection will have between 100 and 100 000 organisms per ml. Some authors (Rubin *et al.* 1992) therefore suggest a diagnostic criterion of more than 1000 organisms per ml of midstream urine (MSSU). While proteinuria and haematuria are often associated with bacteriuria, there are many coexisting reasons why protein or blood may be present in the urine during pregnancy. Their presence is therefore of no diagnostic value.

The pregnant woman may have difficulty in performing a clean catch of voided urine, such that vulval or vaginal contamination of MSU samples often occurs. It is generally accepted that a single mid-stream urine has a false positive rate of up to 20 per cent from such contamination (Kass 1962*b*). In some cases (e.g. a patient admitted with abdominal pain), an appropriate specimen may be taken following passage of a urinary catheter. To eliminate contamination suprapubic aspiration of urine has been used in some studies in antenatal patients (McFadyen and Eykyn 1968; Campbell-Brown *et al.* 1987; Stray-Pedersen *et al.* 1990). However, in many units the house officers or registrars who see women when they are admitted acutely are reluctant to perform suprapubic aspiration of the urine, for fear that the aspirating needle may enter the uterus. In such instances a catheter specimen will provide a safer alternative.

Brumfitt and Hamilton-Miller (1990) have advocated the need for rapid tests (e.g. mixing urine with broth and assessing by optical density or production of certain enzymes), to allow early confirmation of the diagnosis of UTI and acute admission during pregnancy is a good example of where such testing is desirable. Others (MacMillan and Grimes 1991) have commented on the limited usefulness of urine and blood cultures in treating pyelonephritis in pregnancy, pointing out that the cost in the United States of urine culture is $45, and $92 for blood culture plus sensitivities. They calculated that the cost of investigations per patient was $358, which was some 6 to 19 times the cost of antibiotic therapy. They observed that only 3 per cent of pre-treatment cultures led to any change in antibiotic regimen, and suggested that a more cost-effective strategy would be to culture only the urine of those patients who failed to respond to treatment. They calculated that a lack of response and therefore the need for culture in some 10 per cent of patients would still save $18 million a year. Current practice in Britain still is to send urine for culture before commencing treatment.

The other area of diagnostic difficulty in UTI during pregnancy involves the definition of asymptomatic bacteriuria, and the inaccuracy of a single voided midstream specimen of urine. It is recognized that even in early pregnancy, when women attend the antenatal clinic, there are difficulties in collecting an uncontaminated urine specimen. In the study by Turner (1961) the urine was collected after a nurse had washed the vulva with liquid soap and water, and instructed on the collection of a midstream urine (MSSU) into a sterile wide-mouthed jar. Despite these precautions there was still an incidence of contamination. Therefore, most clinics do not use vulval cleansing, and the patient attempts a clean catch, with or without labial separation, during voiding. More than 100 000 organisms per ml of urine on two consecutive MSSUs is regarded as bacteriuria. This may miss some organisms present in lower concentrations such as staphylococci and streptococci. Some studies have made the diagnosis based on a single urine specimen. If the MSU at booking visit is not reported as sterile or without significant growth it should be repeated.

Impact of bacteriuria on pregnancy

On 25 January 1961, Dr Edward Kass participated in a panel discussion of the Special Committee on Infant Mortality for the Medical Society of the County of New York at the New York Academy of Medicine. Kass observed that bacteriuria was found in various patient groups in the Boston City Hospital, ranging from 98 per cent of those patients with inlying catheters for more than 96 hours, to 6 per cent of pregnant women presenting for their first antenatal visit. He described how patients with asymptomatic bacteriuria of pregnancy were studied in two groups. The first group was treated with placebo and the second with a long-acting sulphonamide or, in the 20 per cent where this first-line therapy failed, with nitrofurantoin, and followed with urine cultures at weekly intervals until delivery. In the 48 patients who were given placebo, 20 developed pyelonephritis before term or during the first three months post-partum; 24 per cent had prematurely born infants, and there was a 14 per cent perinatal mortality rate. In the 43 patients who were treated there were no cases of pyelonephritis, there was no perinatal mortality, and the prematurity rate was 10 per cent. In 1000 non-bacteriuric patients, there were no cases of pyelonephritis, perinatal mortality was 2 per cent and the prematurity rate was 9 per cent. The untreated bacteriuric group had a greater likelihood of having babies dying of prematurity, hyalinosis, pulmonary congestion, or atalectasis, but not of sepsis. Kass urged the meeting that if asymptomatic bacteriuria was detected and treated perinatal death could be reduced some 20–30 per cent and that some 10–20 per cent premature births could be prevented.

Asymptomatic bacteriuria and pyelonephritis

Obstetricians had recognized for many years the dangers of pyelonephritis during pregnancy. Many of these studies were performed before antibiotics were available, but more recent epidemiological studies have linked acute UTI with increased fetal mortality and prematurity (Gilstrap *et al.* 1981*b*; McGrady *et al.* 1985).

There is little doubt that asymptomatic bacteriuria will become symptomatic in a proportion of cases, ranging from 14 per cent (Swapp 1973) to 57 per cent (McFadyen and Eykyn 1968). Some of the variation is due to lack of confirmatory microbiology in all patients presenting with typical symptoms or when treatment has been commenced before the patient reaches hospital. In larger series, where some of the asymptomatic bacteriuria patients were not treated (Little 1965), progression to symptoms occurred in 36 per cent of the untreated patients compared to 5 per cent of those treated. Pyelonephritis was also more likely to develop if treatment failed to clear asymptomatic bacteriuria (Gruneberg *et al.* 1969). Those who progressed from asymptomatic to symptomatic infection had a similar incidence of upper and lower tract infection (Pinkerton *et al.* 1965).

What is more doubtful is whether screening for and treating asymptomatic bacteriuria is a useful way of preventing pyelonephritis during pregnancy.

Whereas some studies (Gilstrap *et al.* 1981*a*) found that the majority (66 per cent) of those who presented with acute pyelonephritis had earlier had asymptomatic bacteriuria, others (Dixon and Brant 1967; Lawson and Miller 1971) found this to be the case in only a third of patients. Lawson and Miller (1973) calculated that the test sensitivity of a single MSSU to predict subsequent symptomatic infection was only 54 per cent. Thus, of every 100 patients developing acute pyelonephritis during pregnancy, only 54 would have had asymptomatic bacteriuria, and of these only three-quarters were likely to have infection prevented by treatment at the time of the initial screen. Similarly, Chng and Hall (1982) reported that screening for bacteriuria had a 33 per cent sensitivity in predicting acute infection during pregnancy. The additional information of a previous UTI was no more sensitive. A combination of asymptomatic bacteriuria on screening and a previous history of infection increased the likelihood of infection in pregnancy, but the sensitivity remained low at only 18 per cent.

Routine urine culture in the antenatal clinic is expensive in laboratory time and costs. An acute episode of UTI in pregnancy which is treated appropriately rarely harms the mother or fetus. There are economic and other arguments for abandoning routine urine culture in favour of prompt effective treatment and careful follow-up (recognizing the increased recurrence rate during pregnancy) of those women who do develop acute infection during pregnancy.

Pre-term labour

Early studies were inconsistent in their diagnosis of pre-term labour or prematurity, usually relying on birthweight (less than 2.5 kg) rather than gestational age. Nowadays, pre-term delivery is defined as delivery before 37 weeks, and it is recognized that infants may be inappropriately small for gestational age (e.g. weigh less than 2.5 kg at term). It is interesting to note that the early Australian and American studies (Kincaid-Smith and Bullen 1965; Stuart *et al.* 1965; Savage *et al.* 1967) showed increased prematurity rates among asymptomatic women with bacteriuria, but the majority of British studies (Sleigh *et al.* 1964; Little 1966; Dixon and Brant 1967; Swapp 1973) did not. The study of Savage *et al.* (1967) only sustained a significant difference if twins were included, a similar bias to that in the figures of Kass (1962*b*) which included three sets of twins in his placebo-treated group.

Kass (1962*a*) believed that the link between bacteriuria, symptomatic or not, and pre-term or premature delivery was the release of endotoxins, causing uterine hyper-irritability. The evidence that infection causes pre-term labour has been reviewed by MacLean (1991), and it appears that locally or systematically released prostaglandins are the important mediators of uterine activity.

Thomsen *et al.* (1987) noted a link between group B streptococcus in the urine and pre-term labour. It was postulated that heavy genital tract colonization both led to contamination of urine specimens and produced ascending infection, causing penetration of the fetal membrane and chorioamnionitis. This could explain the observation among Australian aboriginal women (Schultz *et al.* 1991) that low birthweight was associated with genital and UTI in 51 per cent of cases, compared with 13 per cent of controls. Organisms were cultured from the urine in 12.6 per cent of patients compared with 3 per cent of controls. It may also explain the findings in a remarkable study when tetracyclines were given to pregnant women with and without asymptomatic bacteriuria (Elder *et al.* 1971). The prematurity rate was 10 per cent in women with bacteriuria who were treated and thereafter remained clear, and was 18.5 per cent in those with bacteriuria who were treated with placebo and developed pyelonephritis. In those non-bacteriuric patients who were treated with six weeks of tetracycline the prematurity rate went down to 5.4 per cent, compared with 15.2 per cent in the untreated but non-bacteriuric patients, suggesting that infection or organisms in the genital tract but not in the urine may be equally as important.

Two groups have performed meta-analysis on the relationship between asymptomatic bacteriuria and pre-term delivery at low birthweight. Romero *et al.* (1989) reviewed 31 studies, rejected 12 for various reasons, and focused on 19. There were 17 cohort studies which allowed comparison of prematurity in untreated bacteriuria patients and non-bacteriuria patients; five showed significantly fewer low birthweight infants in the non-bacteriuric versus the bacteriuric group, and 14 of the 17 showed the same trend (Relative Risk 0.65; 95 per cent confidence intervals 0.56, 0.74). In four studies with information on gestational age, meta-analysis again showed a significant difference in the rate of pre-term delivery. In eight randomized clinical trials of treatment versus placebo, four showed a significant reduction in prevalence of low birthweight in the antibiotic-treated group (Relative Risk 0.56; 95 per cent confidence intervals 0.42, 0.73). In the one case-control study analysed, the prevalence of asymptomatic bacteriuria was significantly higher in the group delivering before 36 weeks compared with a matched control group delivering after 36 weeks.

The results presented in the other meta-analysis (Wang and Smaill 1990) addressed whether treatment with antibiotic versus no treatment of asymptomatic bacteriuria influenced pre-term delivery or low birthweight and found an Odds Ratio of 0.89 and 95 per cent confidence intervals that traversed unity (i.e. treatment did not influence pre-term delivery). It is of interest that three of the eight randomized studies in the Romero *et al.* (1989) meta-analysis were included in this analysis, but the three other studies included one by Gold *et al.* (1966), which reversed the trend. In this study, performed in Brooklyn, New York, two premature deliveries occurred among the 35 (5.7 per cent) treated patients and none among the 30 control patients. The incidence of prematurity among 1216 non-bacteriuric patients was 13.9 per cent. Whether these data are relevant to modern British practice, with pre-term delivery rates between 3 and 7 per cent (MacLean 1991), remains uncertain.

On balance, the evidence that identification and treatment of asymptomatic bacteriuria significantly alters the incidence of pre-term labour remains unconvincing.

Hypertension

This term is used increasingly to describe hypertension that occurs in later pregnancy, usually associated with oedema and less often with proteinuria. Other terms include pre-eclampsia, pre-eclamptic toxaemia (PET), HOP, or EPH (hypertension, oedema, proteinuria) syndrome, and gestosis.

Early studies of asymptomatic bacteriuria noted an association with hypertension (Kass 1962*a*). Stuart *et al.* (1965), using a definition of hypertension as diastolic pressure greater than 100 mmHg, found 40 per cent of bacteriuric patients of 35 years of age or older developed hypertension, compared with only 5 per cent of control non-bacteriuric patients.

Kincaid-Smith and Bullen (1965), using a blood pressure recording of greater than 140/90 mmHg plus oedema and proteinuria, found an increased incidence of bacteriuria which was not reduced with antibiotic treatment. Savage *et al.* (1967) commented that their bacteriuric group were more likely to be hospitalized for various reasons, including pre-eclamptic toxaemia.

Other studies have been unable to find an increased prevalence of hypertension developing among the bacteriuric patients (Little 1966; Swapp 1973). Norden and Kass (1968) reviewed the literature to that date and concluded that there was some relationship between bacteriuria and hypertension of pregnancy, but that it might be indirect and relate to other factors, including socioeconomic group and patient population. It is unlikely that screening for bacteriuria in early pregnancy contributes to the anticipation or diagnosis of later hypertension of pregnancy.

Anaemia

An Edinburgh study (Robertson *et al.* 1968) found anaemia of pregnancy, with haemoglobin levels less than 10 g per 100 ml, in 14 per cent of treated and 18 per cent of untreated patients with asymptomatic bacteriuria compared with 8 per cent in non-infected controls. In those patients where bacteriuric treatment failed, 88 per cent had anaemia. They suggested that subsequent investigation for chronic pyelonephritis or other renal disease should be carried out. However, it is unlikely that the anaemia is due to renal impairment, as altered function sufficient to cause anaemia is usually not compatible with fertility. Other studies have not commented on rates of anaemia. As anaemia of pregnancy may be associated with many factors, including socioeconomic status, diet, and compliance in taking iron tablets it is difficult to establish where bacteriuria is an independent contributing factor.

Therapy

Certain antibiotics are unsuitable for use during pregnancy (MacLean and McAllister 1990). Sulphonamides cross the placenta, and their use in late pregnancy may increase the risk of kernicterus by displacing bilirubin bound to albumin. Tetracyclines will be incorporated into teeth and bones to cause dysplasia and discoloration. Trimethoprim is an anti-folate agent and its use should be avoided in early pregnancy during neural tube development. There is evidence that prolonged aminoglycoside use (streptomycin) may produce 8th-nerve damage in the fetus but this should not detract from their use for serious infection during pregnancy. Quinolones have been associated with alterations in the joint cartilage of puppies, and should not be used in pregnancy. Some of the more recent semi-synthetic penicillins and cephalosporins, plus imipenem and aztreonam, are too new for significant experience of use in pregnancy to comment on safety. Similarly, the addition of clavulanic acid to amoxycillin, as Augmentin, has meant that the drug carries a caution on use in pregnancy unless considered essential by the clinician. Finally, drug use in pregnancy may have less predictable effects because of altered pharmacokinetics, including absorption. Allergic reactions may occur that will threaten the fetus as well as the mother, and care must be taken for certain individuals such as those women with glucose-6-phosphate dehydrogenase deficiency in whom there is a risk of haemolysis following nitrofurantoin use.

Recommended choice of antibiotics for asymptomatic bacteriuria include amoxycillin, cephradine or a similar oral cephalosporin, nitrofurantoin, nalidixic acid, or sulphonamide. Pyelonephritis should be treated with a second- or third-generation cephalosporin, or a short course of an aminoglycoside (MacLean and McAllister 1990).

Debate continues on the duration of therapy in pregnant women. Little and de Wardener (1966) described treatment of 53 pregnant women with acute pyelonephritis with either short-term treatment for 7 to 14 days, or long-term treatment for 1 to 18 months and found that duration did not affect the rate of re-infection. There is now enthusiasm for single-dose treatment, because of the benefits of reduced fetal exposure and less chance of developing bacterial resistance (McFadyen *et al.* 1987; Bailey 1990). Comparisons with 3-, 5-, and 7-day courses of the identical antibiotic show no advantage over single dose for cephalexin, cotrimoxazole, and amoxycillin (McFadyen *et al.* 1987; Bailey *et al.* 1983; Masterton *et al.* 1985). Failure or re-infection rates for single-dose treatment may be as high as one in three (Harris *et al.* 1982; McFadyen *et al.* 1987) but it appears that those who do not respond are more likely to have urinary tract abnormalities. Wilkie *et al.* (1992), suggested that short-course antimicrobial chemotherapy should never be used for pregnant women, but their statement is not supported by any evidence and has been challenged in subsequent correspondence. Those women who get recurrent bacteriuria during pregnancy should be given prophylactic nitrofurantoin, 50 mg at night, until delivery.

Follow-up

Kass (1962*a*) found that about two-thirds of those with asymptomatic bacteriuria of pregnancy still had organisms present up to one year after delivery. The need for follow-up has been stressed because of the association with subsequent renal failure (Parker and Kunin 1973). Radiological abnormalities, including calyceal changes with blunting or papillary necrosis, reduced cortical thickness and irregular renal contour, the presence of calculi, or congenital anatomical anomalies (Whalley *et al.* 1965; Kincaid-Smith and Bullen 1965; Leigh *et al.* 1968, Gilstrap *et al.* 1981*a*), have been reported in up to 50 per cent of patients. It is suggested that those who have symptomatic infection (Gower *et al.* 1968), evidence of upper urinary tract infection (Fairley *et al.* 1966), failure to respond to single-dose therapy (Bailey 1990), or identification of an unusual organism (Wilkie *et al.* 1992) should have further investigation following delivery. Although earlier studies used intravenous pyelography or urography to investigate selected patients, it is suggested that they rarely provide information that is important in subsequent management (Engel *et al.* 1980; Fowler and Pulaski 1981). An easier method to assess these patients is renal ultrasound for length, shape, and contour of each kidney.

Conclusions

Urinary tract infection is a common complication of pregnancy. Asymptomatic bacteriuria occurs in 5 per cent of women, but prevalence varies. There is uncertainty as to whether it is still valuable to screen for bacteriuria, as the majority of patients becoming symptomatic later in pregnancy would not have been predicted from such screening. Furthermore, if women with clinical features of pyelonephritis are started promptly on antibiotics, serious complications are rare. Pre-term labour continues to be a challenge and has a link with infection, but screening for urinary tract organisms may be less logical than screening for bacterial colonization of the lower genital tract. Women who develop hypertension of pregnancy with proteinuria should be followed-up in the puerperium and investigated if hypertension and/or proteinuria persist, irrespective of whether there has been bacteriuria.

Women with asymptomatic bacteriuria should be offered a single-dose or short court of treatment. The urine should be reassessed later. If infection persists or recurs, or becomes symptomatic, an ultrasound scan of the kidneys will detect those with gross renal pathology. Excretion urology may be indicated following pregnancy to define the detailed anatomy (Chapter 4).

References

Bailey, R. R. (1972). Urinary tract infection—some recent concepts. *Can. Med. Assoc. J.*, **107**, 316–30.

Bailey, R. R. (1990). Review of published studies on single dose therapy of urinary tract infections. *Infection*, **18**(Suppl. 2), S53–6.

Bailey, R. R., Bishop, V., and Peddie, B. A. (1983). Comparison of single dose with a 5 day course of co-trimoxazole for asymptomatic (covert) bacteriuria of pregnancy. *Aust. N.Z. J. Obstet. Gynaec.*, **23**, 139–41.

Beard, R. W. and Roberts, A. P. (1968). Asymptomatic bacteriuria during pregnancy. *Brit. Med. Bull.*, **24**, 44–8.

Brumfitt, W. and Hamilton-Miller, J. M. T. (1990). Urinary tract infection in the 1990's: the state of the art. *Infection*, **18**(Suppl. 2), S34–9.

Campbell-Brown, M., McFadyen, I. R., Seal, D. V., and Stephenson, M. L. (1987). Is screening for bacteriuria in pregnancy worth while? *BMJ*, **294**, 1579–82.

Chng, P. K. and Hall, M. N. (1982). Antenatal prediction of urinary tract infection in pregnancy. *Br. J. Obstet. Gynaecol.*, **89**, 8–11.

Dixon, H. G. and Brant, H. A. (1967). The significance of bacteriuria of pregnancy. *Lancet*, **1**, 19–20.

Elder, H. A., Santamarina, B. A. G., Smith, S., and Kass, E. H. (1971). The natural history of asymptomatic bacteriuria during pregnancy: the effect of tetracycline on the clinical course and the outcome of pregnancy. *Am. J. Obstet. Gynec.*, **111**, 441–62.

Engel, G., Schaeffer, A. J., Grayhack, J. T., and Wendel, E. F. (1980). The role of excretory urography and cystoscopy in the evaluation and management of women with recurrent urinary tract infection. *J. Urol.*, **123**, 190–1.

Fairley, K. F., Bond, A. G., and Adey, F. D. (1966). The site of infection in pregnancy bacteriuria. *Lancet*, **1**, 939–41.

Fowler, J. E. and Pulaski, E. T. (1981). Excretory urography, cystography and cystoscopy in the evaluation of women with urinary tract infection. *New Engl. J. Med.*, **304**, 462–5.

Gilstrap, L. C., Cunningham, F. G., and Whalley, P. J. (1981*a*). Acute pyelonephritis in pregnancy: an anterospective study. *Obstet. Gynecol.*, **57**, 409–13.

Gilstrap, L. C., Leveno, K. J., Cunningham, F. G., Whalley, P. J., and Roark, M. L. (1981*b*). Renal infection and pregnancy outcome. *Am. J. Obstet. Gynec.*, **141**, 709–16.

Gold, E. M., Traub, F. B., Daichman, I., and Terris, M. (1966). Asymptomatic bacteriuria during pregnancy. *Obstet. Gynecol.*, **27**, 206–9.

Gower, P. E., Haswell, B., Sidaway, M. E., and de Wardener, H. E. (1968). Follow up of 164 patients with bacteriuria of pregnancy. *Lancet*, **1**, 990–4.

Gruneberg, R. N., Leigh, D. A., and Brumfitt, W. (1969). Relationship of bacteriuria in pregnancy to acute pyelonephritis, prematurity and fetal mortality. *Lancet*, **2**, 1–3.

Harris, R. E., Gilstrap, L. C., and Pretty, A. (1982). Single-dose antimicrobial therapy for asymptomatic bacteriuria during pregnancy. *Obstet. Gynecol.*, **59**, 546–9.

Kass, E. H. (1962*a*). Material urinary tract infection. *New York State J. Med.*, 2822–6.

Kass, E. H. (1962*b*). Pyelonephritis and bacteriuria. A major problem in preventive medicine. *Ann. Int. Med.*, **56**, 46–53.

Kincaid-Smith, P. and Bullen, M. (1965). Bacteriuria in pregnancy. *Lancet*, **1**, 395–9.

Kunin, C. M. and McCormack, R. C. (1968). An epidemiologic study of bacteriuria and blood pressure among nuns and working women. *New Engl. J. Med.*, **278**, 635–42.

Lawson, D. H. and Miller, A. W. F. (1971). Screening for bacteriuria in pregnancy. *Lancet*, **1**, 9–11.

Lawson, D. H. and Miller, A. W. F. (1973). Screening for bacteriuria in pregnancy. *Arch. Int. Med.*, **132**, 904–8.

Leigh, D. A., Gruneberg, R. N., and Brumfitt, W. (1968). Long-term follow up of bacteriuria in pregnancy. *Lancet*, **1**, 603–5.

Leigh, D. A., Emmanuel, F. X. S., Sedgwick, J., and Dean, R. (1990). Post-operative urinary tract infection and wound infection in women undergoing caesarean section: a comparison of two study periods in 1985 and 1987. *J. Hosp. Infect.*, **15**, 107–16.

Little, P. J. (1965). Prevention of pyelonephritis of pregnancy. *Lancet*, **1**, 567–9.

Little, P. J. (1966). The incidence of urinary infection in 5000 pregnant women. *Lancet*, **2**, 925–8.

Little, P. J. and de Wardener, H. E. (1966). Acute pyelonephritis—incidence of re-infection in 100 patients. *Lancet*, **2**, 1277–8.

McGrady, G. A., Daling, J. R., and Peterson, D. R. (1985). Material urinary tract infection and adverse fetal outcomes. *Am. J. Epidemiol.*, **121**, 377–81.

MacLean, A. B. (1991). Infection and pre-term labour. *Curr. Obstet. Gynaecol.*, **1**, 67–71.

MacLean, A. B. and McAllister, T. (1990). Antimicrobial therapy in obstetrics and gynaecology. In *Clinical infection in obstetrics and gynaecology*, (ed. A. B. MacLean), pp. 210–23, Blackwell, Oxford.

MacMillan, M. C. and Grimes, D. A. (1991). The limited usefulness of urine and blood cultures in treating pyelonephritis in pregnancy. *Obstet. Gynecol.*, **78**, 745–8.

McFadyen, I. R. and Eykyn, S. J. (1968). Suprapubic aspiration of urine in pregnancy. *Lancet*, **1**, 1112–14.

McFadyen, I. R., Campbell-Brown, M., Stephenson, M., and Seal, D. V. (1987). Single-dose treatment of bacteriuria in pregnancy. *Eur. Urol.*, **13**(Suppl. 1), 22–5.

Masterton, R. G., Evans, D. C., and Strike, P. W. (1985). Single-dose amoxycillin in the treatment of bacteriuria in pregnancy and the puerperium—a controlled clinical trial. *Br. J. Obstet. Gynaecol.*, **92**, 498–505.

Norden, C. W. and Kass, E. H. (1968). Bacteriuria of pregnancy—a critical appraisal. *Ann. Rev. Med.*, **19**, 431–70.

Parker, J. and Kunin, C. (1973). Pyelonephritis in young women. A 10 to 20 year follow up. *J. Am. Med. Assoc.*, **224**, 585–90.

Pinkerton, J. H. M., Houston, J. K., and Gibson, G. L. (1965). Significant bacteriuria during pregnancy. *Proc. Roy. Soc. Med.*, **58**, 1041–2.

Robertson, J. G., Livingstone, J. R. B., and Isdale, M. H. (1968). The management and complications of asymptomatic bacteriuria in pregnancy. *J. Obstet. Gynaec. Br. Cwlth.*, **75**, 59–65.

Romero, R., Oyarzun, E., Mazor, M., Sirtori, M., Hobbins, J. C., and Bracken, M. (1989). Meta-analysis of the relationship between asymptomatic bacteriuria and pre-term delivery/low birth weight. *Obstet. Gynecol.*, **73**, 576–82.

Rubin, R. H., Beam, T. R., and Stamm, W. E. (1992). An approach to evaluating antibacterial agents in the treatment of urinary tract infection. *Clin. Infect. Dis.*, **14**(Suppl. 2), S246–51.

Savage, W. E., Hajj, S. N., and Kass, E. H. (1967). Demographic and prognostic characteristics of bacteriuria in pregnancy. *Medicine*, **46**, 385–407.

Schultz, R., Read, A. W., Straton, J. A. Y., Stanley, F. J., and Morich, P. (1991). Genitourinary tract infections in pregnancy and low birth weight: case-control study in Australian Aboriginal women. *BMJ*, **303**, 1369–73.

Sleigh, J. D., Robertson, J. G., and Isdale, M. H. (1964). Asymptomatic bacteriuria in pregnancy. *J. Obstet. Gynaec. Br. Cwlth.*, **71**, 74–81.

Stray-Pedersen, B., Blakstad, M., and Bergan, T. (1990). Bacteriuria in the puerperium. Risk factors, screening procedures and treatment programmes. *Am. J. Obstet. Gynecol.*, **162**, 792–7.

Stuart, K. L., Cummins, G. T. M., and Chin, W. A. (1965). Bacteriuria, prematurity and the hypertensive disorders of pregnancy. *BMJ*, **1**, 554–6.

Swapp, G. H. (1973). Asymptomatic bacteriuria, birthweight and length of gestation in a defined population. In *Urinary tract infection*, (ed. W. Brumfitt and A. W. Asscher), pp. 92–102. Oxford University Press, London.

Thomsen, A. C., Morup, L., and Hansen, K. B. (1987). Antibiotic elimination of group B streptococci in urine in prevention of pre-term labour. *Lancet*, **1**, 591–3.

Turner, G. C. (1961). Bacilluria in pregnancy. *Lancet*, **2**, 1062–4.

Wang, E. and Smaill, F. (1990). Infection in pregnancy. In *Effective care in pregnancy and childbirth*, (ed. I. Chalmers, M. Enkin, and M. J. N. C. Keirse), pp. 535–8. Oxford University Press.

Whalley, P. J., Martin, F. G., and Peters, P. C. (1965). Significance of asymptomatic bacteriuria detected during pregnancy. *J. Am. Med. Assoc.*, **193**, 107–9.

Wilkie, M. E., Almond, M. K., Marsh, F. P. (1992). Diagnosis and management of urinary tract infection in adults. *BMJ*, **305**, 1137–41.

10

Urinary tract infection in diabetes mellitus

Alasdair D. R. Mackie and Paul L. Drury

Introduction

It is widely held that infection, including that of the urinary tract, is more common in subjects with diabetes mellitus. Although there are relatively few recently published data the evidence does suggest that bacteriuria is more common in females with diabetes but not in males. Certain renal tract infections, including emphysematous pyelonephritis and cystitis, perinephric abscess, and candidiasis show a close association with diabetes mellitus. These, together with renal papillary necrosis, form the basis of this chapter. Further detailed discussion of individual problems is to found in Mogensen (1988).

Urinary tract infection

Autopsy studies suggest that urinary tract infection (UTI) is more common in diabetes mellitus (Robbins and Tucker 1944; Barnard *et al.* 1953). Such studies, which primarily examined upper renal tract disease, are, by virtue of case selection, open to bias. In one study, 6.8 per cent of diabetic individuals had pyelonephritis compared to 1.6 per cent of normal subjects (Robbins and Tucker 1944). Even this difference may be an overestimate as other conditions, for example, ischaemia, renal papillary necrosis, and reflux nephropathy may mimic pyelonephritis (Taft *et al.* 1990).

Controlled clinical studies suggest that bacteriuria is more common in diabetic females, but not males. Table 10.1, adapted from Wheat (1980), summarizes these studies. The proportion of females with diabetes and bacteriuria is consistent in these studies (9–20 per cent) and, with two exceptions (O'Sullivan *et al.* 1961; Williams *et al.* 1975), is two- to threefold greater than in non-diabetic females. For males, only Bahl *et al.* (1970) observed a difference.

From a restrospective hospital-based survey of infection, MacFarlane *et al.* (1986) concluded that diabetes mellitus increased the risk of bacteraemia. *Escherichia coli* was the most common pathogen and the principal source was the urinary tract. In a similar prospective study in diabetic individuals Leibovici *et al.* (1991) confirmed the importance of the urinary tract as a source for bacteraemia. In this study Klebsiella spp. was a more frequent isolate in diabetic

Table 10.1 Summary of available studies on the occurrence of urinary tract infection in diabetic subjects

Study	Diabetic		Non-diabetic	
	Total	Bacteriuric (%)	Total	Bacteriuric (%)
Women				
Kass (1957)	54	18	337	6
O'Sullivan *et al.* (1961)	91	20	91	19
Hansen (1964)	152	16	152	5
Vjelsgaard (1966*a*)	128	19	114	8
Bahl *et al.* (1970)	97	11	100	3
Ooi *et al.* (1974)	81	18	81	4
Williams *et al.* (1975)	44	16	27	15
Schmitt *et al.* (1986)	341	9	100	5
Men				
O'Sullivan *et al.* (1961)	59	3	59	2
Hansen (1964)	154	1	154	1
Vjelsgaard (1966*a*)	141	1	146	2
Bahl *et al.* (1970)	97	11	100	3
Ooi *et al.* (1974)	67	8	67	3
Harkonen *et al.* (1977)	37	5	102	4
Schmitt *et al.* (1986)	411	1	100	0

(25 per cent) than non-diabetic individuals (12 per cent) when the urinary tract was the source of infection.

In an uncontrolled study, Forland *et al.* (1977) examined the localization of infection in the renal tract in diabetic subjects. They found that 19 per cent of women and 2 per cent of men had a UTI. Using antibody-coated bacteria, 43 per cent of a selected group of 42 patients had evidence of renal parenchymal disease, which rose to nearly 80 per cent over a 7-week period in the absence of treatment. Out of the total group of 333 patients, 22 had recurrent infections following treatment; 14 were re-infections (recurrence with a different organism or serotype), and eight were relapses (recurrence with the same organism or serotype).

Prior instrumenation may increase the risk of bacteriuria in diabetic and non-diabetic patients (Stamm *et al.* 1977): This paper suggested a doubling of the risk of bacteriuria after cystoscopy or catheterization. In diabetic patients 88 per cent of all UTI may be asymptomatic (Pometta *et al.* 1967), but a significant proportion of these may lead to more severe infection (Wheat 1980).

The factors that predispose diabetic individuals to infection are ill-understood. Many factors may combine to increase the frequency of infection, including autonomic neuropathy leading to delayed bladder emptying (Ellenberg 1976), diabetic nephropathy, and impaired host defence mechanisms (Rayfield *et al.* 1982). The prevalence of UTI in diabetic nephropathy is reported to be 13 per cent (Korzeniowski 1991). Sawers *et al.* (1986) found bacteriuria more common in diabetic women with autonomic neuropathy, but surprisingly no evidence of an increased residual urine volume after micturition. The duration of diabetes (Vejlsgaard 1966*b*) and the presence of complications (Schmitt *et al.* 1986) have been related to increased bacteriuria in diabetes. In alloxan-induced diabetic rats, Obana *et al.* (1991) found greater adherence of *Serratia marescens* to bladder epithelial cells than in control animals. Contrary to what one might expect, poor glycaemic control does not contribute to the frequency of UTI. Schmitt *et al.* (1986) found no relationship between Hb A_1 and bacteriuria in 752 individuals with non-insulin dependent diabeties mellitus (NIDDM). In a second study mean Hb A_1 was 11.5 per cent in bacteriuric and 11.4 per cent in non-bacteriuric diabetic women (Rayfield *et al.* 1982).

Pathogens

Escherichia coli is the most common organism isolated. Schmitt *et al.* (1986) found this to be the case from 75 per cent of isolates from female diabetics. No significant difference in the bacterial isolates is seen between diabetic subjects and controls, although the bacterial counts are generally higher in the former (Wheat 1980). Group B streptococcus is said to be more common in diabetic subjects with pyelonephritis (Korzeniowski 1991).

Therapy

Positive urine cultures (i.e. $>10^5$ organisms per ml) should be treated in the diabetic individual even if asymptomatic. The choice of antibiotic should reflect the sensitivity of the organism and treatment does not differ between diabetic and non-diabetic individuals, although some authorities prefer a longer duration of treatment in diabetic patients (Leibovici *et al.* 1992). A 14-day course of antibiotics is recommended for pyelonephritis (Hooton and Stamm 1991). A cephalosporin, given intravenously for 48 hours, is suitable. Where relapse occurs a six-week treatment is advocated (Turck *et al.* 1966).

Conclusion

Asymptomatic bacteriuria is common in diabetic women, particularly the older age group and *E.coli* the organism most frequently isolated. Untreated infections may lead to renal parenchymal infection which may impair renal function (Ooi *et al.* 1974). In consequence, all UTIs, regardless of symptoms should be treated. Recurrent UTI should lead to imaging of the renal tract to exclude an underlying pathology (e.g. renal papillary necrosis), and may indicate the need for prolonged antibiotic therapy. Treatment for at least 6 weeks may be required.

Infective tubulo-interstitial nephritis

This poorly recognized cause of infection and, sometimes, acute renal failure in unobstructed kidneys was initially documented in two series by Richet and Mayaud (1978), of 30 cases, and Baker *et al.* (1979) in five cases. The larger series included histological evidence of an acute infection with micro-abscesses. The condition has been reviewed by Cattell (1992). From published series it appears that diabetes is a risk factor for acute renal failure in this group (Cattell *et al.* 1985; Cattell 1992) along with analgesic abuse, non-steroidal use, sickle-cell disease (or trait), and possibly alcoholism.

Acute renal failure

Although hard data are lacking, there is an impression that diabetic patients may be more likely than the non-diabetic to suffer acute renal failure as a result of UTI and subsequent pyelonephritis and septicaemia. Apart from infective tubulo-interstitial nephritis, described above, this may result from the failure of auto-regulation of renal blood flow with falls in blood pressure in patients with even moderate degrees of diabetic nephropathy (Parving *et al.* 1984).

Renal tract candidiasis

Diabetes appears more common in individuals with fungal UTI. It is present in up to 90 per cent of patients with *Candida glabrata* (formerly *Torulopsis glabrata*) (Marks *et al.* 1970; Kaufmann and Tan 1974), and *C. albicans* was cultured from the urine of 35 per cent of patients with diabetes mellitus as compared to only 9 per cent of controls without glycosuria (B. Mehnert and H. Mehnert 1958). Candida gives rise to a wide variety of infections of the renal tract. Although many are asymptomatic, they may lead to cystitis, pyelonephritis, renal abscesses, and fungal ball formation (Marks *et al.* 1970, Wise *et al.* 1976).

What constitutes a significant candidal infection in the urinary tract remains to be fully established (*Lancet* 1988). A value of $> 10^4$ organisms per ml is currently taken to reflect infection (Kozinn *et al.* 1978; Goldberg *et al.* 1979). Infection may originate from the genital region, the gastrointestinal tract, or by haematogenous spread.

There is no agreement as to whether, in diabetic subjects, all infections should be treated. Indeed, control of blood sugar may be all that is required to clear the urine. Symptomatic individuals and those with candiduria accompanied by pyuria should receive antifungal therapy. Patients with indwelling catheters that cannot be removed may be treated with intermittent instillations of amphotericin B. Where oral therapy is adequate, flucytosine is advocated (Davies and Reeves 1971). Alternatively, fluconazole may be used (Grant and Clissold 1990). Most lower UTIs clear within two to three weeks (*Lancet* 1988). Renal candidiasis often requires a more aggressive approach, including irrigation of the renal pelvis with antifungal drugs, oral or parenteral therapy, and, sometimes, surgical interventation. Amphotericin B alone or in combination with flucytosine is the treatment of choice (Francis and Walsh 1992).

Perinephric abscess

This type of abscess generally develops in the renal parenchyma and then breaches the surrounding fascia. Diabetes is present in 30–40 per cent of cases (Obrant 1949; Salvatierra *et al.* 1967; Thorley *et al.* 1974). Bilateral abscesses are rare, occurring in only 2 per cent in one series (Salvatierra *et al.* 1967); a single case report in association with type 1 diabetes mellitus is described (Bevan *et al.* 1989). The infection may arise from an ascending UTI or by haematogenous spread. The onset is frequently insidious with symptoms often present for more than five days. These include flank discomfort, nausea, vomiting, dysuria, and, occasionally, haematuria. Two-thirds of patients have flank tenderness or a mass (Atcheson 1941).

Laboratory investigations may show an elevated white cell count or erythrocyte sedimentation rate (ESR) but are not helpful in diagnosis. However, if abscess, blood, and urine cultures are examined then more than 90 per cent show a positive culture (Thorley *et al.* 1974). The intravenous urogram (IVU) is often abnormal, but ultrasound (US) or computed tomography (CT) scan offer the best hope of a positive diagnosis. Sometimes a delay and repeat scanning is necessary before the abscess becomes apparent. US or CT scan-guided aspiration of the abscess may then follow. As in other renal tract disease Gram-negative organisms are most commonly isolated. Anaerobes and Gram-positive cocci, including *Staphylococcus aureus*, are also frequently found.

Treatment includes intravenous antibiotics and control of hyperglycaemia if present. Surgery includes percutaneous drainage of the abscess or nephrectomy. Relief of obstruction caused by renal calculi may be required. The mortality associated with this condition is falling and is now less than 20 per cent (Korzeniowski 1991). Early diagnosis with the increasing use of isotope scans and direct imaging techniques should help to reduce this figure further, but increased awareness of the diagnosis by the non-specialist is required.

Renal papillary necrosis

The pathogenesis of this condition is poorly understood. Infarction of the renal papilla is most likely, with infection probably a contributory factor. Autopsy studies indicate that renal papillary necrosis (RPN) is more common in diabetic subjects (Robbins and Tucker 1944; Edmondson *et al.* 1947). Of 859 diabetic patients autopsied in the first series 29 (3.4 per cent) showed papillary or pyramidal necrosis, and 16 out of 307 (5.2 per cent) in the second study. The prevalence in cases of pyelonephritis was much higher at 25 per cent (Robbins *et al.* 1946; Edmondson *et al.* 1947). The prevalence of RPN in non-diabetic subjects was 0.07 per cent in these two studies.The prevalence of RPN based on autopsy studies may be an underestimate. A prospective study of 76 insulin-dependent diabetes mellitus (IDDM) individuals showed a prevalence of 23.7 per cent (Groop *et al.* 1989). Given that the upper limit of creatinine in the individuals in this study was 200 μmol per litre even this may be an underestimate.

The relationship between RPN and diabetes can be traced back to Turner (1888). However, Froboese (1937) and Gunther (1937) are credited with firmly establishing the link with diabetes mellitus. Of their combined series of 20 subjects, 17 (85 per cent) had diabetes mellitus. Drawing extensively on the German literature, Mandel (1952) identified a total of 160 cases of RPN prior to 1950. Of these 96 (60 per cent) were diabetic. More recent estimates suggest the proportion may be nearer 30 per cent, with other conditions such as analgesic nephropathy, sickle-cell disease, and possibly obstructive uropathy accounting for the remainder.

Clinical presentation

The presentation of RPN may be acute or chronic. The former may be fulminant with flank pain, fever, and septicaemia. It is generally unilateral. Papillae may slough, leading to renal colic. The affected kidney may be enlarged (Fry 1986). The chronic indolent form is more commonly observed. Here changes are often bilateral. Unilateral papillary necrosis suggests the presence of renal artery stenosis or atrophy associated with previous ureteric obstruction. The changes in the kidney may be patchy with the papillae exhibiting differing degrees of necrosis.

RPN is most usually seen in the 6th and 7th decades (Mandel 1952), with women affected more often than men (3:1) (Mujais 1984). Microscopic haematuria is a common finding, occurring in 44 per cent of diabetic subjects with RPN (Groop *et al.* 1989). A previous history of UTI was found in 68 per cent of cases (Groop *et al.* 1989). Renal insufficiency develops in 15 per cent (Lauler *et al.* 1960). The diagnosis should be suspected in a diabetic subject with a UTI who responds poorly to antibiotics, or develops unexplained renal failure (Mujais 1984).

Diagnosis and treatment

The diagnosis of RPN depends on the demonstration of papillary/calyceal abnormalities without focal loss of renal tissue (Fry 1986). The radiological abnormalities are described in Chapter 4.

The IVU is the most sensitive investigation for RPN but is not usually carried out today because of the adverse effect of contrast media on renal function in diabetic subjects. Contrast studies have been recorded as contributing to worsening of renal function in 50 per cent of diabetic subjects with pre-existing renal impairment (Harkonen and Kjellstrand 1977). However, a more recent assessment in IDDM individuals using the newer non-ionic contrast agents (Isopaque and Omnipaque) where the creatinine was below 200 μmol per litre, failed to demonstrate any adverse effect (Groop *et al.* 1989).

Clinically apparent RPN is now relatively rare (Freidman 1990). The reasons for this are unclear, but early identification and treatment of UTI, together with a reduced frequency of IVU examinations may contribute to both a real and an apparent decline. Improved metabolic control cannot be discounted.

Treatment involves aggressive antibiotic therapy when infection is demonstrated. Relief of obstruction may also be required. The prognosis for this condition is not well defined. Patients may have well-preserved renal function, despite extensive papillary damage (Bending 1990). In others, progression to renal failure may be inexorable, although this may be due to the underlying parenchymal disease (e.g. diabetic glomerulosclerosis), rather than renal papillary necrosis.

Emphysematous renal tract disease

Introduction

The presence of gas in the renal tract is relatively uncommon, but shows a strong association with diabetes mellitus. Pneumaturia was first described as early as 1671 (cited in Taussig 1907), but this and subsequent observations often failed to specify the origin of the gas, which may arise in three ways:

(1) prior instrumentation;

(2) vesicocolic or vesicovaginal fistula; and

(3) spontaneous gas formation in the bladder.

Raciborski (1860) is credited with the first description of spontaneous gas formation. An earlier much quoted case described by Brierre de Bosmont (cited in Kelly and MacCallum 1898) is open to doubt. The link with diabetes mellitus was recognized from an early stage with Guiard (1883) publishing four cases describing pneumaturia in association with glycosuria. The first substantive literature review by Kelly and McCallum (1898) recorded that 9 of the 16 cases of pneumaturia had glycosuria. The validity of certain of these cases is questioned by Turman and Rutherford (1971) and Zabbo *et al.* (1985).

The classification of emphysematous renal tract disease (ERTD) presents a problem. That of Turman and Rutherford (1971) is the most logical and comprehensive and is presented in Table 10.2. However, certain of these (e.g. emphysematous ureteritis), may not exist as distinct entities, whilst two or more, such as emphysematous pyelonephritis and peri-renal gas may occur in combination. It is proposed to concentrate on the three conditions most commonly seen, namely emphysematous pyelonephritis with peri-renal gas, emphysematous pyelitis, and emphysematous cystitis. All the early descriptions of pneumaturia, where a fistula was excluded, probably relate to emphysematous cystitis as emphysematous pyelonephritis rarely gives rise to this symptom.

The pathogenesis of ERTD is incompletely understood. Early theories (Senator 1883) that the gas, usually CO_2, although N_2, H_2, O_2, and CH_4 (methane) also present, is a product of glucose fermentation still hold today

Table 10.2 A classification of emphysematous renal tract disease

	Collecting system	Tissue	Outwith renal tract
Kidney	—	Emphysematous pyelonephritis	Peri-renal gas
Pelvis	Intra-pelvic gas	Emphysematous pyelitis	—
Ureter	Intra-ureteral gas	Emphysematous ureteritis	Periurethral gas
Bladder	Intra-cystic gas	Emphysematous cystitis	Peri-cystic gas

(Yang and Shen 1990; Huang *et al.* 1991). Obstruction, and perhaps diabetic micro-angiopathy, may facilitate the development of infection. Why occasional cases are seen in non-diabetic individuals is not known. Impaired vascular supply may be important. Schainuck *et al.* (1968) proposed that necrotic tissue may act as a substrate for gas-forming organisms. Subramanyam *et al.* (1980) described a case of emphysematous pyelonephritis following traumatic renal infarction and tissue necrosis.

Emphysematous pyelonephritis

This is defined as the presence of gas in the renal parenchyma and is often asociated with peri-renal gas. It is a severe life-threatening necrotizing infection with a mortality in excess of 60 per cent. No substantive series of this condition exists, although there are over 80 case reports in the literature several of which are accompanied by a literature review (Spagnola 1978; Michaeli *et al.* 1984; Evanoff *et al.* 1987).

Clinical features

Ninety per cent of cases of emphysematous pyelonephritis are associated with diabetes mellitus (Evanoff *et al.* 1987), although no breakdown of the type of diabetes is given. The mean age reported is 54 years (range 19–81) and women are affected twice as often as men. In contrast to earlier findings that the left kidney was more commonly affected (Michaeli *et al.* 1984; Schultz and Klorfein 1962) a more recent survey (Evanoff *et al.* 1987) found no difference. Bilateral involvement in association with diabetes has been described in rare cases (Gillies and Flocks 1941; Kumar and Rao 1982; Zabbo *et al.* 1985) and in several cases in transplanted kidneys (Brenbridge *et al.* 1979; Parameswaran and Feest 1977; Potter *et al.* 1985).

The clinical presentation is often suggestive of severe acute pyelonephritis, but it may also have an indolent course over several months. In 43 cases the average duration of symptoms was 21 days, ranging from less than a day to eight months (Michaeli *et al.* 1984). Nausea, vomiting (40 per cent), and abdominal pain (55 per cent) are common symptoms. Fever is seen in 80 per cent (Evanoff *et al.* 1987). A palpable mass is rare as is crepitus, although abdominal tenderness is common. Pneumaturia is not found unless there is coincidental emphysematous cystitis.

Laboratory investigations

A neutrophil leucocytosis is observed in the majority of cases. Pyuria is found in 96 per cent (Evanoff *et al.* 1987). Pre-existing renal function was abnormal in 82 per cent of 36 subjects (Michaeli *et al.* 1984). Microbiological investigation shows *E. coli* to be the most common causal organism. In one series, 68 per cent of cases were due to this organism and 9 per cent to Klebsiella (Klein *et al.* 1986). Multiple organisms were found in 14 per cent. Other organisms are rare and many are reported as single cases. *Candida albicans* (Zabbo *et al.* 1985), *C. tropicalis* (Seidenfield *et al.* 1982), cryptococcus (Kumar and Rao 1982), and anaerobic streptococcus (Kass 1957) have been recorded. Clostridium spp. has not been described (Michaeli *et al.* 1984). Pathological examination of the tissue will often reveal an acute inflammation of the interstitium with multiple micro- and macro-abscesses.

Diagnosis

Renal tract emphysema is a radiological diagnosis as the symptoms and signs are little different from other renal infections. The diagnosis should be suspected in any diabetic patient with nausea, vomiting, and abdominal pain, particularily where antibiotic therapy fails to improve an 'acute pyelonephritis' in three to four days. Plain abdominal X-ray or an IVU will reveal gas in 50–80 per cent of cases (Michaeli *et al* 1984; Evanoff *et al.* 1987). Contrast studies should be used judiciously in diabetic subjects with impaired renal function. Langston and Pfister (1970) describe the radiological features of emphysematous pyelonephritis and highlight three patterns. An initial mottling with gas in the renal parenchyma is followed by the development of a crescent of gas surrounding the parenchyma. Finally, extra-vasation of gas occurs through Gerota's fascia into the retroperitoneal space. Such X-ray features are, however, seen in relatively few cases. A simplified classification is suggested by Michaeli *et al.* (1984) :

Stage 1: gas in the renal parenchyma or peri-renal tissue
Stage 2: gas in the kidney and surrounding tissues
Stage 3: extension of gas through Gerota's fascia.

Where there is some doubt, or where delineation is important, the patient should have a CT scan.

Therapy and prognosis

The prognosis for emphysematous pyelonephritis depends on the mode of therapy and the extent of the infection. The highest mortality, 80 per cent, is seen in individuals where the infection extends into the peri-renal space and who receive medical treatment alone (Banks *et al.* 1969; Rosenberg *et al.* 1973). Mortality rates of 60 per cent occur where infection is confined to the renal parenchyma and is treated with antibiotics plus local drainage. The combination of fluid resuscitation, intravenous antibiotics, and nephrectomy may reduce the mortality rate to 20 per cent. Comparison of these data should allow for im-

Table 10.3 Mortality in emphysematous renal tract disease. Comparison of treatment modality between the periods 1898–1970 and 1970–82

	1898–1970		1970–82	
	No. patients	Mortality (%)	No. patients	Mortality (%)
Medical therapy	9	78	4	75
Surgical therapy	12	42	9	11
Combined therapy	7	40	14	7
Overall	28	54	27	21

Adapted from Michaeli *et al.* (1984).

proved diagnostic techniques and resusucitation, but it is evident that there has been little change in mortality from medical therapy alone over the years, as shown in Table 10.3 (compiled from Michaeli *et al.* 1984). It should be noted, however, that the number of cases is small.

Emphysematous pyelitis

In this condition, gas is limited to the collecting system. Evanoff and colleagues (1987) found the condition to be more common in women (3:1), with an overall mean age of 51 years (range less than one to 79 years). In contrast to emphysematous pyelonephritis only 59 per cent of subjects had diabetes, presumably due to a higher proportion of patients with obstruction in this group (64 per cent as against 37 per cent). For reasons that are not clear the left kidney was affected more commonly than the right (53 per cent vs. 36 per cent), and bilateral gas was rarely observed (Soteropolous *et al.* 1957; Ohba *et al.* 1984). The total number of cases is not documented. The symptoms are similar to those in emphysematous pyelonephritis. *Escherichia coli* is again the most common organism. Radiology reveals gas in the collecting system. US or IVU may demonstrate an obstruction. Gas occurs rarely in the bladder in association with emphysematous pyelitis (Ohba *et al.* 1984).

Histopathological studies in this condition are rare, although acute inflammation with submucosal haemorrhage of the renal pelvis and ureter is seen. The renal parenchyma may show an acute interstitial reaction (Harrow and Sloane 1963). Treatment for this condition involves antibiotic therapy with relief of obstruction where necessary. The reported mortality is 18 per cent (Evanoff *et al.* 1987).

Emphysematous cystitis

The early descriptions of pneumaturia in the absence of fistulous communication or instrumentation almost certainly were of this condition. Prior to the review of Bailey (1961), gas production was arbitarily described as primary pneumaturia

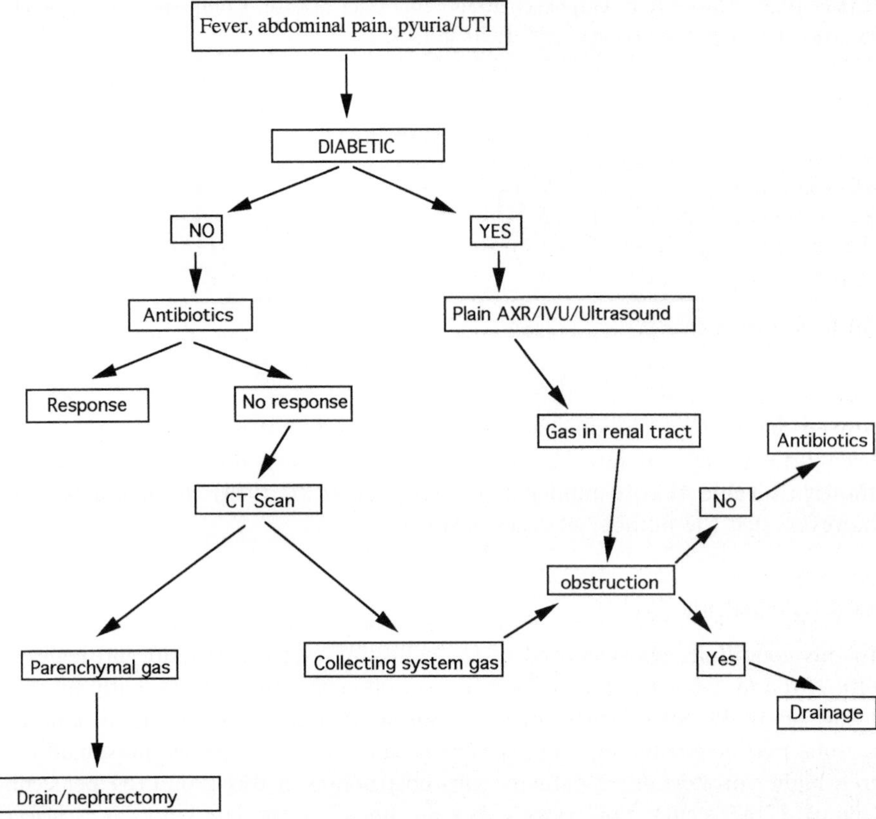

Fig. 10.1 Management plan for renal tract emphysema. (Adapted from Evanoff *et al.* 1987.)

(46 cases) or cystitis emphysematosa (52 cases). Bailey, who considered them to be the same entity added a further 19 cases to the literature. Diabetes mellitus was recorded in 29/46, 13/52, and 15/19 cases respectively—in total 51 per cent of the combined series. Why the proportion of diabetes should be so low in the second group is not clear. Women were more common (2:1) in Bailey's series. Mean age was 54 years (range 25–83). The mean duration of diabetes was 14 years (0–35).

Escherichia coli is the most common infecting organism. Enterobacter is also relatively common, and there are occasional reports of Proteus species, *Staphylococcus aureus*, Streptococcus species, and yeasts (Bailey 1961). Gross haematuria is a common finding. Eleven of 19 cases had gas in the lumen and in the bladder wall, two in the wall, and six in the lumen alone. Autopsy studies in two patients showed acute and chronic submucosal inflammation with vesicles and ulcerated areas in the mucosa. X-rays of the bladder are characteristic with a narrow radiolucent line of gas bubbles outlining the bladder wall that may resemble cobblestones (Fry 1986). An IVU or US may demonstrate an obstruction (e.g. prostatic hypertrophy).

In contrast to the earlier discussed conditions, the prognosis for emphysematous cystitis is good and no death as a direct consequence of infection was seen in Bailey's series.

Figure 10.1 outlines the management of emphysema of the upper renal tract (adapted from Evanoff *et al.* 1987).

Conclusion

ERTD, although uncommon, may be associated with a high mortality. Many cases are associated with diabetes mellitus. A high index of suspicion, appropriate radiological assessment, and early surgical intervention offer the best hope of a cure for emphysematous pyelonephritis. Emphysematous pyelitis and and cystitis are more benign and are treated with antibiotics alone or the combination of antibiotics and relief of obstruction.

References

Atcheson, D. W. (1941). Perinephric abscess with a review of 117 cases. *Journal of Urology*, **46**, 201–8.

Bahl, A. L., Chugh, R. N., and Sharma, K. B. (1970). Asymptomatic bacteriuria in diabetics attending a diabetic clinic. *Indian Journal of Medical Science*, **24**, 1–6.

Bailey, H. (1961). Cystitis emphysematosa. *American Journal of Roentgenology*, **86**, 850–62.

Baker, L. R. I., Cattell, W. R., Fry, I. K. F., and Mallinson, W. J. W. (1979). Acute renal failure due to bacterial pyelonephritis. *Quarterly Journal of Medicine*, **48**, 603–12.

Banks, D. E., Persky, L., and Mahoney, S. A. (1969). Renal emphysema. *Journal of Urology*, **102**, 390–2.

Barnard, D. M., Story, R. D., and Root, H. F. (1953). Urinary-tract infections in diabetic women. *New England Journal of Medicine*, **248**, 136–41.

Bending, J. J. (1990). The kidney and renal tract. In *Diabetes clinical management*, (ed. R. B. Tattersall and E. A. M. Gale), pp. 281–92. Churchill Livingstone, Edinburgh.

Bevan, J. S., Griffiths, G. J., Williams J. D., and Gibby, O. M. (1989). Bilateral renal cortical abscesses in a young woman with type 1 diabetes. *Diabetic Medicine*, **6**, 454–7.

Brenbridge, A. N. A. G., Buschi, A. J., Cochrane, J. A., and Lees, R. F. (1979). Renal emphysema of the transplanted kidney: sonographic appearance. *American Journal of Roentgenology*, **132**, 656–8.

Cattell, W. R. (1992). Urinary tract infection and acute renal failure. In *Advanced renal medicine*, (ed. A. E. G. Raine), pp. 302–13. Oxford University Press.

Cattell, W. R., Greenwood, R. N., and Baker, L. R. I. (1985). Reversible renal failure due to interstitial infection of the kidney. In *Recent advances in chemotherapy*, (ed. J. Ishigami), pp. 225–8. University of Tokyo Press.

Davies, R. R. and Reeves, D. S. (1971). 5-Fluoro-cytosine and urinary candidiasis. *British Medical Journal*, **1**, 577–9.

Edmondson, H. A., Martin, H. E., and Evans, N. (1947). Necrosis of renal papillae and acute pyelonephritis in diabetes mellitus. *Archives of Internal Medicine*, **79**, 148–75.

Ellenberg, M. (1976). Diabetic neuropathy: clinical aspects. *Metabolism*, **25**, 1627–55.

Evanoff, G. V., Thompson, C. S., Foley, R., and Weinman, E. J. (1987). Spectrum of gas within the kidney. *American Journal of Medicine*, **83**, 149–54.

Forland, M., Thomas, V., and Shelokov, A. (1977). Urinary tract infections in patients with diabetes mellitus. *Journal of the American Medical Association*, **238**, 1924–6.

Francis, P. and Walsh, T. J. (1992). Evolving role of flucytosine in immunocompromised patients; new insights into safety, pharmacokinetics, and antifungal therapy. *Clinics in Infectious Disease*, **15**, 1003–18.

Freidman, E. A. (1990). Diabetic renal disease. In *Diabetes mellitus*, (ed. H. Rifkin and D. Porte, jun.), pp. 684–709. Elsevier, New York.

Froboese, C. (1937). Über sequestrierende Marknekrosen der Nieren bei Diabetes mellitus. *Verhandl. d. Deutsch. Gesellch. Path.* **30**, 431–43.

Fry, I. K. (1986). Renal parenchymal disease. In *Diagnostic radiology*, (ed. R. G. Grainger and D. J. Allison), pp. 1115–35. Churchill Livingstone, Edinburgh.

Gillies, C. L. and Flocks, R. (1941). Spontaneous renal and perirenal emphysema. *American Journal of Roentgenology*, **46**, 173–4.

Goldberg, P. K., Kozinn, P. J., Wise, G. J., Nouri, N., and Brooks, R. B. (1979). Incidence and significance of candiduria. *Journal of the American Medical Association*, **241**, 582–4.

Grant, S. M. and Clissold, S. P. (1990). Fluconazole: a review of its pharmacodynamic and pharmacokinetic properties, and therapeutic potential in superficial and systemic mycoses. *Drugs*, **39**, 877–916.

Groop, L. C., Laasonen, L., and Edgren, J. (1989). Renal papillary necrosis in subjects with IDDM. *Diabetes Care*, **12**, 198–202.

Guiard, F-P. (1883). Du dévéloppment spontane de gaz dans la vessie. *Annals d. mal. d. org. genitourin.* **1**, 846–8.

Gunther, G. W. (1937). Die Pepillennekrosen der Niere bei Diabetes. *München. Med. Wochnschr.*, **84**, 1695–9.

Hansen, R. O. (1964). Bacteriuria in diabetic and non-diabetic outpatients. *Acta Medica Scandinavica*, **176**, 721–30.

Harkonen, S. and Kjellstrand, C. M. (1977). Exacerbation of diabetic renal failure following intravenous pyelolography. *American Journal of Medicine*, **63**, 939–46.

Harrow, B. R. and Sloane, J. A. (1963). Ureteritis emphysematosa; spontanoeous ureteral pneumatogram; renal and perirenal emphysema. *Journal of Urology*, **89**, 43–8.

Hooton, T. M. and Stamm, W. E. (1991). Management of acute uncomplicated UTI in adults. In *Urinary tract infections*, (ed. Donald Kaye), pp. 339–57. Medical Clinics of North America, Philadelphia.

Huang, J-J., Chen, K-W., and Ruaan, M-K. (1991). Mixed acid fermantation of glucose as a mechanism of emphysematous urinary tract infection. *Journal of Urology*, **146**, 148–51.

Langston, C. S. and Pfister, R. C. (1970). Renal emphysema. A case report and review of the literature. *American Journal of Roentgenology*, **110**, 778–86.

Kass, E. H. (1957). Bacteriuria and the diagnosis of infections of the urinary tract. *Archives of Internal Medicine*, **100**, 709–14.

Kauffman, C. A. and Tan, J. S. (1974). *Torulopsis glabrata* renal infection. *American Journal of Medicine*, **57**, 217–24.

Kelly, H. A. and MacCallum, W. G. (1898). Pneumaturia. *Journal of the American Medical Association*, **31**, 375–80.

Klein, F. A., Smith, M. J., Vick, C. W., and Schneider V. (1986). Emphysematous pyelonephritis; diagnosis and treatment. *South African Medical Journal*, **79**, 41–6.

Korzeniowski, O. M. (1991). Urinary tract infection in the impaired host. In *Urinary tract infections*, (ed. Donald Kaye), pp. 391–404. Medical Clinics of North America, Philadelphia.

Kozinn, P. J., Taschdjian, C. L., Goldberg, P. K., Wise, G. J., Toni, E. F., and Seeling, M. S. (1978). Advances in the diagnosis of renal candidiasis. *Journal of Urology*, **119**, 184–7.

Kumar, D. and Rao, B. R. (1982). Case profile: bilateral emphysematous pyelonephritis. *Urology*, **20**, 96.

Lancet (1988). Editorial. Urinary tract candidosis. *Lancet*, **2**, 1000–1.

Langston, C. S. and Pfister, R. C. (1970). Renal emphysemia. A case report and review of the literature. *American Journal of Roentgenology*, **110**, 778–86.

Lauler, D. P., Schreiner, G. E., and David A. (1960). Renal medullary necrosis. *American Journal of Medicine*, **29**, 132–56.

Leibovici, L., Samra, Z., Konisberger, H., Kalter-Leibovici, O., Pitlik, S. D., and Drucker M. (1991). Bacteraemia in adult diabetic patients. *Diabetes Care*, **14**, 89–94.

Leibovici, L., Greenshtain, S., Cohen, O., and Wysenbeek, A. J. (1992). Toward improved empiric management of moderate to severe urinary tract infections. *Archives of Internal Medicine*, **152**, 2481–6.

MacFarlane, I. A., Brown, R. M., Smyth, R. W., Burdon, D. W., and Fitzgerald, M. G. (1986). Bacteraemia in diabetics. *Journal of Infection*, **12**, 213–19.

Mandel, E. E. (1952). Renal medullary necrosis. *American Journal of Medicine*, **13**, 322–7.

Marks, M. I., Langston, C., and Eickhoff, T. C. (1970). *Torulopsis glabrata*- an opportunistic pathogen in man. *New England Journal of Medicine*, **283**, 1131–5.

Mehnert, B. and Mehnert, H. (1958). Yeasts in urine and saliva of diabetic and non-diabetic patients. *Diabetes*, **7**, 293–7.

Michaeli, J., Mogle, P., Perlberg, S., Heiman, S., and Caine, M. (1984). Emphysematous pyelonephritis. *Journal of Urology*, **131**, 203–8.

Mogensen, C. E. (ed.) (1988). *The kidney and hypertension in diabetes mellitus.* Kluwer, Boston.

Mujais, S. K. (1984). Renal papillary necrosis in diabetes mellitus. *Seminars in Nephrology*, **4**, 40–7.

Obana, Y., Shibata, K., and Nishino, T. (1991). Adherence of *Serratia marcescens* in the pathogenesis of urinary tract infections in diabetic mice. *Journal of Medical Microbiology*, **35**, 93–7.

Obrant, O. (1949). Perirenal abscess. *Acta Chirurgica Scandinavica*, **97**, 338–53.

Ohba, S., Tsuchiya, H., Kohno, S., and Hamazaki, M. (1984). Ureteritis and pyelitis emphysematosa in a neonate. *Paediatric Radiology*, **14**, 116–7.

Ooi, B. S., Chen, B. T. M., and Yu, M. (1974). Prevalence and site of bacteriuria in diabetes mellitus. *Postgraduate Medical Journal*, **50**, 497–9.

O'Sullivan, D. J., Fitzgerald, M. G., Meynell, M. J., and Malins, J. M. (1961). Urinary tract infection. *British Medical Journal* **1**, 786–8.

Parameswaran, R. and Feest, T. (1977). Gas nephrogram: an unusual complication of renal transplantion. *British Journal of Radiology*, **50**, 438–40.

Parving, H-H., Kastrup, H., Smidt, U. M., Andersen, A. R., Feldt-Rasmussen, B., and Sandahl-Christiansen J. (1984). Impaired autoregulation of glomerular filtration rate in Type I (insulin-dependent) diabetic patients with nephropathy. *Diabetologia*, **27**, 547–52.

Pometta, D., Rees, S. B., Younger, D., and Kass, E. H. (1967). Asymptomatic bacterium in diabetes mellitus. *New England Journal of Medicine*, **276**, 1118–21.

Potter, J. L., Sullivan, B. M., Flournoy, J. C., and Gerza, C. (1985). Emphysema in the renal allograft. *Radiology*, **155**, 51–2.

Raciborski. (1860). Exemple de pneumaturie du urine gazeuse chez une malade affecté d'une nevropathie proteiforme avec prédominance des symptomes de hypochondrie. *Gaz. d'Hôp., Paris*. [Cited in Kelly and MacCallum 1898.]

Rayfield, E. J., Ault, M. J., Keusch, G. T., Brothers, M. J., Nechemias, C., and Smith, H. (1982). Infection and diabetes: the case for glucose control. *American Journal of Medicine*, **72**, 439–50.

Richet, G. and Mayaud, C. (1978). The course of acute renal failure in pyelonephritis and other types of interstitial nephritis. *Nephron*, **22**, 124–7.

Robbins, S. L. and Tucker, A. W. (1944). The cause of death in diabetes. *New England Journal of Medicine*, **231**, 865–8.

Robbins, S. L., Mallory, G. K., and Kimsey, T. D. (1946). Necrotising renal papillitis: a form of acute pyelonephritis. *New England Journal of Medicine*, **235**, 885–93.

Rosenberg, J. W., Quader, A., and Brown, J. S. (1973). Renal emphysema. *Urology*, **1**, 237–9.

Salvatierra, O., Bucklew, W. B., and Morrow, J. W. (1967). Perinephric abscess: a report of 71 cases. *Journal of Urology*, **98**, 296–302.

Sawers, J. S. A., *et al.* (1986). Bacteriuria and autonomic nerve function in diabetic women. *Diabetes Care*, **9**, 460–4.

Schainuck, L. I., Fouty, R., and Cutler, R. E. (1968). Emphysematous pyelonephritis: A new case and review of the literature. *American Journal of Medicine*, **44**, 134–9.

Schmitt, J. K., Fawcett, C. J., and Gullickson, G. (1986). Asymptomatic bacteriuria and haemoglobin A_1. *Diabetes Care*, **9**, 518–20.

Schultz, E. H. and Klorfein, E. H. (1962). Emphysematous pyelonephritis. *Journal of Urology*, **87**, 762–6.

Seidenfeld, S. M., Lemaistre, C. F., Setiawan, H., and Munford, R. S. (1982). Emphysematous pyelonephritis caused by *Candida tropicalis*. *Journal of Infectious Disease*, **146**, 569.

Senator, H. (1883). Über Pneumaturia im allgemeinen und bei diabetes mellitus insbesondere. *Internat. Beitr. z. Wissensch. Med.*, **3**, 317. [Cited in Bailey 1961.].

Soteropoulos, C., Kawashima, E., and Gilmore, J. H. (1957). Cystitis and ureteritis emphysematosa. *Radiology*, **68**, 866–8.

Spagnola, A. M. (1978). Emphysematous pyelonephritis. *American Journal of Medicine*, **64**, 840–4.

Stamm, W. E., Martin, S. M., and Bennett, J. V. (1977). Epidemiology of nosocomial infections due to gram negative bacilli: aspects relevant to development and use of vaccines. *Journal of Infectious Disease*, **136** (Suppl.), S151–60.

Subramanyam, B. R., Lefleur, R. S, and Van Natta, F. C. (1980). Renal emphysema secondary to traumatic renal infarction. *Urologic Radiology*, **2**, 53–4.

Taft, J. L., Billson, V. R., Nankervis, A., Kincaid-Smith, P., and Martin, F. I. R. (1990). A clinical-histological study of individuals with diabetes mellitus and proteinuria. *Diabetic Medicine*, **7**, 215–21.

Taussig, A. E. (1907). Pneumaturia with report of a case. *Boston Medical and Surgical Journal*, **156**, 769–74.

Thorley, J. D., Jones, S. R., and Sandford, J. Y. (1974). Perinephric abscess. *Medicine*, **53**, 441–51.

Turck, M., Anderson, K. N., and Petersdorf, R. G. (1966). Relapse and reinfection in chronic bacteriuria. *New England Journal of Medicine*, **275**, 70–3.

Turman, A. E. and Rutherford, C. (1971). Emphysematous pyelonephritis with perinephric gas. *Journal of Urology*, **105**, 165–70.

Turner, F. C. (1888). Necrosis of the pyramids of one kidney. *Transactions of the Pathological Society of London*, **39**, 159–61 .

Vjelsgaard, R. (1966*a*). Studies on urinary infection in diabetics. I. bacteriuria in patients with diabetes mellitus and in control subjects. *Acta Medica Scandinavica*, **179**, 173–82.

Vejlsgaard, R. (1966*b*). Studies on urinary infection in diabetics. II. significant bacteriuria in relation to long-term diabetic manifestations. *Acta Medica Scandinavica*, **179**, 183–8.

Wheat, L. J. (1980). Infection and diabetes mellitus. *Diabetes Care*, **3**, 187–97.

Williams, D. N., Knight, A. H., King, H., and Harris, D. M. (1975). The microbial flora of the vagina and its relationship to bacteriuria in diabetic and non-diabetic women. *British Journal of Urology*, **47**, 453–7.

Wise, G. J., Goldberg, P., and Kozinn, P. J. (1976). Genitourinary candidiasis: diagnosis and treatment. *Journal of Urology*, **116**, 778–80.

Yang, W-H. and Shen, N-C. (1990). Gas forming infection of the urinary tract: an investigation of fermentation as a mechanism. *Journal of Urology*, **143**, 960–4.

Zabbo, A., Montie, J. E., Popowniak, K. L., and Weinstein, A. J. (1985). Bilateral emphysematous pyelonephritis. *Urology*, **25**, 293–6.

11
Urinary tract infection in the elderly

M. J. Bendall

Introduction

Bacteriuria is very common in the elderly as is symptomatic urinary tract infection (UTI). The importance of significant bacteriuria in the absence of urinary tract symptoms—referred to as asymptomatic bacteriuria in the young—remains unclear. The validity of the concept of asymptomatic bacteriuria in the elderly is also questionable in the context of atypical presentation of disease in this group. The need for treatment of significant bacteriuria in the elderly, in the absence of local or general evidence of infection, is increasingly doubted. The statistical relationship between bacteriuria and death in the elderly may be epiphenomenal and, at a clinical level, raises the question of whether patients die *of* bacteriuria or *with* it.

Epidemiology

In those over 65 years of age the prevalence of bacteriuria is greater in women than in men. Studies of the elderly in different settings demonstrate a prevalence gradient, the lowest levels being in those living in their own homes, the highest in those in long-stay wards (Table 11.1). This gradient primarily reflects increasing levels of physical and mental impairment requiring increasing levels of care by others in different care settings (Boscia *et al.* 1986*b*). Close proximity to other patients, physical care by staff, and the use of communal facilities, such as

Table 11.1 Prevalence of bacteriuria in men and women over the age of 65 years

Study setting	Prevalence (per cent)	
	Men	Women
Subject's own home	6–13	17–33
Residential (rest) home	17–26	23–27
Hospital assessment wards	30–33	32–34
Long-stay hospital wards	34	34–50

Derived from Akhtar *et al.* (1972); Brocklehurst *et al.* (1968); Gladstone and Recco (1976); Kasviki-Charvati *et al.* (1982); Sourander (1966); Sourander and Kasanen (1972).

baths and toilets, may all contribute to the transfer of pathogens from one suspectable individual to another.

In community studies, there is conflicting evidence of increasing prevalence with age. A study in Finland demonstrated prevalences of 2 per cent and 17 per cent respectively in men and women aged between 65 and 69 years rising to 18 per cent and 36 per cent in those aged over 80 years (Sourander 1966; Sourander and Kasanen 1972). Brocklehurst *et al.* (1968, 1972) found an age-related increase only in men and suggested that an increase in the frequency of bacteriuria in women occurred earlier in life and was therefore not detected in studies of those over 65 years old. Boscia *et al.* (1986*b*) demonstrated a significant increase in prevalence of bacteriuria in women but not in men. Akhtar *et al.* (1972) detected no age-related trend in prevalence in either sex.

In elderly inpatients, the evidence for an age-related gradient for bacteriuria is limited and inconclusive. In a study of patients in geriatric wards Walkey *et al.* (1967) reported advancing age to have no effect on the prevalence of bacteriuria in either sex, although a further analysis of the reported data (Bendall 1984) suggests that there may have been an effect of age in men. Bendall (1984) found no effect of age in women but a significant difference in men. Thus, men below the median age of the study population (79 years) had a prevalence of 17.2 per cent and those over the median age, one of 35.4 per cent.

One of the problems in interpreting data from studies of bacteriuria in the elderly is that different criteria have been used to define bacteriuria. In the community-based studies mentioned above only those of Akhtar *et al.* (1972) and Boscia *et al.* (1986*b*) used Kass's bacterial counting method of separating bacteriuria from urinary contamination.

Another issue not addressed in point prevalence studies is the dynamics of bacteriuria—the extent to which bacteriuria comes and goes in individuals studied over time, irrespective of antimicrobial usage. This will be considered later in the chapter.

A further source of information about the epidemiology of UTI in the elderly comes from statistical data collected routinely from clinical services. This has been reviewed by Bendall (1987). General practice consultation rates for cystitis are higher at all ages in women than in men (OPCS 1974). The rate for women is highest during the reproductive years, whereas that for men increases with age. Consultation rates for renal infection show a similar pattern to those for cystitis.

Examination of data from the Hospital Inpatient Enquiry (HIPE) (OPCS 1980*a*) shows an overall increase with age in discharges and deaths due to cystitis in both sexes, and the rate is greater at all ages in women than in men except in those aged 80 to 85 years. This apparent increase in importance of cystitis with age is confirmed by data from death certification (OPCS 1980*b*), which shows mortality due to the condition rising sharply in people aged over 70 years, the rate again being higher in women than in men.

HIPE data (OPCS 1980*a*) for discharges and deaths related to kidney infection shows women to be affected about twice as often as men. The distribution in women is bimodal with an initial peak in the reproductive years—corresponding to the peak in general practice (GP) consultations for cystitis and renal infection—and a second peak in those aged over 80 years. The second peak is not present in GP consultation rates, which, as already discussed, show an apparent lack of age-related prevalence of UTI in elderly women. The discrepancy between these two sets of data may reflect atypical presentation of UTI in elderly women. Brocklehurst *et al.* (1972) found very little association in elderly women between bacteriuria and the presence or absence of symptoms normally associated with UTI in younger women. This has been confirmed in subsequent studies. Thus, elderly women with UTI may not be identified as such but rather present with falling, confusion, or immobility.

In men, there is a sharp peak in incidence of renal infection among those 75 to 80 years of age and the proportion of elderly male hospital patients who die as a result of renal infection is greater than for females. This male distribution almost certainly reflects the increasing impact of prostatic disease with age.

Taking into consideration epidemiological evidence from all the sources discussed it is clear that bacteriuria and UTI increase in frequency and in clinical significance with age and are more common in women than in men. Conditions that affect the urinary tract both directly and indirectly, predispose to infection, and account for the relationship in the elderly between bacteriuria and physical and mental impairment.

Dynamics of bacteriuria

Several studies have shown that in individuals studied over time bacteriuria comes and goes and that many more individuals are affected than suggested by prevalence figures. Sourander's community study (Sourander 1966) showed that 11 per cent of elderly men and 33 per cent of elderly women had bacteriuria when first screened. When followed-up five years later (Sourander and Kasanen 1972), the prevalence in survivors was unchanged but most who were bacteriuric initially were abacteriuric. The rate of reversion from the positive to the negative state was 85 per cent in men and 60 per cent in women. Most of the subjects found to be bacteriuric at five years were originally in the uninfected group.

Boscia *et al.* (1986*b*) conducted a 12-month study of a defined population screened for bacteriuria on three occasions at six-monthly intervals. A rigid definition of bacteriuria was used, based on Kass's criteria, but requiring confirmation of a significant growth by a repeat culture a week later showing significant bacteriuria with the same organism. The cumulative percentage of subjects infected on at least one occasion was high: 30 per cent of women and 10.5 per cent of men. Subjects with impaired activities of daily living or mental status were more likely to have bacteriuria regardless of their place of residence. Persistence of the same organism was infrequent: 6 per cent in women and 1 per cent in men. Persistent bacteriuria was more common in subjects resident in a nursing home, presumably reflecting the greater prevalence of diseases predisposing to the acquisition and persistence of bacteriuria in this group.

In a longitudinal study of residents in a home for the elderly Kasviki-Charvati *et al.* (1982) found a positive conversion rate of 11 per cent in men and 23 per cent in women. The negative conversion rate was 22 per cent in men and 27 per cent in women. Subjects bacteriuric at entry to the study and non-bacteriuric at a 6-month reassessment had re-infection rates at 12 months of 77 per cent for men and 44 per cent for women. A previous history of bacteriuria in a subject with currently sterile urine increased the chance of re-infection by 2 to 7 times that of subjects with no past infection. In long-stay geriatric patients, Brocklehurst *et al.* (1977) found that the positive conversion rate per year was even higher, 46 per cent of previously non-bacteriuric controls becoming positive at one year.

It has been suggested that the more frequently bacteriuria is sought in an elderly individual the more likely will it be detected. It seems probable that most elderly women have episodes of bacteriuria at some time. Boscia *et al.* (1986*b*) concluded that, as the turnover from infected to non-infected status and vice versa was so great, treatment of asymptomatic bacteriuria in the elderly was probably unnecessary.

Significance of bacteriuria

Information about the significance of bacteriuria in the elderly is incomplete and in some respects contradictory. For example, it has often been assumed that bacteriuria represents bladder rather than upper tract infection and because of this is of little importance in terms of patient management. Asscher (1980), on the other hand, has suggested that the major concern in elderly bacteriurics is the possibility of their developing septicaemia. Studies in female inpatients in a geriatric admission ward (Suntharalingham *et al.* 1983) and among elderly women living in an institutional setting (Nicolle *et al.* 1988*b*) suggest that up to two-thirds of elderly females found to have bacteriuria have infections of the upper urinary tract. These subjects are, however, highly selected and the results may not apply to other groups of elderly individuals.

Comparing results and drawing general conclusions from different studies is fraught with difficulty. There are differences between study populations in terms of size, age distribution, and particularly derivation—whether the sample is from the community, a rest home, a nursing home, or a hospital ward. Different derivations lead to different patterns and severity of underlying disease and disability. Some studies showing a lack of association between bacteriuria and other factors such as urinary tract symptoms, hypertension, and renal dysfunction have been based on small sample sizes and may lack the predictive power to demonstrate such relationships.

There is also a lack of consistency in the criteria used to define significant bacteriuria and a failure, in many studies, to recognize the dynamics of bacteriuria over time. The significance of a single isolated episode of bacteriuria in relation to other factors may be totally different from that of persistent or recurrent bacteriuria (Boscia *et al.* 1987*a*).

Morbidity

Diminished glomerular filtration rate and renal plasma flow have been reported in elderly bacteriurics (Marketos *et al.* 1969), but other workers, using less refined measures of renal function, failed to demonstrate any impairment (Akhtar *et al.* 1972; Sourander 1966). In fit elderly individuals there appears to be no relationship between bacteriuria and elevation of blood pressure. In the hospitalized elderly, however, there is some evidence suggesting that patients with bacteriuria tend to have higher blood pressures than controls (Marketos *et al.* 1970). Even if such relationships do exist it does not imply a causal effect. Both may be related to other underlying renal disease.

The possibility of bacteriuria leading to septicaemia has already been mentioned. Though prevalence rates for bacteraemia are 5 to 10 times higher in the old compared to the young (Haley *et al.* 1981) studies in the hospitalized elderly suggest that in geriatric units in which blood cultures are very readily performed, only between 1 and 2 per cent of patients have bacteraemia (Bendall and Bendall 1987; Denham and Godwin 1977; Windsor 1983). In a long-stay care facility the incidence of bacteraemia was 0.3 per 1000 patient care days (Setia *et al.* 1984). Whether screening of the elderly and treatment of those with bacteriuria would prevent deaths due to septicaemia remains to be proved. Bacteriuria is so common in the elderly and the turnover of bacteriuria so high that screening would present enormous logistical and financial problems. Identification of factors particularly associated with septicaemia in the elderly: possibly including diseases of the urinary tract, neurological disorders affecting bladder function, musculoskeletal diseases, dementia, malnutrition, immune compromisation, and perhaps age itself, might allow more appropriate case finding.

Mortality

Several studies have demonstrated a relationship between increased mortality and bacteriuria in the elderly. In their community study Sourander and Kasanen (1972) showed that bacteriuric individuals had a greater five-year mortality than abacteriuric subjects. Dontas *et al.* (1981), in a study of residents in a home for the elderly, showed significant shortening of survival in those with bacteriuria. Similar results have been found in other studies (Evans *et al.* 1982; Platt *et al.* 1982). The mechanism of this relationship is not clear and recent studies that have controlled for confounding influences (age and coexisting disease) have failed to confirm a direct association.

The increased death rate may be due to other underlying disease rather than coexisting bacteriuria. Brocklehurst *et al.* (1977) found a relationship between bacteriuria and dementia. Dontas *et al.* (1981) noted that 'senile cachexia' and cerebrovascular accident were found more commonly in those with bacteriuria. Nordenstam *et al.* (1986) found that other fatal diseases rather than the bacteriuria accounted for the increased mortality in elderly bacteriurics. Thus the relationship between bacteriuria and increased mortality for many elderly patients is probably epiphenomenal rather than causal.

Asymptomatic bacteriuria

The relationship between significant bacteriuria and symptoms normally associated with UTI—dysuria and frequency—is poor. Most elderly patients with significant bacteriuria have no urinary tract symptoms and conversely such symptoms are commonly found in elderly individuals with sterile urine.

Concepts, such as 'significant bacteriuria' and 'asymptomatic bacteriuria', derive mainly from community-based epidemiological studies in younger individuals. Lack of urinary symptoms may have very different connotations in the elderly in whom atypical presentation of disease is common.

Conditions, which in younger individuals present with typical organ or disease-based symptomatology—for example, myocardial infarction presenting with chest pain — in the elderly commonly present in a variety of non-specific ways: falls, immobility, confusion, 'failure to thrive', and incontinence. UTI unaccompanied by urinary symptoms may present in one of these non-specific ways. The presentation may be sudden in onset, indicating that an acute illness is present but equally the symptoms may appear insidiously.

The diagnosis of asymptomatic bacteriuria depends on Kass's criteria of more than 10^5 colony-forming units (CFU) of the same organism per ml of urine. Boscia *et al.* (1986*b*) have used more rigorous criteria in requiring two positive urine culture results with the same organism at 10^5 CFU/ml within one week of each other. Support for this more rigorous approach comes from Nicolle *et al.* (1987*b*) who found that the diagnosis on the basis of a single positive urine culture leads to an over-diagnosis rate of about 10 per cent.

Boscia *et al.* (1986*a*) when screening an ambulant elderly population, found no relationship between asymptomatic bacteriuria and a variety of other non-urinary symptoms. These symptoms were selected as reflecting a sense of impaired well-being and included anorexia, difficulty in falling asleep, difficulty in staying asleep, fatigue, malaise, and weakness. There was also no relationship between bacteriuria and urinary incontinence, a change in frequency of incontinence, urinary frequency, or urgency. They concluded that, in the elderly, bacteriuria in the absence of dysuria is asymptomatic.

The same may not apply to an elderly individual admitted to hospital with recent onset of non-specific symptomatology. In the search for a cause for this presentation, urine culture is commonly performed and if a significant growth of a single organism is found, it may be argued that the physician is already committed to treatment of the bacteriuria by virtue of having sought it in the first place. There is no evidence as to what the clinical outcome would be if bacteriuria were not treated in this situation.

The apparently benign nature of asymptomatic bacteriuria is further supported by studies which demonstrate that the condition does not necessarily progress to symptomatic disease. Indeed, in populations in which asymptomatic bacteriuria is common, symptomatic infection is relatively uncommon (Nicolle *et al.* 1983, 1987*a*).

A question remains as to whether long-term antimicrobial treatment of elderly people with asymptomatic bacteriuria would confer significant benefit in terms of morbidity or mortality. A prerequisite to studies of this question is the development of treatment regimes effective at maintaining subjects bacteriuria-free in the long term. Boscia *et al.* (1987*b*) found that in mobile, community-living elderly women with bacteriuria, 35 per cent of those not treated and 64 per cent of those treated were free from bacteriuria six months after entry to the study. In the light of these results they suggested that regimes to keep individuals bacteriuria-free were a possibility.

Studies of the long-term treatment of asymptomatic bacteriuria are few and confined to subjects in long-stay facilities. In their studies of such subjects Nicolle's group found that treatment of asymptomatic bacteriuria detected by monthly urine culture did not seem to confer significant benefit either in terms of the likelihood of subsequent symptomatic infection or of mortality (Nicolle *et al.* 1983, 1987*b*, 1988*a*). The problem with such studies is that there are many confounding variables which will influence outcome and the subject sample sizes have been low. Nordenstam *et al.* (1986) have suggested that to exclude adequately an effect of bacteriuria on mortality by allowing for clinical variables and to examine the effect of treatment, large multi-centre studies will be necessary.

Two other factors must be considered in the context of long-term antimicrobial treatment. First, the rate of adverse reactions to antibiotics in the elderly is high and may outweigh potential benefits. Secondly, use of antimicrobial agents is associated with the acquisition of often multiply-resistant organisms, which may make treatment of subsequent clinical infection difficult (Bendall and Grüneberg 1979; Grüneberg and Bendall 1979; Bendall 1984; Bendall *et al.* 1986, 1989; Bendall 1987).

At the moment, therefore, asymptomatic bacteriuria is considered to be benign in the elderly and the value of long-term treatment of those with the condition remains to be proven.

Aetiology

A detailed discussion of age-related change in the immune system is beyond the scope of the current text. There is some waning of immune responses but, in the elderly, the role which this plays in the general increase in the incidence of infections is unclear. Impaired immune responses do not of themselves explain the phenomenon (Fox 1992). There is no evidence that local periurethral and vaginal antibodies, which are thought to play a part in local defence mechanisms, decline with age. General debility, and local functional disturbance consequent on age-related change or diseases probably play a major part.

Most infections of the urinary tract occur by organisms ascending the urethra from the perineum. Age-related changes in the urethra result in loss of the physical barrier normally presented by the closed urethra. This predisposes the elderly individual to urinary incontinence and infection. The ageing changes include loss of urethral smooth muscle and replacement by connective tissue, thinning of the urinary epithelium, and mucosal atrophy. The shorter urethra in females may render them more susceptible to infection, although in some studies very elderly men have rates of incontinence and infection approaching those in women of the same age.

Flushing of the lower urinary tract also prevents ascent of contaminating organisms. Many elderly patients, especially those with urinary incontinence, those who live in institutions, and those who are acutely ill from other causes, have a reduced fluid intake and hence reduced urinary output.

Urinary stasis is a problem for many elderly patients. This can arise for a number of reasons including bladder diverticula and trabeculation, prostatic hypertrophy in men, uterine prolapse in women, constipation leading to physical bladder outflow obstruction, or atony of the bladder due to reflex relaxation.

Neurological diseases, in particular, cerebrovascular disease and senile dementia, lead to abnormal bladder function. The patient may have an unstable bladder in which uncontrolled contractions and emptying occur with volumes of urine that would be readily contained by a normal bladder. The patient experiences urge micturition or incontinence. Alternatively, neurological disease may lead to an atonic bladder. In both types of neurological bladder disorder stasis tends to occur with inadequate flushing and an increased predisposition to infection.

Alteration in perineal microbial flora with replacement of commensals by more pathogenic bacteria may increase the risk of infection. This occurs particularly in conditions of poor hygiene, faecal incontinence, in diabetes mellitus, when the patient is exposed to antimicrobial therapy, or is in an environment in which there is extensive use of antimicrobial agents. Faecal incontinence with perineal soiling probably increases the bacterial inoculum size (Brocklehurst *et al.* 1977).

The role of adherence of bacteria to uroepithelial cells, which some studies have suggested is the most important bacterial virulence factor for UTI, may be less in the elderly, being associated with bacteriuria in elderly men only (Sobel and Kaye 1987).

Bacteriology

The most common causative organism is *Escherichia coli*, although infection with other organisms, such as Proteus spp., Klebsiella spp., and *Pseudomonas aeruginosa*, is more common than in younger individuals (Akhtar *et al.* 1972; Lye 1978; Walkey *et al.* 1967; Wolfson *et al.* 1965). In the hospitalized elderly in geriatric wards the pattern of organisms isolated depends on whether the infection is community- or hospital-acquired. *Escherichia coli* accounts for about 80 per cent of isolates in community-acquired infection and for 55 per cent in hospital-acquired infection. The respective figures for Klebsiella spp. are 3.5 and 17 per cent, and for Proteus spp., 3.5 and 4 per cent (Bendall 1984).

The differences in urinary bacterial flora between younger and older individuals and between community- and hospital-acquired infection in the elderly probably reflect the greater likelihood of elderly patients receiving antimicrobial therapy and its effect in changing the indigenous bacterial population within institutional environments. In institutions there is also a much greater risk of contamination of the environment by urinary and faecal material.

Treatment

Little is known about the prevention of UTI in the elderly. As discussed above, use of antimicrobial therapy for eradication and prevention is probably ineffective in the frail elderly living in institutions, nor, in this group, does it seem to affect survival. In the case of fit ambulant individuals living independently in the community the role of antimicrobial prevention is unproven.

It seems probable that measures to improve hygiene, increase fluid intake, and to avoid urinary tract instrumentation would reduce the risk of infection. Prevention of faecal incontinence is possible whether the incontinence is due to constipation with faecal overflow or due to loss of neurological control of rectal function (Tobin and Brocklehurst 1986). Control of faecal incontinence has the dual effect of reducing perineal soiling and reducing environmental soiling. The latter may be of importance in institutions in which use of antimicrobial agents may lead to the patients developing resistant bowel flora.

It has been suggested that in patients requiring long-term hospital care, lactulose therapy may be associated with a decrease in both the numbers of urinary infections and the prescription of antimicrobials (McCutcheon and Fulton 1989). The study was small and retrospective and properly controlled prospective studies are needed to confirm these observations. Whether any effect of lactulose is a result of it preventing constipation and associated faecal incontinence, or a specific property of the drug is unclear. Further work is needed since, if the former is the mechanism, there are other equally effective, more palatable, and cheaper therapies for constipation.

In the elderly, the most common situations in which bacteriuria is detected are when patients present with acute urinary tract symptoms, have general features of infection (fever or rigors), or present in an atypical fashion (falls, confusion, or immobility). As discussed above, when bacteriuria is found it is almost inevitable that the clinician is committed to treating the patient with appropriate antimicrobial therapy. The principles of therapy are the same as those in younger patients and described elsewhere in this book. The main difference is that in the frail elderly intravenous therapy is generally used more readily than in younger patients. The risk of sudden and unpredictable deterioration is also much higher in the elderly, as possibly is the risk of secondary septicaemia. Attention to adequate fluid intake to encourage physical flushing of the urinary tract is essential and if the patient is unable to take sufficient orally then intravenous or subcutaneous fluids should be administered.

As indicated earlier, a therapeutic dilemma occurs when bacteriuria is detected in the context of the initial investigation of an atypical presentation (fall, confusion, incontinence, immobility). If, by the time the positive result of urine culture is available, another cause for the patient's condition has not been identified, the decision whether or not to use antimicrobial chemotherapy depends on the patient's condition. If the patient is still non-specifically unwell a repeat urine specimen should be obtained for microbiology and the patient started on appropriate antimicrobial treatment. If the repeat urine specimen is sterile, therapy should be stopped immediately to prevent morbidity due to the antimicrobial agent. However, when a positive result of an initial urine specimen is available and the patient is much improved no therapy should be given. Some would advocate repeating the urine specimen at this stage in case the patient's condition subsequently deteriorates. In practice, this is of little help. There is no guarantee that an organism so detected would be the same one that caused subsequent infection and if the patient did deteriorate a fresh specimen at the time would be essential.

Catheterized patients

Many elderly patients are permanently catheterized unnecessarily and suffer as a result of it. Permanent catheterization should be a last resort when other methods of management have failed. The most common reason for a catheter in an elderly person is urinary incontinence. This can be investigated and managed in a variety of ways outside the scope of this book. The reader is referred to an excellent monograph on the subject by Smith and Clamp (1991). A permanent catheter is sometimes required if the patient is severely incontinent and not controlled by other means. Patients with severe urinary incontinence may develop masceration of the skin on the perineum, buttocks, and legs, and an indwelling catheter may be the only way of protecting the skin. Some elderly patients suffer with chronic urinary retention which may require a permanent catheter.

Intermittent catheterization is increasingly used in elderly patients with a neuropathic or hypotonic bladder (Consumer's Association 1991; Hunt *et al.* 1993). Both conditions may lead to retention of urine commonly accompanied by overflow incontinence. Many patients perform the procedure several times a day without difficulty. For others a carer can be trained in the technique or the community nurse can visit the patient at home. A full sterile technique is not necessary. It is sufficient for the patient or carer to wash their hands before catheterization and after the procedure to wash the catheter in tap water and either boil it for 30 seconds or leave it immersed in a solution of sodium hypochlorite. The same catheter, if made of plastic, an be used for a month or more. Infection rates are very low. Patients using the technique, who were previously permanently catheterized, prefer intermittent catheterization. It provides greater physical and sexual freedom, and much less discomfort from catheter blockage and infection.

Catheterized patients should be treated with antimicrobial therapy for UTI if they develop general evidence of infection without signs in other systems prone to infection in the elderly, the most common being the respiratory tract. Alternatively, treatment is indicated if the patient develops signs or symptoms related to the urinary tract. The presence of bacteriuria in a catheterized patient who has no local or systemic evidence of infection is not an indication for antimicrobial therapy. Bacteriuria is the rule in elderly patients who have long-term catheters and treatment of asymptomatic bacteriuria in such patients is of no proven benefit. Treatment places the patient at risk of side-effects from antimicrobial agents and leads to colonization of the patient and his or her environment with, often multiply-resistant, organisms.

An adequate fluid intake to flush the catheter is of vital importance in catheterized patients. It helps to prevent catheter blockage, urinary stasis, and an increased risk of systemic infection. It also reduces the frequency of re-catheterization, which in turn, reduces the risk of infection.

In catheterized patients who are asymptomatic there is no indication for repeated or regular urine culture 'in case the patient develops an infection'. Bacteria isolated from catheters vary from specimen to specimen and the last available culture result may be therapeutically misleading if a patient becomes seriously ill with a catheter-induced infection. If this happens it is best to assume ignorance of the infecting organism, to send a fresh specimen, and to treat with a broad-spectrum antimicrobial agent likely to be active against the majority of organisms causing such infections.

References

Akhtar, A. J., Andrews, G. R., Caird, F. I. and Fallon, R. J. (1972). Urinary tract infection in the elderly: a population study. *Age and Ageing*, **1**, 48–54.

Asscher, A. W. (1980). *The challenge of urinary tract infection*, p. 16. Academic Press, London.

Bendall, M. J. (1984). A review of urinary tract infection in the elderly. *Journal of Antimicrobial Chemotherapy*, **13**(Suppl. B), 69–78.

Bendall, M. J. (1987). Bacterial resistance to antimicrobial agents in geriatric medical wards. Unpublished DM thesis. University of Nottingham.

Bendall, M. J. and Bendall, P. (1987). Bacteraemia in the elderly. In *Aging: the universal experience*, (ed. G. L. Maddox and E. W. Busse), pp. 120–6. Springer, New York.

Bendall, M. J. , Ebrahim, S., Finch, R. G., Slack, R. C. B., and Towner, K. J. (1986). The effect of an antibiotic policy on bacterial resistance in patients in geriatric medical wards. *Quarterly Journal of Medicine*, **233**, 849–54.

Bendall, M. J., Ebrahim, S., Finch, R. G., Slack, R. C. B., and Towner, K. J. (1989). Bacterial resistance to trimethoprim in geriatric medical wards. *Gerontology*, **35**, 121–6.

Bendall, M. J. and Grüneberg, R. N. (1979). An outbreak of infection caused by trimethoprim-resistant coliform bacilli in a geriatric unit. *Age and Ageing*, **8**, 231–6.

Boscia, J. A., Kobasa, W. D., Abrutyn, E., Levison, M. E., Kaplan, A. M., and Kaye, D. (1986*a*). Lack of association between bacteriuria and symptoms in the elderly. *American Journal of Medicine*, **81**, 979–82.

Boscia, J. A., Kobasa, W. D., Knight, R. A., Abrutyn, E., Levison, M. E., and Kaye, D. (1986*b*). Epidemiology of bacteriuria in an elderly ambulatory population. *American Journal of Medicine*, **80**, 208–14.

Boscia, J. A., Abrutyn, E., and Kaye, D. (1987*a*). Asymptomatic bacteriuria in elderly persons: to treat or not to treat? *Annals of Internal Medicine*, **106**, 764–6.

Boscia, J. A., Kobasa, W. D., Knight, R. A., Abrutyn, E., Levison, M. E., and Kaye, D. (1987*b*). Therapy vs. no therapy for bacteriuria in elderly ambulatory nonhospitalised women. *Journal of the American Medical Association*, **257**, 1067–71.

Brocklehurst, J. C., Dillane, J. B., Griffiths, L. L., and Fry, J. (1968). The prevalence and symptomatology of urinary tract infection in an aged population. *Gerontologica Clinica*, **10**, 242–53.

Brocklehurst, J. C., Fry, J., Griffiths, L. L., and Kalton, G. (1972). Urinary tract infection and symptoms of dysuria in women aged 45–64 years: their relevance to similar findings in the elderly. *Age and Ageing*, **1**, 41–7.

Brocklehurst, J. C., Bee, P., Jones, D., and Palmer, M. K. (1977). Bacteriuria in geriatric hospital patients: its correlates and management. *Age and Ageing*, **6**, 240–5.

Consumer's Association (1991). Underused: intermittent self-catheterisation. *Drug and Therapeutics Bulletin*, **29**, 37–9.

Denham, M. J. and Goodwin, G. S. (1977). The value of blood cultures in geriatric practice. *Age and Ageing*, **6**, 85–8.

Dontas, A. S., Kasviki-Charvati, P., Papanayiotou, P. C., and Marketos, S. G. (1981). Bacteriuria and survival in old age. *New England Journal of Medicine*, **304**, 939–43.

Evans, D. A., *et al.* (1982). Bacteriuria and subsequent mortality in women. *Lancet*, **1**, 156–8.

Fox, R. A. (1992). Immunology and Ageing. In *Oxford textbook of geriatric medicine*, (ed. J. Grimley Evans and T. Franklin Williams), pp. 51–6. Oxford University Press.

Gladstone, J. L. and Recco, R. (1976). Host factors and infectious disease in the elderly. *Medical Clinics of North America*, **60**, 1225–40.

Grüneberg, R. N. and Bendall, M. J. (1979). Hospital outbreak of trimethoprim resistance in pathogenic coliform bacteria. *British Medical Journal*, **ii**, 7–9.

Haley, R. W., *et al.* (1981). Nosocomial infections in U.S. hospitals, 1975–1976: estimated frequency by selected characteristics of patients. *American Journal of Medicine*, **70**, 947–59.

Hunt, G., Whitaker, R., and Oakeshott, P. (1993). *The user's guide to self catheterisation*. Family Doctor Publications, British Medical Association, London.

Kasviki-Charvati, P., Drolette-Kefakis, B., Papanayiotou, P. C., and Dontas, A. S. (1982). Turnover of bacteriuria in old age. *Age and Ageing*, **11**, 169–74.

Lye, M. (1978). Defining and treating urinary infections. *Geriatrics*, **14**, 71–7.

McCutcheon, J. and Fulton, J. D. (1989). Lowered prevalence of infection with lactulose therapy in patients in long-term hospital care. *Journal of Hospital Infection*, **13**, 81–6.

Marketos, S. G., Papanayiotou, P. C., and Dontas A. S. (1969). Bacteriuria and non-obstructive renovascular disease in old age. *Journal of Gerontology*, **24**, 33–6.

Marketos, S. G., Dontas, A. S., Papanayiotou, P. C., and Economou, P. (1970). Bacteriuria and hypertension in old age. *Geriatrics*, **25**, 136–47.

Nicolle, L. E., Bjornson, J., Harding, G. K. M., and MacDonell, J. A. (1983). Bacteriuria in elderly institutionalised men. *New England Journal of Medicine*, **309**, 1420–5.

Nicolle, L. E., Henderson, E., Bjornson, J., McIntyre, M., Harding, G. K. M., and MacDonell, J. A. (1987*a*). The association of bacteriuria with resident characteristics and survival in elderly institutionalised men. *Annals of Internal Medicine*, **106**, 682–6.

Nicolle, L. E., Mayhew, W. J., and Bryan, L. (1987*b*). Prospective randomized comparison of therapy and no therapy for asymptomatic bacteriuria in institutionalised elderly women. *The American Journal of Medicine*, **83**, 27–33.

Nicolle, L. E., Mayhew, J. W., and Bryan, L. (1988*a*). Outcome following antimicrobial therapy for asymptomatic bacteriuria in elderly women resident in an institution. *Age and Ageing*, **17**, 187–92.

Nicolle, L. E., Muir, P., Harding, G. K. M., and Norris, M. (1988*b*). Localisation of urinary tract infection in elderly, institutionalised women with asymptomatic bacteriuria. *Journal of Infectious Diseases*, **157**, 65–70.

Nordenstam, G. R., Brandberg, C. A., Oden, A. S., Svanborg-Edén, C. M., and Svanborg, A. (1986). Bacteriuria and mortality in an elderly population. *New England Journal of Medicine*, **314**, 1152–6.

OPCS (Office of Population Censuses and Surveys) (1974). *Morbidity statistics from general practice. Second national study 1970–71*. Studies on medical and population subjects, No. 26. HMSO, London.

OPCS (Office of Population Censuses and Surveys) (1980*a*). *Hospital inpatient enquiry*. HMSO, London.

OPCS (Office of Population Censuses and Surveys) (1980*b*). *Mortality statistics*. HMSO, London.

Platt, R., Polk, B. F., Murdock, B., and Rosner, B. (1982). Mortality associated with nosocomial urinary-tract infection. *New England Journal of Medicine*, **307**, 637–42.

Setia, U., Serventi, I., and Lorenz, P. (1984). Bacteraemia in a long-term care facility: spectrum and mortality. *Archives of Internal Medicine*, **144**, 1663–5.

Smith, N. and Clamp, M. (1991). *Continence problems in general practice. Practical guides for general practice*, No. 13. Oxford University Press.

Sobel, J. D. and Kaye, D. (1987). The role of bacterial adherence in urinary tract infection in elderly adults. *Journal of Gerontology*, **42**, 29–32.

Sourander, L. B. (1966). Urinary tract infection in the aged—an epidemiological study. *Annales medicine internea Fennae*, **55**(Suppl. 45), 7–55.

Sourander, L. B. and Kasanen, A. (1972). A five year follow-up of bacteriuria in the aged. *Gerontologica Clinica*, **14**, 274–81.

Suntharalingam, M., Seth, V., and Moore-Smith, B. (1983). Site of urinary tract infections in elderly women admitted to an acute geriatric assessment unit. *Age and Ageing*, **12**, 317–22.

Tobin, G. W. and Brocklehurst, J. C. (1986). Faecal incontinence in residential homes for the elderly: prevalence, aetiology and management. *Age and Ageing*, **15**, 41–6.

Walkey, F. A., Judge, T. G., Thompson, J., and Sarkari, N. B. S. (1967). Incidence of urinary infection in the elderly. *Scottish Medical Journal*, **12**, 411–14.

Windsor, A. C. M. (1983). Bacteraemia in a geriatric unit. *Gerontology*, **29**, 125–30.

Wolfson, S. A., Kalmanson, G. M., Rubini, M. E., and Guze, L. B. (1965). Epidemiology of bacteriuria in a predominantly geriatric male population. *American Journal of Medical Science*, **250**, 168–73.

12

The role of the urologist in urinary tract infection

Hugh Whitfield

Introduction

Although urologists may be called upon to treat patients with uncomplicated urinary tract infections there is a wide variety of clinical situations when a surgical contribution is of particular importance. Infection in either the upper or the lower urinary tract can have devastating consequences if not recognized or if managed incorrectly. It is, therefore, a fundamental part of their training that urologists should be taught to recognize those situations when patients are particularly at risk.

Urologists must also have a comprehensive understanding of microbiology and antibiotics. It is well known that organisms are becoming resistant to many of the common antibiotics and that morbidity and mortality rise dramatically if patients are treated inappropriately (Dunagen *et al.* 1989). The need to treat patients with newer and often more expensive antibiotics may well be valid. However, the urologist faces an extra responsibility in that if such antibiotics are used indiscriminately, bacterial resistance may develop at a faster rate than in other clinical situations. This is because of the difficulty in eradicating infection in the presence of a foreign body, such as a catheter, stent, or stone, which encourages the development of resistance. The local bacteriological flora and its bacteriological sensitivity varies in different hospitals and it is essential that the urologist liaises closely with his microbiologist colleagues to formulate a policy for prophylaxis and treatment in any given clinical situation.

Lastly, it is always essential to provide the microbiology laboratory with the correct specimen. One of the difficulties that can be encountered in urological practice is that the correct specimen may be difficult to obtain, for example, from an ileal conduit or in patients with a ureterosigmoidostomy. In addition, bladder organisms may be absent in the presence of an obstructed, infected kidney and bacteria may only be released from within an infection stone following treatment. A combined approach between urologist and microbiologist is the most reliable way to manage such patients.

In this chapter the emphasis will be on urinary tract infection (UTI) occurring in particular urological situations which are not covered elsewhere in this monograph.

UTI in endoscopic urological surgery

Any endoscopic manipulation in either the upper or the lower urinary tract carries with it a risk of introducing infection. Since upper tract infection causes severe systemic symptoms, which on occasions may be life-threatening, more attention and care is paid towards the prophylaxis and treatment of infection during endoscopic surgery in the ureter or the kidney. However, endoscopic procedures in the bladder and urethra are far more common and for this reason alone merit more consideration than often afforded. Since no consensus has been reached about prophylaxis and treatment in such situations it is mandatory for the urologist to know the incidence of infective complications and to be aware of the arguments raised when discussing their management.

One of the difficulties in comparing the results of different studies of UTI in relation to endoscopic urological surgery is that the definition of urinary tract infection is not uniform. In some cases the presence of a pure growth of an organism in the absence of pyuria is not regarded as evidence of infection whilst others do not regard the presence of white cells as a prerequisite for the diagnosis of infection. Most investigators use $> 10^5$ colony-forming (CFU) units per ml of urine as an indication of significant bacteriuria but some studies have used $> 10^4$ per ml.

Cystoscopy

There are so many different indications for cystoscopy that it is not relevant to identify overall pre- and post-cystoscopy infection rates. Rather, certain patients must be regarded as being at higher risk than others. It is almost universal urological practice to cystoscope any patient who has had haematuria for which no cause has been found on urine culture, urine cytology, and intravenous urography. Such investigations are now most commonly performed under local anaesthesia using a flexible cystoscope. Whether or not bacteriuria was identified, many of these patients may have had UTI as a provocative cause for their haematuria. Clark and Higgs (1990), in a series of 161 patients undergoing flexible cystoscopy, found that of those uninfected prior to the examination 12 (7.5 per cent) yielded a pure growth of an organism three days after the cystoscopy. Fowler (1984) reported an incidence of 10 per cent in a small series of patients undergoing both flexible and rigid cystoscopy. In previous studies involving rigid cystoscopy alone, infection rates between 2.8 and 5.0 per cent have been reported (Chodak and Plaut 1979). Some series report a higher incidence of infection in women but the case for prophylactic antibiotic administration in both men and women remains controversial. Some subgroups have been identified who appear to be at greater risk: those in whom there is a proven history of UTI and those in whom a procedure is performed during the cystoscopy. The dilemma is heightened by the realization that what might be best for an individual on an isolated occasion might prove detrimental to the population at large from a wider bacteriological perspective. The indiscriminant use of antibiotics can only encourage more organisms to become resistant to a wider range of antibiotics.

The author's own practice is to treat patients prophylactically only if they fall into a high risk group by virtue of a previous urinary track infection, an intra-operative procedure (e.g. removal of [1]JJ stent, [2]bladder biopsy, [3]or diathermy), or a residual urine of more than 50 ml. Ideally, the first dose should be given at least one hour prior to the cystoscopy. The antibiotic chosen must be influenced by previous bacteriology and local bacteriological sensitivity patterns.

Transurethral prostatectomy

All over the world the number of patients undergoing transurethral prostatectomy (TURP) has risen rapidly over the last 10 years in spite of the new modalities of treatment which have yet to stand the test of time. Although the operation is recognized as being very safe, with a mortality of less than 1 per cent, infections contribute to a significant proportion of the morbidity and mortality. At worst, infection can be manifested as septicaemia and death. Upper tract infection with loin pain and fever and lower tract infection with epididymitis, scrotal pain, and fever are two of the more acute and severe manifestations of infection. The dysuria which accompanies 'uncomplicated' lower tract infection may be severe. Lastly, as in so many other surgical situations, infection can provoke secondary haemorrhage and this itself is a major complication of prostatectomy, often or usually occurring when the patient has been discharged from hospital.

The majority of patients who present with acute retention of urine, and who therefore have an indwelling catheter, will develop a urinary infection by the time of their TURP. These patients need appropriate antibiotic treatment. In a comprehensive review of the literature, Grabe (1987) identified a high complication rate in patients with pre-existing bacteriuria, with bacteraemia in up to 60 per cent and septicaemia in up to 6–10 per cent. Even when antibiotic treatment was continued for a full course there was a significant rate of relapse. This is hardly surprising in view of the fact that there is a raw prostatic fossa, an indwelling urethral catheter, and the possibility that infection has taken hold within the remaining prostatic capsule.

Patients who have a significant residual urine volume secondary to prostatic obstruction are prone to develop a urinary infection. Such infections should be treated by an appropriate antibiotic prior to surgery. The potential for recurrent infection in such patients provides a strong medical indication for recommending TURP. Because organisms may be suppressed rather than eliminated in this group of patients, and because organisms may be present within the prostate, a history of urinary infection is an indication for prophylactic antibiotic treatment at the time of surgery. The temperature chart of a patient who underwent elective transurethral prostatectomy is shown in Fig. 12.1. A pre-operative urine culture had been sterile and a urine specimen taken immediately prior to the removal of the catheter also showed no infection. However, the patient developed

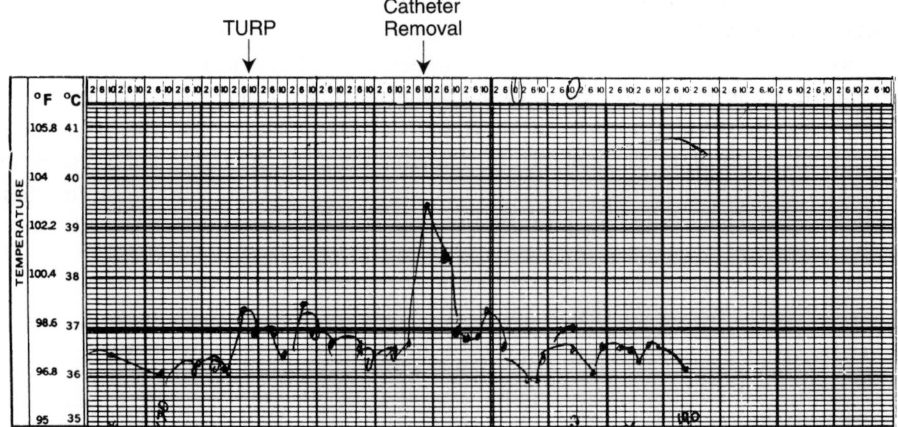

Fig. 12.1 The temperature chart of a patient who developed a pyrexia following transurethral prostatectomy, when the urethral catheter was removed.

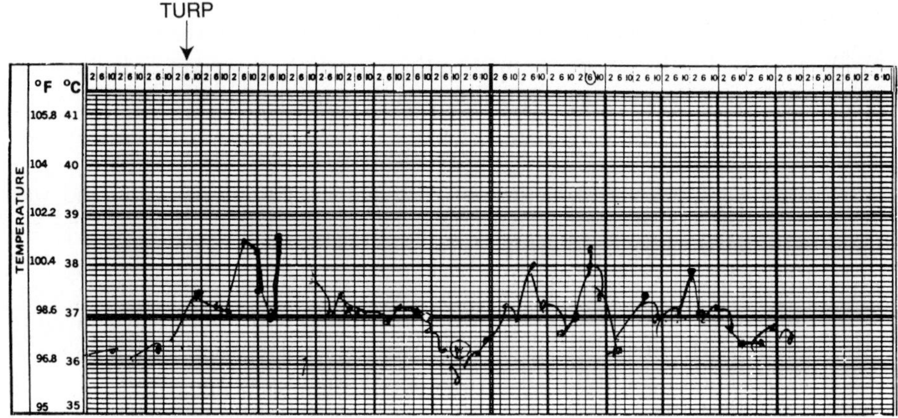

Fig. 12.2 The temperature chart of a patient with a prolonged pyrexia after a transurethral prostatectomy.

a high fever within an hour of catheter removal. Blood cultures were taken but no organisms grown. Nevertheless, the patient was started on parenteral antibiotics since it is not possible to predict the subsequent course of such a fever. Fig. 12.2 is the temperature chart of a patient who also underwent elective prostatectomy in whom there was no evidence of pre-operative urinary infection. However, following the surgery he became pyrexial and although blood and urine cultures showed no growth the pyrexia was slow to settle, even with prolonged parenteral antibiotics. It is such events which raise the possibility that on occasions the presence of infection, perhaps in residual prostatic tissue, may not be revealed by standard urine cultures. Alternatively, endotoxin release during surgery or during bladder irrigation may provoke the pyrexia.

In the majority of patients undergoing elective TURP in whom no infection has been identified prior to surgery, the urethral catheter is removed after 48–72 hours. This period is critical from a bacteriological point of view, since catheter induced infection rates rise steeply after 72 hours. There is, therefore, much logic in initiating prophylactic antibiotic treatment after the catheter has been removed. A catheter specimen of urine should be taken immediately prior to the catheter removal and before the first dose of the antibiotic, which should be continued for five days. Alternatively, the first dose of prophylactic antibiotic may be given one hour before catheter removal but following a catheter specimen of urine. Other authors have recommended that prophylaxis should begin prior to surgery and continued either until the catheter is removed or for 48–72 hours after catheter removal.

When a TURP is performed on a patient who is bacteriuric (e.g. those with an indwelling urethral catheter or bladder stones), antibiotic treatment should begin immediately prior to surgery and continue for a minimum of five days. If there is a pre-existing history of proven bacteriological prostatitis or histological evidence of acute or chronic prostatitis an antibiotic should be continued for six weeks.

The choice of antibiotic in the elective TURP group will be governed by local bacteriological sensitivities, by any patient allergy and by cost. A bactericidal antibiotic is to be preferred to a bacteriostatic one. Trimethoprim or nitrofurantoin (formulated as Macrodantin to reduce nausea) are the author's choice. Second-generation cephalosporins are not recommended as they are only bacteriostatic. In the high-risk group, a parenteral antibiotic should be administered, the first dose either with the pre-med or at the time of induction of anaesthesia. An aminoglycoside is effective, economical, and very safe when renal function is not impaired. In a patient who requires long-term antibiotic treatment it will be necessary to change to an oral antibiotic after 3–5 days.

These regimes, together with a fluid intake of 3 litres in 24 hours, should minimize the incidence of urinary infections following TURP. The vogue for performing a bilateral vasectomy at the time of the prostatectomy has largely disappeared, having been shown to be ineffective.

Part of the audit of any urological department should include a review of infection rates following prostatectomy. Meticulous attention to nursing procedures is essential to prevent contamination. Catheter care should be performed regularly, cleaning the external urethral meatus and the exposed catheter to prevent encrustations of congealed blood. Sterile saline or a very weak water-based antiseptic solution (e.g. Savlon) should be used to clean the catheter and meatus at least twice a day).

A suprapubic catheter is sometimes used instead of a urethral one. One advantage is that the potential for causing urethral trauma in the male by inexpert catheterization is avoided. However, they are more prone to be pulled out inadvertently unless inserted as a formal open cystotomy. With long-term use the infection rate is no different from an indwelling urethral catheter. A suprapubic catheter may be required in females with neuropathic bladder disorders in whom the unstable bladder contractions tend to expel the balloon. As the urethra becomes progressively more and more dilated no urethral catheter can be retained. To be effective in this situation suprapubic catheterisation must be accompanied by urethral closure, a difficult surgical procedure requiring general anaesthesia.

The length of time for which a urethral or a suprapubic catheter can be left varies from patient to patient. Some seem to encrust their catheters more rapidly than others and can require changing every week, whereas others can last for three months. The material from which the catheter is made seems to be of less importance than the individual's own susceptibility to encrust catheters.

Although there is no controversy about the need for antibiotics in patients with proven bacteriuria the case for prophylactic antimicrobials remains unproven. The best interests of an individual may not always coincide with the interests of the community at large. If antibiotics are to be administered the policy should be based on a consensus between surgeon and microbiologist in the light of risk factors, local bacteriological flora, and economic considerations.

Ureteroscopy

The most common ureteroscopic procedure performed is the endoscopic removal of a ureteric calculus. The majority of such stones are composed of calcium oxalate, and although theoretically metabolic stones are not infective in origin, it is not uncommon for stone analysis to reveal bacteria within them (see also Fig. 12.3). In many patients there is a degree of urinary stasis above a ureteric stone which will encourage infection. The endoscopic manoeuvre itself may provoke ureteric oedema and a degree of obstruction and stasis. If the stone needs to be fragmented, organisms that exist within the matrix of even metabolic stones may be released and increase the risk of infection. For all these reasons antibiotic prophylaxis is mandatory. In patients without bacteriuria with uncomplicated ureteric stones who are often cared for on a day case basis, one parenteral dose of an antibiotic on induction of anaesthesia may suffice. In more complicated cases, for example, those with prostatic enlargement and a residual urine or patients who have a JJ stent prior to or following endoscopy, prophylaxis for 24–72 hours should be given. In the most complex cases with large stones, ureteric dilatation or pre-existing infection a parenteral antibiotic in full dosage is required for 3–5 days before reverting to a full course of an oral antibiotic. It is essential that following any endoscopic procedure in these complex cases urinary drainage is established. The insertion of an intra-luminal JJ stent has been advocated to avoid temporary ureteric obstruction from oedema that may be provoked by the procedure. If the attempt to remove a stone is unsuccessful a percutaneous nephrostomy tube should be inserted. This will provide free drainage to the obstructed kidney and minimize the chances of infective complications.

During endoscopic procedures on the ureter high pressure irrigation is often used. Ureteric perforation is not uncommon and if infection also exists there is experimental evidence that ureteric stricture formation is more common than in the absence of infection (Boddy *et al.* 1989).

Renal stone surgery

The management of renal stones has been revolutionized in the last 10 years by the introduction of percutaneous nephrolithotomy (PCNL) and extra-corporeal shockwave lithotripsy (ESWL). Although there remains a place for open surgery for stone disease this is now reserved for stag-horn calculi in which the main stone burden lies within calices. Occasionally, the combination of a renal stone and renal outflow obstruction may be best treated by an open operation, although percutaneous procedures are described for the treatment of pelviureteric junction obstruction and the results are very satisfactory.

Whatever the method of stone removal the principles of antibiotic prophylaxis remain the same. Stones are either metabolic or infective in origin. Those that are infective will clearly carry a much higher potential for provoking subsequent infection than the metabolic variety. Nevertheless, even metabolic stones can contain organisms. An example of this is shown in Fig. 12.3; electron microscopy reveals microorganisms within the organic matrix of a decalcified calcium oxalate stone.

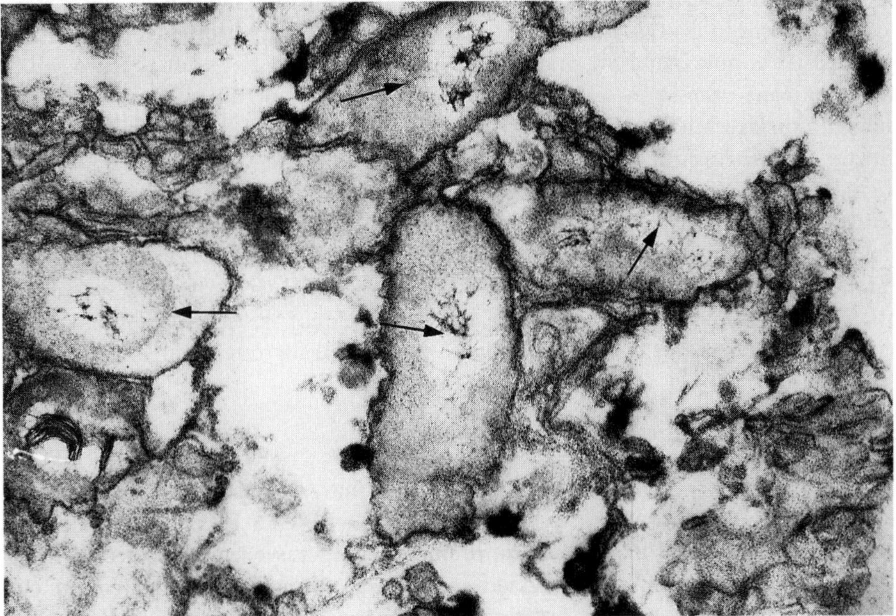

Fig. 12.3 An electron photomicrograph showing organisms (arrowed) within the matrix of a decalcified calcium oxalate stone.

Midstream urine cultures are usually positive in patients whose stones are infective in origin. Antibiotic sensitivities can be identified and appropriate treatment given. The situation is more difficult when the urine is sterile but experience has shown that organisms may be released during stone treatment and prophylactic antibiotics should be given.

Open renal surgery

An appropriate antibiotic must be given for all patients who have a positive urine culture pre-operatively. It is well recognized that the incidence of stone recurrence is related to infection (Sleight and Wickham 1977). Because of peri-operational oedema and temporary ischaemia, the elimination of infection requires a 6-week course of post-operative antibiotics in a kidney which has been rendered stone-free. Culture of a stone fragment removed at the time of open surgery may help to identify the most appropriate antibiotic. The removal of stones and the elimination of infection may result in significant renal functional improvement even in kidneys which have been so badly damaged that the patient is in chronic renal failure (Witherow and Wickham 1980). The techniques developed during the 1970s to conserve renal function during prolonged periods of intra-operative renal ischaemia remain important and relevant in the 1990s for a few selected patients.

Percutaneous nephrolithotomy (PCNL)

This was first described by Fernström and Johannson in 1976. Over the next 10 years the technique was streamlined and purpose-built instruments were manufactured. It is now standard practice to perform the two stages of the procedure under one anaesthetic. A track is dilated to a diameter of some 10 mm between the skin surface and the collecting system of the kidney. During the dilatation process and during the subsequent irrigation of the intra-renal collecting system there is a potential for infection to be disseminated intra-vascularly. Most surgeons therefore recommend prophylactic antibiotics. As for open renal surgery, stones that are infective in origin will tend to recur unless infection is completely eliminated. Again, this will require a 6-week post-operative course of an appropriate antimicrobial agent. Culture of a stone fragment is, as with open surgery, valuable in identifying the right antibiotic to be used for treatment.

Extra-corporeal shockwave lithotripsy (ESWL)

Although extracorporeal shockwave lithotripsy has an excellent safety record, complications can undoubtedly arise. Bacteriuria following ESWL was described by Michaels *et al.* (1988). In a more recent report, Gasser and Frei (1993) studied 23 patients, obtaining between four and seven blood cultures. In one patient small numbers of two different microorganisms were found but were thought to represent contamination. Their conclusion was that only high-risk patients (e.g. those with a risk of developing bacterial endocarditis) should be considered for prophylatic antibiotics. In this study, three of their patients were shown to have urinary infections prior to treatment. Since the results were not available at the time of ESWL they had not received antibiotic prophylaxis. Only one developed a significant illness and this was associated with urinary obstruction caused by a stone fragment in the ureter. As in all clinical situations, it is the combination of infection plus obstruction that poses the greatest threat. Other authors, however, have recommended prophylactic antibiotics. In a study of 181 patients, Claes *et al.* (1989) found a significant reduction in fever, bacteriuria, and leucocyturia in patients given amoxycillin/clavulanate prophylaxis compared to placebo. As with transurethral prostatectomy, studies have shown conflicting results. The dangers of infection following lithotripsy, which is usually performed on an outpatient basis, are such that the author recommends antibiotic prophylaxis for all patients.

Intestine in the urinary tract

Since the beginning of this century, bowel segments have been used as a substitute for diseased parts of the urinary tract. Most commonly, the underlying pathology involves the bladder but also on occasion the ureter. Ureterosigmoidostomy remained a well-established technique for many years despite the complications that could occur. The principle of diverting the urine to a cutaneous urostomy via an ileal conduit was popularized by Bricker (1950). The long-term results are well established. There is almost inevitably a steady deterioration of renal function, which occurs for a variety of reasons. With the original Bricker technique it was impossible to prevent ureteric reflux. To overcome this disadvantage the use of an isolated colonic segment was described in which an anti-reflux anastomosis could be achieved (Richie *et al.* 1974). However, patients with a colonic conduit diversion also experience renal damage. It seems that several factors, such as reflux, obstruction, and infection, either alone or in combination, may contribute (Elder *et al.* 1979).

In an attempt to overcome these problems there has been an upsurge of interest in the use of bowel in the urinary tract itself. A segment of large or small intestine can be used to augment or to replace the bladder. Alternatively, if the patient's own sphincter mechanism is compromised because of, for example, neurological dysfunction or malignant disease, a continent urinary diversion may be performed. A continent urinary diversion consists of two parts; a reservoir and a continent stoma brought to the skin surface on the abdominal wall. The reservoir is fashioned from a segment of bowel which has been detubularized by incising longitudinally along the antimesenteric border. The reservoir is then fashioned by folding the detubularized segment into a W-configuration and joining together the adjacent bowel margins. Continence is achieved in one of several ways. A segment of small bowel may be intussuscepted, or the appendix, a Fallopian tube, or even a ureter may be used and fashioned in a way that creates a continent stoma. The patient will then catheterize the stoma and empty the reservoir every 3–4 hours.

At first sight, enthusiasts for the very many varied techniques described could seem to be advocating replacement or augmentation of the urinary tract with bowel as if no significant difference existed between the behaviour of transitional cell epithelium and intestinal mucosa. This is far from reality. A clear distinction must be drawn between the anatomical configurations that have been described and the functional results. There is widespread agreement that detubularized bowel provides a better reservoir than an intact bowel segment. Small and large intestine, caecum, and stomach can be utilized alone or in combination. Great ingenuity has been displayed in creating variations on a theme. These are chiefly of surgical interest, but can be grouped into a few principal types (Table 12.1). In terms of function there are significant differences between different intestinal segments. For example, the low pH of stomach can provoked quite severe dysuria. Electrolyte disturbances are a well-recognized hazard, particularly in patients with impaired renal function. Long-term metabolic effects have also been described (Woodhouse 1994). Whatever the anatomical configuration, the incorporation of bowel into the urinary tract will risk provoking infection for two main reasons. First, intestinal mucosa reacts to the presence of urine by producing excess mucus, which may act as a foreign body to encourage infection. Secondly, there is almost inevitably a degree of urinary stasis, the degree of which depends on the particular procedure.

Table 12.1 The use of intestine in the urinary tract

Procedure	Pathology	Gastrointestinal tract
Augmentation/substitution cystoplasty	Carcinoma of the bladder Interstitial cystitis Tuberculosis Bladder instability	Small intestine Large intestine Small and large intestine Stomach
Continent urinary diversion	Post DXR contraction. Congenital anomalies Intractable incontinence	
Conduit diversion	Carcinoma of the bladder Congenital anomalies (e.g. exstrophy, neuropathy) Intractable incontinence	
Ureteric replacement	Injury (e.g. trauma, stone, DXR)	Ileum
Ureterosigmoidostomy	Carcinoma of the bladder Congenital anomalies (e.g. exstrophy)	Colon

Ureterosigmoidostomy

The earliest form of urinary diversion was performed by implanting the ureters into the sigmoid colon. This technique remained popular for a long time, despite the well-recognized complications. Hyperchloraemic acidosis was a common electrolyte disturbance which was particularly dangerous in patients with impaired renal function. Although techniques are now commonly used to prevent ureteric reflux this was not always the case. In some patients, the presence of infected reflux, often associated with a high pressure reservoir for urine and therefore high-pressure reflux, led to devastating renal damage and septicaemia. Moreover, the risk of malignant change occurring at the site of ureteric implantation is greatest when the urinary and faecal streams are mixed. The increased risk has been estimated at being between 100 and 7000 times that in the normal population (Gittes 1981; Stewart 1986). It is therefore essential that any patient who has this form of urinary diversion undergoes regular colonoscopy since, in most cases, a frankly malignant tumour is preceded by an adenoma which can be visualized and biopsied. Obtaining an uncontaminated specimen of urine for bacteriological assessment is impossible and patients requiring antibiotic treatment because of the symptoms of a urinary tract infection may have to be treated blindly. For these reasons, the operation has become less popular and is performed infrequently. However, patients who have this form of diversion are usually very pleased with the results since no appliances are needed. With the use of anti-reflux techniques, alkalinizing agents, and appropriate antibiotics where necessary, the quality of life can be very good (Silverman *et al.* 1986).

Conduit urinary diversion

Bacteriuria is an almost inevitable sequel to any form of conduit diversion and may cause no symptoms (Bergman 1978). Controversy surrounds the importance of such infection, some authors maintaining that there is a direct correlation between renal damage and the presence of infection, whereas others find no such association (Pernet and Jonas 1985; Philp *et al.* 1980). This may partly be due to the heterogeneous patient population groups. In most series there is a clear distinction between the renal functional results in patients who have been diverted because of a bladder neuropathy and those who are diverted following a cystectomy. In this latter group, renal function seems to be better maintained than in patients who are diverted because of a neuropathic bladder (e.g. those with spina bifida). This may relate to the fact that in the latter group, the condition has existed since infancy when high pressures and recurrent infections are more likely to affect the developing kidney. This may be compounded by neurogenic abnormality of the bowel.

Studies have been performed correlating the presence of bacterial growth in the conduit and the serum levels of C-reactive protein (CRP). Bergman (1978) found no correlation between the presence of bacterial infection and the level of CRP. This result was contradicted by Kiker *et al.* (1982) who found increased CRP levels in all patients with an ileal conduit with bacterial infection $> 10^5$ organisms per ml. In a recent study (Åkerlund *et al.* 1994), no correlation was found between the CRP levels and serum antibody titres against *E. coli* and Proteus, raising the possibility that the CRP levels did not depend on renal parenchymal infection. They concluded that bacterial growth from an ileal conduit was only of clinical importance when a consistently raised antibody level against *E. coli* was found. The only valid method for collecting a urine sample from a patient with a conduit diversion is to remove the stoma appliance and to pass a small well-lubricated catheter to the bottom of the loop, thereby collecting urine from a site as proximal as possible.

Augmentation/substitution cystoplasty

To try to overcome some of the problems associated with ureterosigmoidostomy and conduit diversion and to offer patients a continent form of diversion there has been a bewildering variety of operations described during the last 15 years. There is a general consensus of opinion that a low-pressure reservoir is required and the best way to achieve this is by detubularizing the segment of bowel which is chosen. Such a detubularized reconstructed reservoir can be used either to augment or to substitute the urinary bladder. If the urethra is not involved with neoplastic or neuropathic disease and if a bladder neck or distal sphincter mechanism is available to achieve continence, then the urethra can be anastomosed to the reservoir. On other occasions, a continent stoma can be achieved by one of a variety of techniques mentioned above. The surgical, metabolic, and neoplastic complications of these procedures are very real, but not of relevance to this chapter. Problems arising because of infection are both important and common.

Intestinal mucosa responds to the presence of urine by secreting a thick mucopolysaccharide mucus. This can cause mechanical problems, particularly in men in whom it may cause urinary retention. Although the amount of mucus secreted tends to diminish with time there is some evidence that oral cranberry juice may reduce mucus production (Rosenbaum *et al.* 1989). The presence of mucus may also increase the incidence of infection. Patients with a continent stoma need to self-catheterize their reservoir every four hours or so. This procedure can itself encourage infection although conversely, by reducing the residual urine volume it may reduce the potential for infection. Because augmented and substituted bladders empty incompletely, patients in whom the reservoir is attached to their urethra may also require to self-catheterize intermittently. Residual urine together with the presence of mucus is a potent combination encouraging infection. However, in most patients long-term antibiotic prophylaxis is not needed.

The presence of infection increases the chances of urinary tract stones. Patients with bladder reservoirs have a higher incidence of stone both in the reservoir and in the upper urinary tract. The incidence of renal stones varies between 1.6 and 6.8 per cent (Woodhouse 1994). This incidence is the same as is found in patients who have had a conduit diversion. Some techniques of continent urinary diversion involve the use of metal staples and in such patients the incidence of stones has been reported between 16.7 and 52.5 per cent (Ginsberg *et al.* 1991).

Other situations

Long-term indwelling catheters

It has been known for a long time that patients who, for whatever reason, require permanent urethral catheterization tend to encrust their catheters. This encrustation occurs at a very variable rate. Since infection is almost invariably present this alone cannot be implicated. Although the manufacturers of catheters made from different substances would promote one or other material there is no consistent difference between, for example, Silastic and latex Foley catheters (J. C. Brocklehurst and S. Brocklehurst 1978). Even when antibiotics are given organisms can be grown in 76 per cent of patients. Bladder washouts with or without an antiseptic can reduce the infection rate to between 6 and 9 per cent, but chemical cystitis can occur if washouts are given very frequently. Brocklehurst and Brocklehurst concluded that there was no relationship between catheter material, infection, urinary pH, and encrustation. However, they confirmed the findings of Bruce and Clark (1974) of a very variable patient susceptibility to encrustation and subsequent catheter blockage and urinary leakage.

Nothing has changed significantly in the materials used for catheter manufacturer during the last 20 years. It remains impossible to show any advantage from intermittent or continuous antibiotics although bladder washouts may help. A recent study (Capewell and Morris 1993) reported the result of a postal audit on the management of long-term indwelling catheters. Marked variations were found and much of the care was less than ideal. These authors recommended that community-based nurses should develop protocols for catheter management.

Intermittent catheterization

There are a number of patients who are best managed by intermittent, often self-catheterization. These include patients with neurological disorders affecting the bladder (e.g. spina bifida, acquired traumatic cord lesions resulting in paraplegia, multiple sclerosis). The bladder may function as a satisfactory reservoir, with or without the use of surgical augmentation or the use of anticholinergic drugs such as oxybutynin. Patients may then learn to catheterize themselves every four hours to empty their bladder. If they themselves are unable to master the technique then a carer can perform the procedure for them. The incidence of urinary infections may be reduced (Whitfield and Mayo 1976). The technique was re-popularized in the 1950s and 1960s in the early management of patients with traumatic paraplegia and tetraplegia by Guttmann and Frankel (1966). Since patients who have augmented or substituted bladders using intestine may fail to empty their neo-bladders completely, intermittent catheterization is often required in this group post-operatively. A useful guide to intermittent catheterization has been published by the British Medical Association (Hunt *et al.* 1993).

Peri-renal abscess

Percutaneous drainage of abscesses has become increasingly popular and can often be the treatment of choice, particularly in frail old, ill patients. Since the kidney is extra-peritoneal this approach is particularly appropriate. Under ultrasound (US) or computed tomography (CT) guidance a small drainage tube can be inserted under local anaesthesia, thus avoiding the need for a general anaesthetic and a more traumatic surgical intervention. The only drawback to this approach is that abscesses may be multi-locular and it is difficult to break down septae percutaneously.

The underlying cause of a peri-renal abscess may subsequently require open surgery but this can be performed electively when the patient is as fit as possible (Fig. 12.4). Irrigation of the catheter with saline to maintain drainage is sometimes necessary. An antibiotic solution, such as ampicillin or gentamicin, can also be used and provides an effective way of ensuring high levels of antibiotic in the appropriate place. Acetylcystine has been used to reduce the viscosity of pus and to improve drainage. Resolution of the abscess can be monitored either sonographically (US) or with CT scanning (Rosen and Roven 1984).

Miscellaneous causes of infection

Vesicointestinal fistulae

The most common cause of a fistulous communication between the bowel and the bladder is diverticulitis. Colonic tumours, Crohn's disease, bladder tumours, pelvic radiotherapy, and appendix abscess may also cause such fistulae. There is often a history of pneumaturia and a mixed growth of faecal flora will be found. The diagnosis can be confirmed by contrast studies of the small and large bowel, although a CT scan is probably the most sensitive diagnostic investigation and will demonstrate contrast from the intestine within the bladder. Occasionally, intravenous urography, retrograde ureterography, or antegrade ureterography may be helpful. Surgical repair can usually be performed in one stage when the use of interposed momentum is advantageous (Mileski *et al.* 1987).

Congenital and acquired abnormalities

Congenital anomalies which may result in relapsing bacteriuria include non-functioning duplications, pericaliceal diverticula, urachal cysts, medullary sponge kidney, and pelviureteric junction obstruction. Acquired anomalies predisposing to infection include unilateral cortical atrophy secondary to calculus obstruction, and non-refluxing ureteric stumps following nephrectomy. The surgical correction of these problems is, except in the case of medullary sponge kidney, perfectly straightforward. The diagnosis of infection in such situation may be confirmed by localization studies described by Stamey *et al.* (1965). These localization techniques are, however, only necessary when surgery is contemplated. Stamey himself is on record as saying that it makes no difference therapeutically whether the infection is in the upper or lower urinary tract if surgery is not contemplated (Stamey *et al.* 1965).

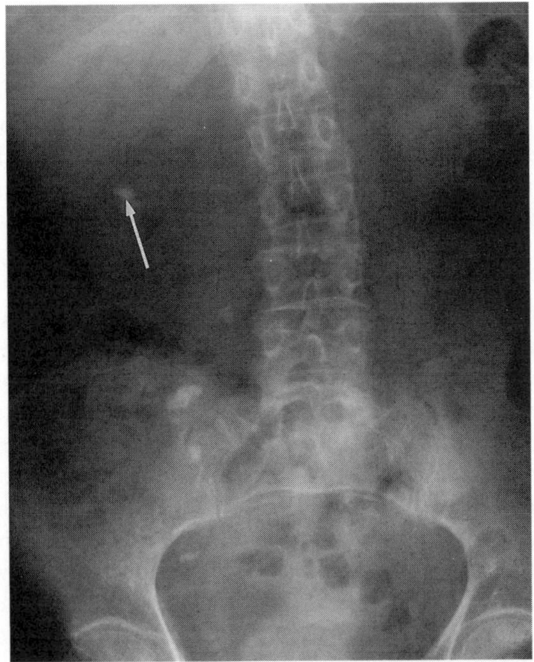

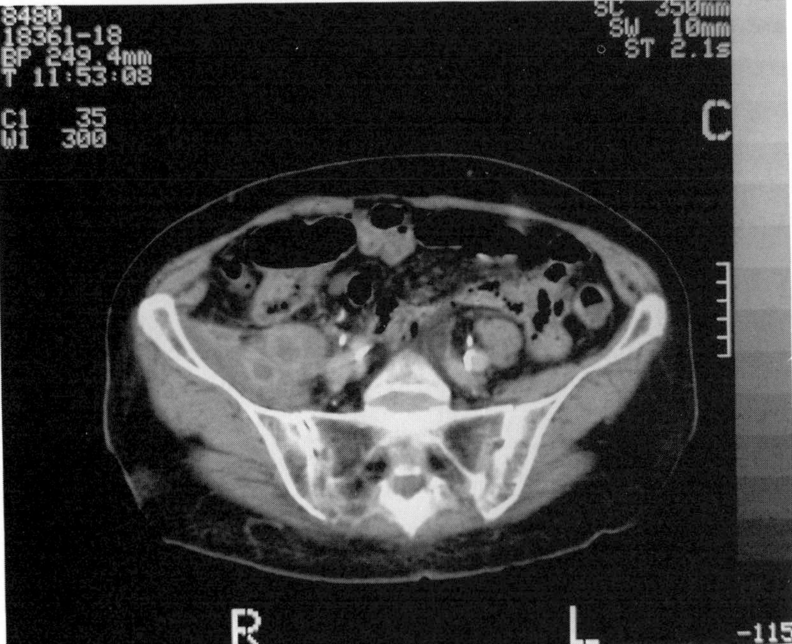

Fig. 12.4 (a) A plain X-ray showing a small collection of stones (arrowed) in the lower pole of the right kidney. (b) A CT scan of the same patient showing a retroperitoneal and sacral abscess which had arisen from the pyonephrosis secondary to the renal stones.

Prostatic biopsy

The advent of a more reliable biochemical marker for prostatic disease, prostatic-specific antigen (PSA), together with the availability of accurate imaging of the prostate by transrectal ultrasound (TRUS) and magnetic resonance imaging (MRI), have increased the number of indications for transrectal biopsy of the prostate. However, prostatic biopsy can provoke infective complications the incidence of which is related to the size of the needle used. Fine-needle aspirates for cytology are associated with a significantly lower rate of complication than a core biopsy (Hendry and Williams 1971). A recent report suggests that the newer type of more automated biopsy needle which can be either 14 or 18 gauge, which makes biopsy more reliable and reduces the number of specimens that need to be taken from any individual patient, is associated with a lower morbidity than previously described. In a series of 670 men who underwent transrectal biopsy Desmond *et al.* (1993) reported a fever/prostatitis rate of 0.6 per cent of whom half required hospitalization. Early in the series, 51 patients (7.6 per cent) received enemas before the biopsy but this practice was subsequently abandoned. The majority of patients (86.6 per cent) received oral ciprofloxacin for 1–3 days, starting prior to the biopsy. This large but retrospective study suggests that the morbidity associated with transrectal biopsy under these conditions is minimal. To try to reduce the complication rates still further Webb *et al.* (1993) have advocated a transperineal approach with transrectal ultrasound guidance.

Lower urinary tract stents

During the last five years polyurethane and metal stents have been designed to relieve bladder outflow obstruction due either to a urethral stricture or to benign prostatic hypertrophy. When used in the urethra the stent is designed to become epithelialized, thereby reducing the chance of encrustation and infection. Chapple *et al.* (1991) have reported good results. Stents used to overcome prostatic obstruction have been used in patients considered unfit for surgery. Epithelialization of the stent tends to be incomplete, increasing the risks of encrustation and infection but the results are acceptable in this difficult group of patients (Williams *et al.* 1993).

Conclusions

The urologist needs to know when his or her patients are at risk from the complications of urinary tract infection, and to know how best to prevent these. The management of patients with established infections, which can sometimes be life-threatening, needs to be undertaken in collaboration with the urologist's colleagues: the nephrologist and bacteriologist.

References

Åkerlund, S., Capanello, M., Kaijser, B., and Jonsson, O. (1994). Bacteriuria in patients with a continent ileal reservoir for urinary diversion does not regularly require antibiotic treatment. *British Journal of Urology*, **74**, 171–81.

Bergman, B. (1978). Studies on patients with ileal conduit diversion with special regard to renal infection. *Scandinavian Journal of Urology and Nephrology*, **47**(Suppl.), 1–32.

Boddy, S-A. M., *et al.* (1989). Irrigation and acute ureteric dilatation—as for ureteroscopy. *British Journal of Urology*, **63**, 11–13.

Bricker, E. M. (1950). Bladder substitution after pelvic evisceration. *Surgical Clinics of North America*, **30**, 1511–21.

Brocklehurst, J. C. and Brocklehurst, S. (1978). The management of indwelling catheters. *British Journal of Urology*, **50**, 102–5.

Bruce, A. W. and Clarke, A. F. (1974). The problem of catheter encrustation. *Canadian Medical Journal*, **III**, 238–41.

Capewell, A. E. and Morris, S. L. (1993). Audit of catheter management provided by district nurses and continence advisers. *British Journal of Urology*, **71**, 259–64.

Chapple, C. R., Rickards, D., and Milroy, E. J. G. (1991). Permanently implanted urethral stents. *Seminars in Interventional Radiology*, **8**, 284–92.

Chodak, G. W. and Plaut, M. E. (1979). Systemic antibiotics for prophylaxis in urological surgery: a critical review. *Journal of Urology*, **121**, 695–9.

Claes, H., Vandeursen, R., and Baert, L. (1989). Amoxycillin/Clavulanate prophylaxis for extracorporeal shockwave lithotripsy—a comparative study. *Journal of Antimicrobial Chemotherapy*, **24**(Suppl. B), 271–20.

Clark, K. R., and Higgs, M. J. (1990). Urinary infection following out-patient flexible cystoscopy. *British Journal of Urology*, **66**, 503–5.

Desmond, P. M., Clark, J., Thompson, I. M., Zeidman, E. J. and Mueller, E. J. (1993). Morbidity with contemporary prostate biopsy. *Journal of Urology*, **150**, 1425–6.

Dunagen, W. M., Woodward, R. S., and Medoff, G. (1989). Anti-microbial misuse in patients with positive blood cultures. *American Journal of Medicine*, **87**, 253–9.

Elder, D. D., Moisey, C. U., and Rees, R. W. M. (1979). A long-term follow-up of the colonic conduit operation in children. *British Journal of Urology*, **51**, 462–5.

Fernström, I. and Johannson, B. (1976). Percutaneous pyelolithotomy: a new extraction technique. *Scandinavian Journal of Urology and Nephrology*, **4**, 257–9.

Fowler, C. G. (1984). Fibrescope urethrocystoscopy. *British Journal of Urology*, **56**, 304–7.

Gasser, T. C. and Frei, R. (1993). Risk of bacteraemia during extracorporeal shockwave lithotripsy. *British Journal of Urology*, **71**, 17–20.

Ginsberg, D., Huffman, J. L., Liestovsky, G., Boyd, S., and Skinner, D. G. (1991). Urinary tract stones: a complication of the Kock pouch continent urinary diversion. *Journal of Urology*, **145**, 956–9.

Gittes, R. F. (1981). Carcinogens in ureterosigmoidostomy. *Urological Clinics of North America*, **13**, 201–5.

Grabe, M. (1987). Anti-microbial agents in transurethral prostatic resection. *Journal of Urology*, **138**, 245–52.

Guttmann, L. and Frankel, H. (1966). The value of intermittent catherisation in the early management of traumatic paraplegia and tetraplegia. *Paraplegia*, **4**, 63–84.

Hendry, W. F. and Williams, J. P. (1971). Transrectal prostatic biopsy. *British Medical Journal*, **4**, 595–7.

Hunt, G., Whitaker, R., and Oakeshott, P. (1993). *The user's guide to intermittent catheterisation*. Published in association with the British Medical Association, London.

Kiker, J. D., Woodside, J. R., Reed, W. P., Borden, T. A., and Woodside, M-D. (1982). Urinary lactic dehydrogenase and serum C-reactive proteins as a means of localizing the site of urinary tract infection in patients with ileal conduits. *Journal of Urology*, **128**, 749–51.

Michaels, E. K., Fowler, J. E., and Mariano, M. (1988). Bacteriuria following extracorporeal shockwave lithotripsy of infection stones. *Journal of Urology*, **140**, 254–6.

Mileski, W. J., Joehlrjrege, V., and Nahrwold, D. L. (1987). One stage resection and anastomosis in the management of colo-vesical fistulae. *American Journal of Surgery*, **153**, 75–9.

Pernet, F. P. P. M. and Jonas, U. (1985). Ileal conduit urinary diversion: Early and late results of 132 cases in a 25-year period. *World Journal of Urology*, **3**, 140–4.

Philp, N. H., Williams, J. L., and Byers, C. E. (1980). Ileal conduit urinary diversion: Long-term follow-up in adults. *British Journal of Urology*, **52**, 515–19.

Richie, J. P., Skinner, D. G., and Waisman, J. (1974). The effect of reflux on the development of pyelonephritis in urinary diversion: an experimental study. *Journal of Surgical Research*, **16**, 256–61.

Rosen, R. J. and Roven, S. J. (1984). Percutaneous drainage of abscesses and fluid collections. *Urology*, **23**(5a), 54–8.

Rosenbaum, T. P., Shah, P. J. R., Rose, G. A., and Lloyd-Davies, R. W. (1989). Cranberry juice helps the problem of mucus production in entero-uroplasties. *Neurology and Urodynamics*, **8**, 344–5.

Silverman, A. H., Woodhouse, C. R. J., Strachan, J. R., Cumming, J., and Keighley, M. R. B. (1986). Long-term management of patients who have had urinary diversions into the colon. *British Journal of Urology*, **58**, 634–9.

Sleight, M. W. and Wickham, J. E. A. (1977). Long-term follow-up 100 cases of renal calculi. *British Journal of Urology*, **49**, 601–4.

Stamey, T. A., Govan, D. E., and Palmer, J. M. (1965). The localisation and treatment of urinary tract infections: the role of bactericidal urine levels as opposed to serum levels. *Medicine* (Baltimore), **44**, 1.

Stewart, M. (1986). Urinary diversion and bowel cancer. *Annals of the Royal College of Surgeons of England*, **68**, 98–102.

Webb, J. A. W., Shanmuganathan, K., and McLean, A. (1993). Complications of ultrasound guided transperineal prostate biopsy. A prospective study. *British Journal of Urology*, **72**, 775–7.

Whitfield, H. N. and Mayo, M. E. (1976). Intermittent self-catheterisation. *British Journal of Urology*, **63**, 330–2.

Williams, G., Coulange, C., Milroy, E. J. G., Sarramon, J. P., and Rubben, H. (1993). The Urolume, a permanently implanted prostatic stent for patients at high risk for surgery—results from five collaborative centres. *British Journal of Urology*, **72**, 335–40.

Witherow, R. O'N. and Wickham, J. E. A. (1980). Nephrolithotomy in chronic renal failure; saved from dialysis. *British Journal of Urology*, **52**, 419–21.

Woodhouse, C. R. J. (1994). The infective, metabolic and histological consequences of enterocystoplasty. *European Urology Update Series*, **3**, 10–15.

13
Urinary tract infection in men

David J. Riden and Anthony J. Schaeffer

Introduction

Men have fewer urinary tract infections (UTIs) than women despite having less stringent criteria for diagnosis and a higher prevalence of anatomical and functional abnormalities of the urinary tract. Different organisms infect men and the prevalence of bacteriuria varies at different ages. Recurrent infections are common and urological evaluation and treatment is frequently required and beneficial. Studies over the last decade have delineated differences between male and female populations in regard to epidemiology, microbiology, diagnosis, and treatment of UTI. In particular, the diagnosis, classification, and treatment of prostatitis has been clarified so that a unified approach is possible to this common and often confusing clinical problem.

Epidemiology

Bacteriuria is much more common in females than males at all ages of life except in the first year when the prevalence in boys (less than 1 per cent) is four times greater than in girls (Bergstrom *et al.* 1972; Jodal 1987). It has been estimated that at least 30 per cent of all women experience a UTI during their lifetime (Grapey and Schaeffer 1994). This compares with a recent United States survey of persons aged 14–61 years in which 12 per cent of men reported a past history of kidney, bladder, or urinary infections (Kunin 1987). Approximately 40 per cent of all male office visits for urogenital problems are infection related, the majority being related to prostatitis (25 per cent) and cystourethritis (10 per cent) (Lipsky 1989; Kunin 1987).

Male infants have a higher rate of UTI than female infants, possibly related to two factors: a higher rate of congenital genitourinary anomalies and the presence of a prepuce. Forty to 85 per cent of bacteriuric boys will have some demonstrable genitourinary abnormality, a rate twice that seen in bacteriuric girls (Burbige *et al.* 1984). Additionally, several studies have shown that uncircumcised male infants have a significantly higher rate of UTI than those who are circumcised (Winberg 1989).

Uncomplicated infection (i.e. community-acquired infection occurring in individuals with normal urinary tracts) is rare in men but does occur in association with lack of circumcision or HIV infection. Anal intercourse, particularly in homosexual males, may increase the risk of infection by exposing the urethra to large quantities of faecal *Escherichia coli* (Barnes *et al.* 1986).

Most infection in boys and men is complicated; that is, the individuals have an anatomical or urological abnormality, a recent catheterization, or have had urological surgery. Vesicoureteric reflux and urethral valves are commonly found in infant boys with bacteriuria and infection, and may lead to renal scarring and chronic renal disease. The most common cause of complicated infection in men is nosocomial introduction of urinary pathogens. Instrumentation of the urinary tract, such as peri-operative catheterization with a break in sterile technique, accounts for the majority of infections.

The incidence of infection in men is less than 1 per cent until the sixth decade, when prostatic hyperplasia frequently develops leading to urinary tract obstruction, residual urine, and instrumentation for the evaluation and management of the condition.

The acquisition of functionally disabling conditions, such as paraplegia, arthritis, or neurological impairment, are statistically related to the acquisition and maintenance of bacteriuria. Frequently, such conditions result in an increased incidence of catheterization and nosocomial urinary tract infections. As many as 10 per cent of hospitalized patients have urinary catheters and approximately 20 per cent of those with catheters develop bacteriuria. As a result, urosepsis secondary to catheter-associated bacteriuria is the most common source of Gram-negative bacteraemia and septicaemia in hospitalized patients.

Pathophysiology

The male urethra, usually 14–20 cm in length, is substantially longer than the female urethra, and provides a natural barrier from the colonized skin of the perineum and anus. Penetration of this urethral defence is required in order for bacteruria to develop. The issue of bacterial seeding by prostatic infections is covered in subsequent sections. Urinary tract infections occur because of a breakdown of a functional or structural aspect of the normal host defence mechanisms. Such breakdown can have a myriad of causes: instrumentation, bladder outlet obstruction, bladder tumours or stones, urethral strictures, or foreign bodies (chiefly catheters). Structural defects in the genitourinary tract, usually acquired rather than congenital, may predispose to UTI. Neurogenic bladder conditions cause stagnation of urine and potentiate bacteriuria, as do alterations of intrinsic or extrinsic bladder anatomy due to surgery, radiation, or trauma. External compression of the bladder by tumour or inflammatory processes or internal hypertrophy and trabeculation of detrusor musculature, and, in particular, formation of diverticula predispose to bacteriuria. Introduction of few bacteria may lead to multiplication to high concentration, especially in the bladder environment associated with outlet obstruction, or any of the preceding causes. Normal bladder flushing with urine may be impaired, and consequent breakdown of host barriers, such as the glycosaminoglycan layer of the bladder, may begin a cascade of events leading to infection. Systemic immunodeficiency, and in particular, diabetes mellitus, predispose to bacteriuria and the subsequent events leading to UTI.

Escherichia coli and other Enterobacteriaceae are the predominant uropathogens in men. *Escherichia coli.*, Proteus spp., and other Gram-negative bacilli are cultured in boys with UTI, especially those who are uncircumcised (Wiswell and Smith 1985). In elderly men, *E. coli* continues to be the predominant organism but Proteus, Klebsiella, Serratia, Pseudomonas species, and enterococci have become increasingly prevalent. As hospitalization or institutionalization of elderly males is increasingly common, so too is the diversity of bacteria seen with nosocomial bacteriuria (Teillac 1991).

Urethritis in sexually active men is commonly caused by *Neisseria gonorrhea*, *Chlamydia trachomatous*, and possibly *Ureaplasma urealyticum*. Enterococcal infection has become far more frequent in young sexually active males presenting with uncomplicated UTI. Insertional anal intercourse could predispose to inoculation with coliform organisms and subsequent infection.

Clinical manifestations

The clinical manifestations of UTI range from assymptomatic bacteriuria in boys and elderly men to classic signs of acute cystitis, febrile illness, and Gram-negative septicaemia. Typical symptoms include dysuria, frequency, urgency, and suprapubic pressure. Gross haematuria and voiding dysfunction are common. A febrile illness, if associated with flank or abdominal pain, suggests pyelonephritis or, if associated with prostatic tenderness, prostatitis. Approximately 20 per cent of patients with acute pyelonephritis or acute prostatitis develop Gram-negative bacteraemia. Recurrent infections, particularly at close intervals and with the same or an unusual organism, strongly suggest structural abnormalities of the urinary tract or chronic bacterial prostatitis.

The majority of elderly patients have asymptomatic bacteriuria (Wolfson *et al.* 1965). Non-specific symptoms, such as lethargy, confusion, anorexia, and incontinence, frequently cause missed or delayed diagnosis and may lead to significant morbidity and mortality. Even severe UTI in the elderly may not be associated with fever.

Diagnosis

A presumptive diagnosis of UTI can be made by dip-sticks and microscopic urinalysis and confirmed via urine culture. The dip-stick test can detect leucocyte esterase activity, indicating the presence of neutrophils and urinary tract inflammation. Similarly, the presence of nitrites can indicate the presence of Gram-negative bacteria, since these organisms can reduce nitrate to nitrite. These tests are quite accurate for detection of large numbers of bacteria, but less so for fewer numbers of bacteria, despite the fact that very few bacteria can be associated with clinical symptoms of infection. Examination of Gram-stained slides of urinary sediment may identify Gram-negative bacilli and guide antimicrobial selection. (Fair *et al.* 1976) We do not recommend Gram-stain procedures for routine screening but in the setting of acute pyelonephritis or suspicious febrile illness, Gram's stain of urinary sediment may guide early antimicrobial intervention.

Microscopic evaluation of urine is easily accomplished and, when properly carried out, is remarkably useful in the diagnosis of UTI. No preparation is necessary in collecting urine samples in boys and men who are circumcised. For those who are uncircumcised, the foreskin should be retracted, the glans penis washed with soap, and rinsed with water prior to specimen collection. A two-glass collection is routinely collected (i.e. the first 10 ml of urine and a mid-stream specimen should be obtained). This collection technique permits evaluation of a urethral urine specimen and a bladder specimen. If pyuria and bacteriuria are present in the first voided specimen in contradistinction to the second, urethral pathology, such as stricture or diverticula, should be suspected and evaluated via urethroscopy or retrograde urethrography. Most patients with UTI have pyuria. Men are less likely than women to contaminate voided urine specimens, and therefore colony counts in voided specimens one to two orders of magnitude lower are considered to represent significant bacteriuria. Specimens from such patients may be positive on dip-sticks for leucocyte esterase activity but not for nitrites, given the lower colony counts present. In a study of older men with irritative urethral symptoms who were evaluated by first void, mid-stream, and suprapubic aspirate urine collections, Lipsky *et al.* (1987) found that midstream urine cultures, which grew 1000 colony-forming units per millilitre of a predominant species, best differentiated infection from no infection (sensitivity 0.97 and specificity 0.97). In asymptomatic patients, at least two cultures growing the same organism in quantities greater than or equal to 100 000 colony-forming units per ml are required to confirm the diagnosis. Since most infections in boys and men are complicated, a thorough evaluation of the urinary tract by radio-logical, laboratory, and urological testing should be pursued. Fever, haematuria, and relapsing infection with the same strain at close intervals suggest a focus of bacterial persistence within the urinary tract, and diligent work-up is essential. Radiographic assessment in a setting of uncomplicated cystitis, particularly with low clinical suspicion of anatomic or foreign body abnormalities, is often unrevealing and unlikely to yield useful data. Characteristic radiographic findings of acute pyelonephritis are seen on excretion urography and computed tomography (Chapter 4).

Bacteriological localization studies differentiating upper from lower tract infection may be useful in determining the aetiology of UTI in men and direct its treatment. As with most infections of the urinary tract, most data collection and research on localization studies has been performed in female patients and thus little information is available that is male-specific. However, there is no reason to believe that the accuracy of such data is gender dependent. The value and role of localization studies is dealt with in Chapter 6.

Treatment

Selection of antimicrobial therapy for treatment of UTI in boys and men should take into consideration the age of the patient, the severity of the infection, the probable pathogen, and the possibility of an underlying abnormality that could complicate treatment. Acute uncomplicated cystitis in boys should be treated with a 7-day course of trimethoprim, trimethoprim-sulphamethoxazole, or nitrofurantoin. We currently recommend 3- or 7-day therapy in men, with these antimicrobials or one of the newer fluoroquinolones (Table 13.1). Generally, fluoroquinolones are expensive and offer no clear superiority over trimethoprim-sulphamethoxazole. Fluoroquinolones are not recommended in children except in rare circumstances mainly because animal studies have shown chondrocyte and cartilage abnormalities with the use of fluoride-chemical-based agents.

Algorithms regarding length of treatment for acute uncomplicated UTI are based upon the treatment of women. It is generally accepted that women with typical symptoms of acute uncomplicated UTI and corroborating evidence on dip-stick and microscopic urinalysis can be treated without pre-therapy urine culture. Treatment decisions are made and therapy nearly completed before urine culture and sensitivity results are available. In addition, the literature is now replete with clinical trials touting much shorter courses of therapy. Norrby (1990) reviewed 28 separate clinical trials of short-term therapy (single-dose or 3-day therapy) for women with acute uncomplicated UTI. Three-day therapy emerged as the treatment of choice when trimethoprim, trimethoprim-sulphamethoxazole, or fluoroquinolones were used. Cephalosporins required 5-day therapy for equivalent efficacy. Post-therapy cultures were reserved for those who did not respond to treatment after 3 days of antimicrobials. It should be emphasized that few clinical trials are available that include significant numbers of male subjects. The few data available suggest that the response to antimicrobials should not be different to that in women with uncomplicated UTI.

Acute pyelonephritis

Infection in patients with acute pyelonephritis (APN) can be subdivided into:

(1) infection that does not warrant hospitalization;

(2) infection in patients who are sufficiently ill to require hospitalization or parenteral therapy; and

(3) infection associated with hospitalization, urological surgery, or urinary tract abnormalities.

In all cases, antimicrobial therapy should be initiated with a drug both active against potential uropathogens and which achieves therapeutic antimicrobial levels in renal tissue as well as urine. As delineated above, Gram's stain of the urinary sediment is helpful to guide selection of the initial empirical antimicrobial therapy.

Table 13.1 Antimicrobial agents in the treatment of urinary tract infection in men and boys

First choice drugs	Dose	Duration	Comments
Oral antimicrobial agents for acute uncomplicated cystitis			
Trimethoprim	200 mg twice daily 10 mg/kg/day Divided twice daily for boys	3–7 days	Low resistance 5–15% in uncomplicated acute cystitis; use in sulpha-allergic patients
Trimethoprim-sulphamethoxazole	1 double strength (160/800) 10 mg/kg/day Divided twice daily for boys	3–7 days	Check sulpha allergy; most *Pseudomonas aeruginosa* resistant as are most enterococci
Nitrofurantoin	100 mg 4 times daily 5–7 mg/kg/day Divided 6 hourly for boys	3–7 days	Ineffective against *P. aeruginosa* and some Proteus species
Ciprofloxacin*	500–750 mg twice daily	3–7 days	Most effective fluoroquinolone against *P. aeruginosa*
Ofloxacin*	200–400 mg twice daily	3–7 days	Effective against Chlamydia and Ureaplasma
Lomefloxacin*	400 mg/day	3–7 days	Benefit of once daily dosing
Enoxacin*	200 mg twice daily	3–7 days	Inhibits theophylline metabolism
Norfloxin*	400 mg twice daily	3–7 days	Usage limited to urinary infections
Parenteral and oral antimicrobial agents for acute pyelonephritis			
Amipicillin	2 g IV 4–6 hourly	48–72 h	Until afebrile or sensitivities return
Gentamicin	1.5 mg/kg, 8–12 hourly	48–72 h	Serum levels for more than 48 hours therapy
Trimethoprim-sulphamethoxazole	160/800 IV, 12 hourly	48–72 h	Not recommended in case of sepsis
Ciprofloxacin	400 mg IV, 12 hourly	48–72 h	For sulpha-allergic patients with intolerance for aminoglycoside therapy

Oral agents are the same as for uncomplicated cystitis; oral therapy is initiated once euthermic state established and tailored to sensitivities from cultures (blood and urine). Parenteral therapy offers little benefit beyond 72 hours if euthermia is maintained.
*NOT for use in boys <18 years old; IV, intravenous.

Patients with flank pain and fever suggestive of APN can be treated on an outpatient basis if they have a straightforward diagnosis and if compliant follow-up care is assured. Fourteen days oral therapy with trimethoprim, trimethoprim-sulphamethoxazole, or a fluoroquinolone is preferred (Ronald 1987). Elderly patients, and those with severe nausea and emesis with concomitant dehydration, or those with subtle or overt signs of septicaemia should be admitted to hospital. Supportive care with intravenous (IV) or oral fluids and IV parenteral antimicrobials should be instituted urgently. IV trimethoprim-sulphamethoxazole, aminoglycoside therapy, or a fluoroquinolone should be given until defervescence and clinical improvement is noted, usually within 72 hours. Oral therapy is then begun. There is no evidence that longer periods of therapy are required in patients with bacteraemia. Between 10 and 30 per cent of individuals with APN relapse following a 14-day course of therapy. Individuals who relapse are usually cured by a second 14-day course of treatment, but occasionally a 6-week course is required (Tolkoff-Rubin and Rubin 1987).

Failure to respond to antimicrobial therapy suggests infection caused by a drug-resistant strain, an anatomical abnormality, urinary obstruction, or an unrecognized focus of infection seeding the urinary tract. Renal imaging by non-invasive means and progressing as necessary to complicated or invasive procedures should be carried out until the situation is defined. Ultrasonography or excretion urography may be required to detect abnormalities and guide further investigation and/or therapy. Relief of obstruction, removal of calcarious material, or correction of stricture disease should be undertaken where indicated.

Patients with indwelling catheters or external catheter devices will continue to develop bacteriuria on a variable basis. Prophylaxis is inappropriate and expensive and leads to selection of resistant strains. Early symptomatic treatment may avert more serious infection.

Prostatitis

Bacterial prostatitis is the most common cause of acute complicated or chronic recurrent UTI in men, and the most common inflammatory entity encountered in urological practice. Despite this, many aspects of prostatitis are still poorly understood, and both patients and clinicians are often frustrated in dealing with this condition. Further classification and more detailed clinical and laboratory strategies in pursuit of diagnosis and new antimicrobial drugs may offer better treatment in the future.

Pathogenesis

Bacterial prostatitis is caused by the usual uropathogens. *Escherichia coli* and other members of the Enterobacteriaceae family, such as Klebsiella and Proteus spp. predominate. Pseudomonas and *Enterococcus faecalis* are less common, occurring more usually in a hospitalized or institutionalized host. Mixed infections involving two or more strains or classes of microorganisms are not uncommon.

The role of Gram-positive bacteria, other than enterococci, as pathogens in prostatitis is controversial. Although uncommon, chronic bacterial prostatitis caused by *Staphylococcus aureus* has been documented, usually as a consequence of a hospital-acquired catheter-associated infection. The aetiological role of other Gram-positive bacteria, chiefly *Staphy. epidermitis* and *saprophyticus*, micrococci, non-group D streptococci, and diptheroids, is doubtful (Jimenez-Cruz *et al.* 1984). These organisms are skin inhabitants, existing as urethral commensals rather than true pathogens. Furthermore, they do not cause relapsing UTI in untreated patients.

The pathogenesis of bacterial prostatitis is unknown. Ascending urethral infection after vaginal or rectal inoculation of the urinary meatus during sexual intercourse presumably plays an important role (Blacklock 1974; Stamey 1973). As such, the prostatitis may represent an extension or complication of urethritis. Evidence of reflux of urine into the prostatic ducts has come from crystallographic analysis of prostatic calculi, where constituents found in urine, but foreign to prostatic secretions, are found (Ramirez *et al.* 1980; Sutor and Wooley 1974). Kirby *et al.* (1982) provided more direct proof of intra-prostatic urinary reflux by instilling 400 ml of a carbon particle suspension in the bladder through a urethral catheter in five patients with pre-existing non bacterial prostatitis. Seventy-two hours later, following voiding, prostatic massage was performed. All patients had carbon containing macrophages in the expressed prostatic fluid (EPS). Other proposed pathogenic mechanisms include direct extension, lymphogenous or haematogenous spread of faecal microorganisms.

The role of prostatic secretions in the pathogenesis of prostatitis is unclear. Normal prostatic secretion has some antibacterial property. Marked changes occur in the prostatic secretions of patients with prostatitis. In bacterial prostatitis, the prostatic secretions become more alkaline and less viscous than normal, and contain decreased levels of zinc (Meares 1980). Interestingly, zinc has been identified as an antibacterial factor. However, oral administration of zinc to patients with documented prostatitis did not alter the serum level of zinc or alter clinical outcome (Fair *et al.* 1976). Prostatic secretory dysfunction may adversely affect the normal antibacterial nature of prostatic secretions and the diffusion of certain drugs into the prostatic fluid.

Recent studies indicate that measurement of the immune response in prostatic fluid provides specific indicators of bacterial prostatitis that easily distinguish it from non-bacterial prostatitis (Shortliffe *et al.* 1981). In acute bacterial prostatitis cured by medical therapy, serum and prostatic fluid antigen-specific IgG are both elevated at the onset of infection but decline slowly during the ensuing 6–12 months. Antigen-specific IgA in prostatic fluid becomes elevated immediately after infection and begins to decline only after about 12 months. In contrast, the initial elevation in serum IgA disappears after only 1 month.

In chronic bacterial prostatitis, although prostatic fluid antigen-specific IgA and IgG are both elevated, neither immunoglobulin is substantially elevated in serum. In chronic bacterial prostatitis cured by medical therapy, prostatic fluid IgA remains elevated for almost 2 years and IgG for 6 months before each begins to decline to normal. In men with bacterial prostatitis that is not cured by medical therapy, prostatic fluid antigen-specific IgA and IgG remain persistently elevated. Shortliffe and Wehner (1986) reported on the immune response of the prostatic fluid of patients with non-bacterial prostatitis. These patients had a weak but definite antibody response to bacterial antigens, as compared to normal healthy controls. Shortliffe *et al.* (1985) also reported insignificant antigen-specific antibody elevations against Ureaplasma and Chlamydia in the prostatic fluid of male patients with non-bacterial prostatitis.

Classification of prostatitis

It is usual to subdivide patients with prostatitis into those with acute or chronic bacterial prostatitis and those with non-bacterial prostatitis (Table 13.2). There is a further subgroup of patients who may have similar symptoms of urinary urgency, dysuria, poor urine flow or prostatic discomfort but do not have evidence of inflammation or bacterial infection within the prostatic fluid. This syndrome has been termed 'prostatodynia' because the symptoms were judged to be of prostatic origin. However, many patients are unable to differentiate prostatic pain from pelvic or perineal syndromes. 'Pelviperineal pain' is therefore a more appropriate term for this condition.

To distinguish these conditions it is necessary to demonstrate evidence of inflammation within the prostate and to culture sequential samples of urethral and bladder urine and prostatic secretions. In order to identify the presence of inflammation in the prostate it is first necessary to define the microscopic findings in normal prostatic fluid. This is done by counting the number of white blood cells per high-power field (hpf) on microscopic examination of expressed prostatic fluid (EPS) (Drach *et al.* 1978). The major formed elements of expressed prostatic fluid are white blood cells, large oval fat macrophages laden with cholesterol particles, and lecithin granules. The majority of white blood cells are polymorphonuclear whereas lymphocytes are uncommon. Oval fat macrophages occur in all sizes ranging from one to several times the diameter of a white blood cell. They are often dark brown and are termed 'oval brown bodies'. Normal prostatic fluid has few white blood cells and few oval bodies. The small granular bodies commonly termed 'lecithin granules' are composed of phospholipids, and are seen to be plentiful in the secretions of healthy adult males. The changes that occur in the prostatic secretion of men with bacterial and non-bacterial prostatitis are an increase in the number of leucocytes, often found in clumps, an increase in oval fat macrophages and a variable decrease in lecithin bodies.

Schaeffer *et al.* (1981) studied 119 consecutive patients with no history, symptoms, or physical findings (excluding prostatic fluid examination) of urinary tract inflammation with a normal prostate gland by digital examination, and fewer than two white blood cells per hpf in the first 10 ml of voided urine and no or insignificant growth on urine culture (Fig. 13.1). Of these patients, 31 were judged to have no urological disease and had prostatic fluid containing 0.7 + 0.41

Table 13.2 Classification of prostatitis

	Pain	Evidence of inflammation (EPS)	Culture-positive (EPS)	Culture-positive (bladder)	Common aetiological bacteria	Rectal examination (prostate)
Acute bacterial prostatitis	+	+	+	+[a]	Enterobacteriaceae	Abnormal
Chronic bacterial prostatitis	±	+	+	+[b]	Enterobacteriaceae	Normal
'Nonbacterial' prostatitis	±	+	0	0	?	Normal
Pelviperineal pain	±	0	0	0	0	Normal

[a]Acute bacterial prostatitis is nearly always accompanied by bladder infection.
[b]Characterized by recurrent bacteriuria, at varying intervals up to several months, after stopping antimicrobial therapy.
EPS, expressed prostatic secretion.
Modified from Stamey (1980).

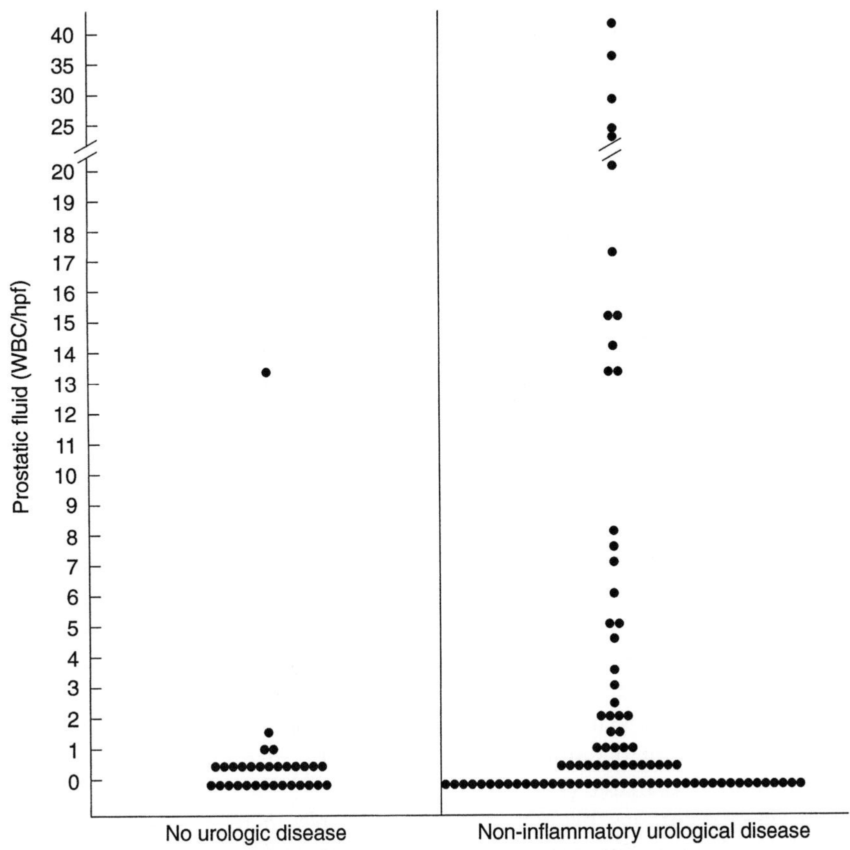

Fig. 13.1 Number of white blood cells per high-power microscopic field (WBC/hpf) in prostatic fluid from patients with no urological disease or non-inflammatory urological disease. (From Schaeffer *et al.* 1981.)

white blood cells per hpf (mean + standard error of mean). Eighty-eight patients with a variety of non-inflammatory urological diseases had 3.8 + 0.83 white blood cells per hpf in the prostatic fluid. There were two white blood cells or less per hpf observed in 97 per cent of the patients with no urological disease and in 75 per cent with non-inflammatory urological disease and normal prostate glands by digital exam. Only 13 of 119 patients in these two groups had 10 white blood cells or more per hpf. Similar results have been reported by Blacklock (1969) and Anderson and Weller (1979).

It appears, therefore, that clinically significant inflammation is present when prostatic fluid contains 10 or more white blood cells per hpf. Urethral inflammation, infertility, and benign prostatic hyperplasia can cause elevated leucocyte counts in EPS. In the same study, Schaeffer *et al.* (1981) found 18 infertile men with average leucocyte counts in EPS of 8.3 per hpf, significantly higher than the value of less than one white blood cell per hpf observed in patients with no urological disease. Indeed, seven infertile but otherwise healthy men had greater than 10 white blood cells per hpf in the prostatic fluid. The white blood cell count in prostatic secretions also rises significantly in healthy men for several hours after sexual intercourse and ejaculation (Jameson 1967).

The distinguishing characteristics of patients with bacterial or non bacterial-prostatitis are summarized in Table 13.2. All patients with bacterial or non-bacterial prostatitis have evidence of inflammation in their expressed prostatic secretions, and therefore cannot be distinguished on this basis. Patients with bacterial prostatitis, both acute and chronic, are distinguished from those with non-bacterial prostatitis by recovery of bacteria from the prostatic secretions. In virtually all patients with bacterial prostatitis, urinary infections with bladder bacteriuria also occurs. Conversely, patients with non-bacterial prostatitis have no such urinary infection, unless concomitant anatomical or risk factors are present.

Quantitative segmental bacteriological localization cultures

Bacterial prostatitis can be differentiated from non-bacterial prostatitis only by sequential, quantitative bacteriological culture of the urethral and bladder urine, and prostatic secretions. The lower tract localization studies described by Meares and Stamey (1968) remain the gold standard for the diagnosis and follow up of prostatitis syndromes. Sequential collection and culture of a urethral specimen (initially voided urine or voided bladder; VB1), a bladder specimen (midstream urine or VB2), or a prostatic specimen (expressed prostatic secretion; EPS), and a urine specimen voided immediately after prostatic massage (VB3) is the best diagnostic strategy available (Fig. 13.2).

When the patient has bladder infection, all specimens will show bacterial growth. In such cases, the patient should be treated with an antimicrobial drug

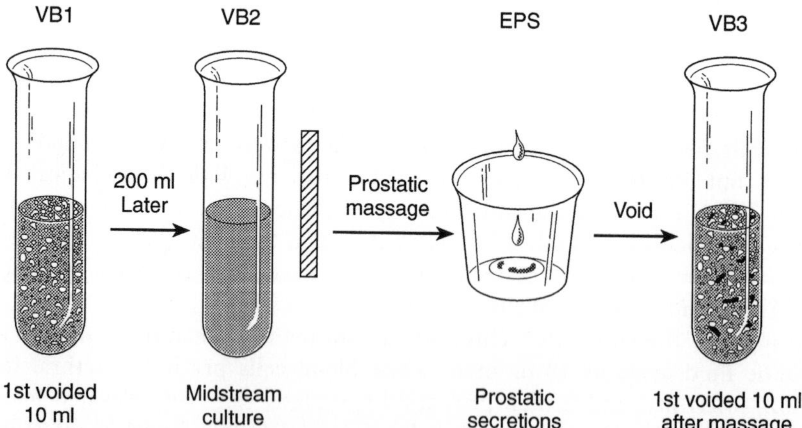

Fig. 13.2 Segmented culture technique for localizing urinary infections in the male urethra or the prostate. VB, voided bladder. (From Meares and Stamey 1968.)

such as nitrofurantoin or a penicillin derivative. These will sterilize the bladder urine and clear the urethra of bacterial organisms without penetrating the prostatic tissue and thus altering its microbial flora. Demonstration of bacteria in the post-prostatic massage urine (VB3) or EPS, when the urethral and midstream urine specimens show no growth, is highly diagnostic of bacterial prostatitis. Alternatively, a bacterial count of tenfold or more in VB3 or EPS compared to that in the urethral specimen is indicative of bacterial prostatitis. The accuracy of this method has been questioned by Pfau (1986), and Fowler and Mariano (1984), based primarily on shortcomings in the contribution and quantification of urethral bacteria. In addition, it is little used by the average clinician because of expense, time, and difficulty in proper performance of the test by patients. In addition, difficulty in obtaining prostatic secretions after massage, previous, often empirical antimicrobial therapy prescribed by referring physicians, and an overall diagnostic yield ranging between 40 and 70 per cent make localization difficult to justify on a routine basis.

Nevertheless, we continue to recommend quantitative localization as the test of choice, even though multiple repeat attempts and meticulous adherence to procedure protocol may be required. This is because we often are asked to consult and treat refractory cases who have been treated with multiple courses of antimicrobials and other different treatments without any hard documentation of UTI with fever.

Prostatic imaging

Recent advances in technology have allowed the common application of transrectal prostate ultrasound (US) in the diagnosis of both benign and malignant prostatic disease. The sonographic features of prostatitis on transrectal prostatic US however, are neither sensitive nor specific enough to allow identification of any one feature as being diagnostic of prostatitis (Doble and Carter 1989). Granulomatous prostatitis, estimated to occur in 0.8 per cent of benign inflammatory prostatic conditions, is a potential sequela of acute bacterial prostatitis, and is often confused with carcinoma of the prostate due to identical features of hypoechogenicity on transrectal US (Bude *et al.* 1990).

The presence of prostatic calcarious material can be imaged via transrectal US and may be associated with bacterial prostatitis, but the incidence of prostatic calculi, estimated at 75 per cent in middle-aged men and nearly 100 per cent in elderly males, far exceeds the incidence of bacterial prostatitis. Prostatic stones usually are tiny and occur in small clusters, which appear as hyperechoic lesions with shadowing on sonographic imaging. These calculi are not normally colonized by bacteria and cause no harm provided they remain confined to the prostate. In certain men with prostate calculi and recurrent UTI, however, the stones have been shown to become colonized and to be the source of bacterial persistence (Eykyn *et al.* 1974; Meares 1974). It is plausible that unrecognized colonized stones are not permeated by antimicrobials and are responsible for the failure of such therapy to cure the condition.

The value of transrectal US of the prostate over computed tomography (CT) of the pelvis in suspected prostatic abscess has not been clearly shown. However, the reduced cost and wider availability of transrectal US, coupled with the ability to provide imaging for perineal drainage, may make US the imaging modality of choice.

Acute bacterial prostatitis

This usually presents with dramatic onset of fever, malaise, low back or perineal pain, and myalgia preceding by several days the onset of urinary frequency, dysuria, urgency, and varying degrees of bladder outlet obstruction. Palpation of the prostate usually reveals a tender, warm, swollen irregular gland that may be partially or totally indurated or 'boggy'. Prostatic massage should be avoided because of the risk of bacteraemia, but gentle pressure on the prostate may induce copious amounts of purulent prostatic secretions. Since cystitis usually accompanies acute bacterial prostatitis, the pathogen can generally be identified by culture of the voided urine.

Supportive care in the form of analgesics, antipyretics, hydration, stool softeners, and bed rest should be instituted. If urine flow is obstructed and the patient cannot urinate, suprapubic needle aspiration or percutaneous suprapubic catheter placement is recommended. Urethral catheterization, although often technically possible, may further exacerbate the inflammatory process and has been shown to increase the risk of complications, such as acute epididymitis. Thus, it is best avoided in favour of suprapubic diversion. Patients with acute bacterial prostatitis respond dramatically to antimicrobial drugs that do not normally achieve therapeutic levels in prostatic fluid.

Rarely, but more often in elderly, debilitated, or immunocompromised patients, the toxicity associated with acute bacterial prostatitis may require admission to hospital and parenteral antimicrobial therapy, using an aminoglycoside-penicillin-derivative combination. If the patient responds to such therapy, a suitable oral antimicrobial agent is substituted and given in full dose for thirty days. If the patient's condition does not warrant parenteral therapy, we initiate treatment with trimethoprim-sulphamethoxazole or carbenicillin inadanyl sodium until the results of the culture and sensitivity testing are known. If the patient is allergic to sulphonamides or penicillin, we begin therapy with trimethoprim alone. Once therapy has been tailored to the known antimicrobial sensitivities and if the clinical response is favourable, therapy is continued for at least 30 days, to avert chronic prostatitis (Meares 1991). Repeat cultures are obtained after the 30-day treatment course. If repeat cultures are positive, two weeks of further therapy is initiated, and cultures are again repeated. (Table 13.3)

Abscess is a potential but rare complication of acute bacterial prostatitis. An abscess can be suggested by a fluctuant prostate on digital rectal examination and confirmed by transrectal US or CT. In addition to antimicrobial therapy, surgical drainage of prostatic abscess is generally required, by either the transurethral or

Table 13.3 Antimicrobial agents used in the treatment of acute and chronic prostatitis

Drug	Dosage	Duration	Comments
Acute prostatitis			
Trimethoprim-sulphamethoxazole	1 double strength tab (160/800)	30 days	Refractory cases may respond to ciprofloxacin or norfloxin (see text)
Trimethoprim	100 mg twice daily	30 days	Reassess once sensitivities known
Carbenicillin indanyl sodium*	2 tabs 4 times a day	30 days	Check sensitivities
Ciprofloxacin	500 mg twice daily	30 days	May be appropriate in ill-appearing patients
Chronic prostatitis			
Ciprofloxacin	500 mg twice daily	14 days	Repeat cultures
Norfloxacin	400 mg twice daily	14 days	Repeat cultures
Ofloxacin	400 mg twice daily	14 days	Repeat cultures
Suppression therapy for refractory cases			
Trimethoprim-sulphamethoxazole	1 single strength daily (80/400)	?	For refractory cases to suppress recurrent urinary infections.
Nitrofurantoin	100 mg daily	?	Inexpensive but may be ill-tolerated due to side-effects
Tetracycline	250 mg daily	?	

*If repeat cultures are positive after 30 days therapy, or clinical failure.

transperineal route. Leport *et al.* (1989) reported on a group of human immunodeficiency virus-infected patients who presented with prostatitis and among whom several had prostatic abscesses demonstrated on transrectal US. Drainage was not performed. The patients were treated with long-term antimicrobial therapy with fluoroquinolones. The average duration of therapy was five months, and two patients had recurrent abscesses. Despite these data, we continue to favour drainage via transurethral or transperineal approaches. Overwhelming sepsis can ensue on rupture of prostatic abscesses, even in the face of oral antimicrobial therapy (Nelson, personal communication).

Finally, the advent of widespread use of radioimmunoassay for the serine-protease prostate-specific antigen (PSA) warrants a special note. In the face of any prostatic inflammatory process, the permeability characteristics of the prostatic cellular wall is altered, resulting in the dispersion of PSA into both the semen and the bloodstream. The serum PSA may be elevated in prostatic inflammation. If prostatic inflammation is suspected as the cause of an elevated PSA, antimicrobial therapy with trimethoprim-sulphamethoxazole, fluoroquinolones, or trimethoprim alone should be initiated and continued for 4–6 weeks, followed by repeat measurement of the serum PSA level. The PSA should fall dramatically. However, no hard data are available to allow specific quantification of the rate, velocity, or percentage of the decrease. The elevated PSA must be carefully correlated with the clinical scenario; specifically, the age, family history, and digital prostate examination. The high incidence of prostatic carcinoma prescribes close follow-up for such patients. Persistent elevation of PSA above 4.0 ng/ml despite a 30-day treatment should necessitate urological consultation. Bacterial prostatitis, acute or chronic, appears to be associated with higher elevation in serum PSA; however, no conclusive prospective studies have evaluated PSA in populations of men with chronic prostatitis, non-bacterial prostatitis, or pelviperineal pain. Despite the lack of efficacy of antimicrobials in the treatment of non-bacterial prostatitis or pelviperineal pain, a trial of antimicrobials seems warranted in the patient with elevated PSA and no overt clinical signs of prostatic carcinoma.

Chronic bacterial prostatitis

This is a rare phenomenon characterized by relatively asymptomatic periods between episodes of recurrent bacteriuria. Diagnosis is nearly impossible by physical examination; lower tract localization cultures must be performed.

The infection is thought to be caused by small numbers of bacteria in the prostatic fluid and is virtually impossible to eradicate with most antimicrobial therapy. The most common pathogens are Enterobacteriaceae, species of Pseudomonas, and *Streptococcus faecalis*. Other Gram-positive organisms have been implicated much less frequently. They rarely cause recurrent bacteriuria and therefore do not fit the classic picture of intermittent symptomatic bacteriuria seen in chronic prostatitis. There is much debate regarding the role, if any, of such Gram-positive bacilli in the aetiology and maintenance of chronic prostatitis. Recent work from multiple centres implicates *Ureaplasma urealyticum* and *Chlamydia trachomitis* in the clinical syndromes associated with chronic prostatitis. Again, the re-culture rate is low and the role of such organisms is the subject of current research and heated debate among investigators.

That said, chronic bacterial prostatitis is one of the most common causes of relapsing UTI in men. In men with recurrent bacteriuria whose excretion urogram is normal, the possibility of chronic bacterial prostatitis should be considered and pursued with localization cultures. Antecedent episodes of acute bacterial prostatitis are often recounted, and nearly as many men will complain of previous mild to moderate irritative voiding symptoms and pain or discomfort involving various sites: the perineum, low back, scrotum, or penis, particularly glandular tingling. Haematasemia and painful ejaculation occur infrequently in the setting of chronic bacterial prostatitis. Urine analysis including dip-slide testing and microscopy, along with EPS examination, should be considered in men with these presenting symptoms.

Men with chronic bacterial prostatitis are usually asymptomatic except for symptoms associated with bacteriuria or acute exacerbation of chronic prostatic infection. Appropriate oral antimicrobial therapy usually controls the acute episode. Hot sitz baths and anti-pyretics are also helpful. Septic episodes requiring hospitalization and parenteral therapy occur rarely.

The pharmacokinetics of drug penetration into the prostate have been studied by using a dog prostate fistula model (Meares 1982; Winningham *et al.* 1968). These studies demonstrated that the most important determinants of antibiotic diffusion into prostatic secretions were lipid solubility and the degree of ionization in plasma. Only non-ionized, non-protein bound, lipid-soluble molecules crossed the lipid barrier or prostatic epithelial cell. The pH of dog prostatic fluid is acidic whereas the pH of prostatic expressate from normal men is alkaline. Furthermore, the pH of prostatic expressate is higher in patients with prostatitis (Meares 1982). Extrapolation of the dog data to humans in the treatment of bacterial prostatitis is therefore questionable. The efficacy of minocycline and carbenicillin has been reported but not reproduced (Paulson and de Vere White 1978; Oliveris *et al.* 1979).

Trimethoprim-sulphamethoxazole (TMP-SMX), 160 mg/800 mg twice daily for 12 weeks, will cure 30 to 40 per cent of patients (Meares 1982). Pfau (1986) reported 50 per cent success rate with intramuscular injection of kanamycin. Direct injection of antimicrobial agents into the prostate with favourable results has been reported in studies performed by Baert and Leonard (1988) and by Jimenez-Cruz *et al.* (1988). The anal submucosal route of antimicrobial delivery was recently reported with a '100 per cent' cure rate documented by a negative culture two to three years post-treatment (Shafik 1991).

One of the most exciting recent developments in the treatment of prostatitis is the use of fluoroquinolones. Although the first quinolone, nalidixic acid, became available in 1963, it was not widely used for several reasons. Blood levels were insufficient to treat all but UTI and organisms developed resistance during therapy. Both *Pseudomonas species* and enterococci were regularly resistant. These problems were overcome with the fluroquinolones. These agents have a broad spectrum of activity against aerobic Gram-negative and Gram-positive bacteria (Schaeffer 1987; Sabbaj *et al.* 1985). They act by inhibiting bacterial gyrases essential to deoxyribonucleic acid replication, transcription, and repair (Wolfson and Hooper 1985). Spontaneous development of resistance is extremely rare. These drugs have small molecular sizes, high lipid solubility, and low protein binding (14–30 per cent) which may facilitate tissue penetration (Hooper and Wolfson 1985). In addition, unlike trimethoprim which is a base, fluoroquinolones are carboxylic acids and thus should undergo 'ion trapping' in the alkaline milieu of the prostatic secretions found in human chronic bacterial prostatitis.

The pharmacokinetics of fluoroquinolones have been described in many studies (Bologna *et al.* 1985; Dan *et al.* 1987; Hoogkamp-Korstanje *et al.* 1984; Scully 1990). Intra-prostatic concentration of norfloxacin and ciprofloxacin were 79 to 250 per cent of simultaneous serum levels. Norfloxacin achieved prostatic levels of 0.78 to 1.63 μg/g. These are inhibitory to ≥ 90 per cent of commonly isolated Enterobacteriaceae, with the exception of some species of Serratia and Providencia (Wolfson and Hooper 1985). The mean ciprofloxacin prostatic levels of 1.28 to 3.49 μg/g are inhibitory to > 90 per cent of Enterobacteriaceae as well as *P. aeruginosa* and enterococci.

Initial studies showed that norfloxacin and ciprofloxacin achieved 60–92 per cent cure rates in the treatment of chronic bacterial prostatitis (Sabbaj *et al.* 1986; Guibert *et al.* 1986; Langemeyer *et al.* 1987; Childs 1990). Patients followed-up for 1–2.5 months had cure rates of 74–92 per cent. Two studies with a minimum follow-up of 6 months reported cure rates of 53–64 per cent (Weidner *et al.* 1987; Schaeffer and Daras 1990).

Weidner *et al.* (1991) treated 17 men with chronic bacterial prostatitis. All had been treated with trimethoprim and/or TMP-SMX for at least 6 weeks without showing improvement. Patients received 500 mg of ciprofloxacin orally twice daily for two weeks. All patients completed the 1-year follow-up. Of 12 patients with *E. coli* prostatitis, treatment with ciprofloxacin was completed in 10 patients. One patient stopped therapy because of severe headaches. No patients had evidence of bacterial infection in a specimen during therapy. Of the 10 patients with *E. coli* prostatitis and 12-month follow-up, *E. coli* was eradicated in five. Two patients had low numbers of *E. coli* on follow-up cultures but, on subsequent examination, signs of *E. coli* infection could not be confirmed. The drug failed in three men, and in all three cases the re-isolated *E. coli* strains were susceptible to ciprofloxacin.

Five patients had prostatitis due to other microorganisms: *Enterococcus faecalis* in three patients: *P. aeruginosa* in one patient; and Enterobacter in one patient. Of these patients, the Enterobacter prostatitis was cured. Ciprofloxacin treatment was not effective in patients with *E. faecalis* and *P. aeruginosa* prostatitis. Overall, eight of 15 patients (53 per cent) with 12-month follow-up were cured.

Weidner *et al.* (1991) reported their re-evaluation of 4 weeks of treatment with ciprofloxacin for chronic bacterial prostatitis due to *E. coli.* After a median follow-up of 30 months (range 21–36 months) 10 of the 16 patients were considered cured as judged by bacteriological results and clinical symptoms. In two men a second ciprofloxacin regimen was successful. In two patients ciprofloxacin therapy failed and in another two patients therapy had to be discontinued due to central nervous system side-effects.

Schaeffer and Darras (1990) assessed efficacy of norfloxacin in the treatment of chronic bacterial prostatitis in 15 men. All patients had bacterial prostatitis refractory to TMP-SMX and/or carbenicillin. They were treated with 400 mg twice a day for 28 days. All the pathogens were sensitive to norfloxacin and absent in prostatic fluid cultures obtained during therapy. One patient had negative post-therapy prostatic fluid cultures but was lost to follow-up at 1 month. Of the 14 patients followed for at least 6 months, nine (64 per cent) were cured of the original infection. Six of these remained uninfected and had negative prostatic secretion and urine cultures for at least 6 months and were uninfected at 2 years follow-up. In three patients, the urinary infections recurred with new pathogens after post-therapy negative prostatic fluid cultures. Bacterial prostatitis with the original pathogen recurred in five patients within 2 months of completing therapy. The bacteria remained susceptible to norfloxacin but could not be eradicated with 30–90 days of additional norfloxacin therapy. Cures were achieved in nine of 12 patients with *E. coli* and two patients with *Pseudomonas prostatitis* did not respond to therapy. No patients experienced significant adverse effects. Overall, these data suggest that both ciprofloxacin and norfloxacin are effective and safe for treatment of chronic refractory bacterial prostatitis. Initial studies on the use of ofloxacin for prostatitis also show promising results (Cox 1989; Remy *et al.* 1988). These two studies suffer from lack of a follow-up and lack of standard localization culture results. Cox reported a 100 per cent bacteriological cure rate using ofloxacin for treatment of a well-defined group of patients with chronic bacterial prostatitis. Unfortunately, the study was terminated with long-term follow-up of only 5 weeks. The natural history of chronic bacterial prostatitis shows relapsing infections even months after treatment. Therefore, the result of this study has to be considered unsatisfactory with regard to the treatment of chronic bacterial prostatitis. Further studies with longer follow-up and proper design will be necessary before the true value of ofloxacin can be appraised.

Toxicity with fluoroquinolone therapy was rare and never caused withdrawal of greater than 10 per cent of patients in any study. At present, the fluroquinolones represent a reasonable alternative to TMP-SMX. Patients who are not cured by prolonged antimicrobial therapy can be managed with suppressive therapy to prevent recurrent UTI. The bacteria usually remain susceptible to many antimicrobial agents. Low-dose TMP-SMX, nitrofurantoin, or tetracycline are appropriate choices for suppressive therapy. Since prolonged treatment with prostate-tissue-penetrating agents rarely clears the pathogen from the prostate, therapy should focus on prevention of bacteriuria and UTI with low-dose, low-cost antimicrobial therapy, or antiseptics. Discontinuation of suppressive therapy eventually leads to recurrent symptoms and bacteriuria.

Surgical treatment of chronic bacterial prostatitis

Transurethral resection of the prostate is the only alternative, short of radical prostatectomy, for surgical management of bacterial prostatitis. About one-third of patients with well-documented bacterial prostatitis have been cured by Meares' technique of transurethral resection (Meares 1980). Transurethral prostatectomy is curative only if all the foci of infected tissue and calculi are removed. Since most inflammation of chronic prostatitis occurs in the peripheral zone of the gland, and all the ducts from the peripheral zone empty into the urethra distal to the verumontanum, transurethral resection beyond the verumontanum is required to remove the infected tissue (Blacklock 1974). Such an extensive resection carries a high risk of urinary incontinence. It is possible that some patients respond to extensive transurethral resection as a result of the incidental resolution of a bladder neck obstruction.

Non-bacterial prostatitis

Non-bacterial prostatitis, also called abacterial prostatitis or prostatitis, is the most common form of the prostatitis syndromes, being approximately eight times more common than bacterial prostatitis. Usually, the symptoms, physical findings, and the microscopic appearance of the prostatic expressates in non-bacterial prostatitis and chronic bacterial prostatitis are indistinguishable. However, the patient with non-bacterial prostatitis typically has no history of documented UTI and has negative localization cultures. Non-bacterial prostatitis is characterized by irritative or obstructive voiding symptoms or pain localized to the pelvic, perineal, scrotal, or low back area. Approximately one-third of the patients with non-bacterial prostatitis are asymptomatic. Since the aetiology is unknown, the treatment is empirical and often unrewarding.

Controversy regarding the role of Chlamydia, Ureaplasma, and Mycoplasma in the pathogenesis of prostatitis continues. Most investigators believe that mycoplasmas and ureaplasmas are not causative agents in non-bacterial prostatitis (Berger *et al.* 1989; Mardh and Collen 1975; Mardh *et al.* 1978; Meares 1973). Brunner *et al.* (1983) found a tenfold or greater increase in quantitative counts of *Ureaplasma urealyticum* in prostatic cultures compared with urethral culture in 82 (13.7 per cent) of 597 patients who appeared to have non-bacterial prostatitis. Most of these patients were said to respond favourably to tetracycline. However, until culture results are substantiated by demonstration of an antigen-specific immune response in the prostatic secretions, *U. urealyticum* remains an unconfirmed pathogen in prostatitis.

Chlamydia trachomatis remains the most controversial putative agent in prostatitis. Both Berger *et al.* (1989) and Mardh *et al.* (1978) studied 50 or more patients with nonbacterial prostatitis and found little or no evidence that *C. trachomatis* was an aetiological agent. In contrast, Poletti *et al.* (1985) performed transrectal aspiration biopsies of the prostate in 30 men with non-bacterial prostatitis and reported isolating *C. trachomatis* in tissue cultures from 10 (33 per cent). Schachter (1985), however, in an accompanying editorial expressed concerns over the authors' methods of identifying Chlamydia and over the observation that all 30 men had positive urethral cultures for Chlamydia, which raised questions about specimen contamination. He therefore concluded that *C. trachomatis* remains an unproven pathogen in prostatitis.

In 1988, Weidner *et al.* found *C. trachomatis* in 43 patients out of 233 with signs and symptoms of chronic prostatitis. Their analysis of the micro-immunofluorescence test against the sera of patients with positive chlamydial cultures and high leucocyte counts in post-prostatic massage urine showed titres of > 1:8 in 13 of 15 patients. This was taken as evidence for the role of Chlamydia in the pathogenesis of chronic prostatitis, although their data on urethral cultures in a relatively small number of patients were not presented.

Subsequently, Doble *et al.* (1989) reported a study of 50 men with non-bacterial prostatitis, only one of whom had Chlamydia detected in the urethra by an immunofluorescence technique. Each patient underwent transperineal prostatic aspiration biopsy under transrectal ultrasonic control. Chlamydia was detected in none of their patients despite use of McCoy tissue culture.

Abdelatiff *et al.* (1991) studied 23 transurethrally resected prostate specimens with 'histological' evidence of chronic abacterial prostatitis by using colorimetric *in situ* hybridization techniques for evidence of *Chlamydia trachomatis*. Intracellular Chlamydia bodies were detected in seven of 23 cases (30.4 per cent). However, this histopathological finding did not correlate with pre-operative clinical and bacteriological results. Indeed their definition of abacterial prostatitis was different from the accepted definition of Drach *et al.* (1978). Lastly, Shortliffe *et al.* (1985, 1986) detected insignificant antigen-specific antibody elevations against Chlamydia in the prostatic secretions of their patients with non-bacterial prostatitis. No unequivocal evidence exists to support the aetiological role of Chlamydia in non-bacterial prostatitis thus far. Chlamydia therefore must be assumed to play an insignificant role in the aetiology of prostatitis.

If Chlamydia or Ureaplasma are a likely cause of urethritis associated with non-bacterial prostatitis, a trial of tetracycline derivatives or erythromycin for seven days is reasonable. Continuation of antimicrobial therapy without clear effectiveness is futile and unwarranted. Management should include a frank discussion with the patient and reassurance about the nature of the entity. Some patients have responded to symptomatic therapy with hot sitz baths, anti-inflammatory drugs, such as ibuprofen, or alpha-blocking agents as discussed below.

Pelviperineal pain

Men who present with pelviperineal pain (prostatodynia) have symptoms of prostatitis but no documented UTI, no pathogenic organism on culture, and generally have normal findings on EPS. As many as 25 per cent, however, will have leucocytes in the urine or EPS.

The typical patient with pelviperineal pain is young to middle-aged and experiences variable signs and symptoms of abnormal urinary flow, irritative voiding dysfunction, and pain in the perineum or lower back. Penile and urethral pain are particularly common.

Physical examination is rarely revealing. Such men often have increased voluntary rectal tone and a tender prostate on rectal examination. Investigation of this group of men has led to considerable evidence that pelviperineal pain results from neuromuscular dysfunction of the bladder outlet and prostatic urethra. Cystoscopic examination often suggests mild bladder neck obstruction and unremarkable bladder findings. Urodynamic studies (cystometrogram or video-urodynamic imaging) performed on patients with pelviperineal pain show spasm and narrowing of the urethra at the bladder neck and just proximal to the external urinary sphincter, with resultant incomplete 'funnelling' (Barbalais *et al.* 1983; Barbalais 1990). Urethral pressure profiles typically show a high maximum urethral closure pressure in the distal prostatic and membranous urethral segments, despite electrical silence of the external sphincter on electromyography. This region of the prostate is known to be rich in alpha-adrenergic receptors. Despite silence on electromyography, this condition seems to fit into a variant category of detrusor internal sphincter dyssynergia. Treatment with alpha-receptor blockers, especially agents selective for the alpha-1 receptors, have relieved symptomotology associated with pelviperineal pain. Currently, prazosin, terazosin, and doxazosin are useful in attempts to palliate the unusual symptom complex associated with pelviperineal complaints.

The recommended prescribing schedule is to begin terazosin, 1 mg orally once daily at bedtime for 3–5 days, then 2 mg at bedtime. There may be an early response, but usually relief is obtained after 2–3 weeks. The dosage can be increased to 5 mg daily depending on tolerance. As such agents affect alpha-receptors in the vasculature, blood pressure must be monitored closely and the dosage must be titrated to individual tolerance to minimize side-effects.

Pelvic floor myalgia has been suggested as an aetiology of pelviperineal pain. However, our own experience indicates this is rarely the cause (Segura *et al.* 1979; Sinaki *et al.* 1977). Stress is thought to have an important, if not pre-eminent role in the aetiology of pelviperineal pain. Most men with pelviperineal pain do admit to stress and emotional tension. Whether such stress is a cause of pelviperineal pain, or a result of it is not certain. Motivated patients who are identified as having significant life stress should be referred to a consulting psychiatrist or psychologist. Lastly, it should be emphasized that despite the predilection for pelviperineal pain occurring in relatively young or middle-aged men, conditions causing irritative voiding, such as benign prostatic hyperplasia, carcinoma-*in-situ* of the bladder, or interstitial cystitis, should be addressed appropriately.

References

Abdelatif, O. M., Chandler, F. W., and McGuire, B. S. jun. (1991). Chlamydia trachomatis in chronic abacterial prostatitis: Demonstration by colorimetric in situ hybridization. *Human Pathology*, **22**, 41–4.

Anderson, R. U. and Weller, C. (1979). Prostatic secretion leukocyte studies in non-bacterial prostatitis (prostatosis). *Journal of Urology*, **121**, 292–4.

Baert, L. and Leonard, A. (1988). Chronic bacterial prostatitis: 10 years of experience with local antibiotics. *Journal of Urology*, **140**, 755–7.

Barbalias, G. A. (1990). Prostatodynia or painful male urethral syndrome? *Urology*, **36**, 146–53.

Barbalias, G. A., Meares, E. M. jun., and Sant, G. R. (1983). Prostatodynia: Clinical and urodynamic characteristics. *Journal of Urology*, **130**, 514–7.

Barnes, R. C., Diafuku, R., Roddy, R. E., and Stamm, W. E. (1986). Urinary tract infection in sexually active homosexual men. *Lancet*, **1**, 171–3.

Berger, R. E., *et al.* (1989). Case-control study of men with suspected chronic idiopathic prostatitis. *Journal of Urology*, **141**, 328–31.

Bergstrom, T., Larsen, K., Lincoln K., and Winberg, J. (1972). Studies of urinary tract infections in infants and childhood. *Journal of Pediatrics*, **80**, 858–66.

Blacklock, N. J. (1969). Some observations on prostatitis. In *Advances in the study of the prostate*, (ed. D. C. Williams, M. H. Briggs, and M. Stanford), pp. 37–55. Heinemann Medical, London.

Blacklock, N. J. (1974). Anatomic factors in prostatitis. *British Journal of Urology*, **46**, 47–54.

Bologna, M., *et al.* (1985). Norfloxacin in prostatitis: Correlation between HPLC tissue concentration and clinical results. *Drugs in Experimental Clinical Research*, **11**, 95–100.

Brunner, H., Weidner, W., and Schiefer, H. G. (1983). Studies of the role of *Ureaplasma urealyticum* and *Mycoplasma hominis* in prostatitis. *Journal of Infectious Diseases*, **147**, 807–13.

Bude, R., *et al.* (1990). Transrectal ultrasound appearance of granulomatous prostatitis. *Journal of Ultrasound Medicine*, **9**, 677–80.

Burbige, K. A., Retik, A. B., Colodny, A. H., Bauer, S. B., and Lebowitz, R. (1984). Urinary tract infection in boys. *Journal of Urology*, **132**, 541–2.

Childs, S. J. (1990). Ciprofloxacin in treatment of chronic bacterial prostatitis. *Urology* (Suppl. 35), 15–18.

Cox, C. E. (1989). Ofloxacin in the management of complicated urinary tract infections, including prostatitis. *American Journal of Medicine*, **87**(Suppl. 6C), 61–8.

Dan, M., *et al.* (1987). Penetration of norfloxacin into human prostatic tissue following single-dose oral administration. *Chemotherapy*, **33**, 240–2.

Doble, A. and Carter, S. S. (1989). Ultrasonographic findings in prostatitis. *Urologic Clinics of North America*, **16**, 763–72.

Doble A., *et al.* (1989). The role of Chlamydia trachomatis in chronic abacterial prostatitis: A study using ultrasound guided biopsy. *Journal of Urology*, **141**, 332–3.

Drach G. W., *et al.* (1978). (Letter to the Editor) Classification of benign diseases associated with prostatic pain: prostatitis or prostatodynia. *Journal of Urology*, **120**, 226.

Eykyn, S., *et al.* (1974). Prostatic calculi as a source of recurrent bacteriuria in the male. *British Journal of Urology*, **46**, 527–32.

Fair, W. R., Couch, J., and Wehner, N. (1976). Prostatic antibacterial factor: Identity and significance. *Urology*, **7**, 169–77.

Fowler, J. E. jun. and Mariano M. (1984). Difficulties in quantitating the contribution of urethral bacteria to prostatic fluid and seminal fluid cultures. *Journal of Urology*, **132**, 471–73.

Grapey, D. S. and Schaeffer, A. J. (1994). Urinary tract infection in females. In *Female urology: female genitourinary dysfunction and reconstruction*, (2nd edn), (ed. S. Raz). W. B. Saunders/Academic Press, Orlando, Florida.

Guibert, J., *et al.* (1986). Ciprofloxacin in the treatment of urinary tract infection due to Enterobacteriaceae. *European Journal of Clinical Microbiology and Infectious Disease*, **5**, 247–8.

Hooper, D. C. and Wolfson, J. S. (1985). The fluoroquinolones: Pharmacology; clinical uses, and toxicities in humans. *Antimicrobial Agents and Chemotherapy*, **28**, 716–21.

Hoogkamp-Korstanje, J. A. A., van Oort, H. J., and Schipper, J. J. (1984). Intraprostatic concentration of ciprofloxacin and its activity against urinary pathogens. *Journal of Antimicrobial Chemotherapy*, **14**, 641–5.

Jameson, R. M. (1967). Sexual activity and the variations of the white cell content of the prostatic secretion. *Investigative Urology*, **5**, 297–302.

Jimenez-Cruz, J. F. *et al.* (1984). Prostatitis: Are the gram-positive organisms pathogenic? *European Urology*, **10**, 311–14.

Jimenez-Cruz, J. F., Tormo, F. B., and Gomez, J. G. (1988). Treatment of chronic prostatitis: Intraprostatic antibiotics. *Journal of Urology*, **139**, 967–70.

Jodal, U. (1987). The natural history of bacteriuria in childhood. *Infectious Disease Clinics of North America*, **1**, 713–29.

Kirby, R. S., *et al.* (1982). Intraprostatic urinary reflux: An aetiological factor in abacterial prostatitis. *British Journal of Urology*, **54**, 729–31.

Kunin, C. M. (1987). *Detection, prevention, and management of urinary tract infections* (4th edn). Lea & Febiger, Philadelphia.

Langemeyer, T. N. M., *et al.* (1987). Treatment of chronic bacterial prostatitis with ciprofloxacin. *Pharmacology Weekly Bulletin (Sci)*, **9**(Suppl.), S78–81.

Leport, C., Rousseau, F., Perronne, C., Salmon, D., Joerg, A., and Vilde J. L. (1989). Bacterial prostatitis in patients infected with the human immunodeficiency virus. *Journal of Urology*, **141**, 334–6.

Lipsky, B. A. (1989). Urinary tract infection in men. *Annals of Internal Medicine*, **110**, 138–50.

Lipsky, B. A., Ireton, R. C., Fihn, S., Hackett, R., and Berger, R. E. (1987). Diagnosis of bacteriuria in men: Specimen collection and culture interpretation. *Journal of Infectious Diseases*, **155**, 847–54.

Mardh, P. A. and Collen, S. (1975). Search for uro-genital tract infections in patients with symptoms of prostatitis. Studies on aerobic and strictly anaerobic bacteria, mycoplasma, fungi, trichomonads and viruses. *Scandinavian Journal of Urology and Nephrology*, **9**, 8–16.

Mardh, P. A., *et al.* (1978). Role of *Chlamydia trachomatis* in non-acute prostatitis. *British Journal of Venereal Disease*, **54**, 330–4.

Meares, E. M. jun. (1973). Bacterial prostatitis versus "prostatosis": A clinical and bacteriological study. *Journal of the American Medical Association*, **24**, 1372–5.

Meares, E. M. jun. (1974). Infection stones of the prostate gland: laboratory diagnosis and clinical management. *Urology*, **4**, 560–6.

Meares, E. M. jun. (1980). Prostatitis syndromes: New perspectives about old woes. *Journal of Urology*, **123**, 141–7.

Meares, E. M. jun. (1982). Prostatitis: Review of pharmacokinetics and therapy. *Reviews in Infectious Disease*, **4**, 475–83.

Meares, E. M. jun. (1991). Prostatitis. *Medical Clinics of North America*, **75**, 405–44.

Meares, E. M. jun. and Stamey, T. A. (1968). Bacteriologic localization patterns in bacterial prostatitis and urethritis. *Investigative Urology*, **5**, 492–518.

Norrby, S. R. (1990). Short-term treatment of uncomplicated lower urinary tract infections in women. *Reviews in Infectious Disease*, **12**, 458–67.

Oliveris, R. A., Sachs, R. M., and Castre, P. G. (1979). Clinical experience with geocillin in the treatment of bacterial prostatitis. *Current Therapeutics Research*, **25**, 415–21.

Paulson, D. F. and de Vere White, R. (1978). Trimethoprim-sulphamethoxazole and minocycline-hydrochloride in the treatment of culture-proved bacterial prostatitis. *Journal of Urology*, **120**, 184–5.

Pfau, A. (1986). Prostatitis: A continuing enigma. *Urologic Clinics of North America*, **13**, 695–715.

Poletti, F., *et al.* (1985). Isolation of Chlamydia trachomatis from the prostatic cells in patients affected by nonacute abacterial prostatitis. *Journal of Urology*, **134**, 691–3.

Ramirez, C. T., *et al.* (1980). A crystallographic study of prostatic calculi. *Journal of Urology*, **124**, 840–3.

Remy, G., *et al.* (1988). Use of ofloxacin for prostatitis. *Reviews in Infectious Disease*, **10**(Suppl. 1), S173–4.

Ronald, A. R. (1987). Optimal duration of treatment for kidney infection. *Annals of Internal Medicine*, **106**, 467–73.

Sabbaj, J., Hoagland, V. L., and Shih, W. J. (1985). Multiclinic comparative study of norfloxacin and trimethoprim-sulfamethoxazole for treatment of urinary tract infections. *Antimicrobial Agents and Chemotherapy*, **27**, 297–301.

Sabbaj, J., Hoagland, V. L., and Cook, T. (1986). Norfloxacin versus cotrimoxazole in the treatment of recurring urinary tract infection in men. *Scandinavian Journal of Infectious Disease*, **48**(Suppl.), 48–53.

Schachter, J. (1985) (Editorial) Is *Chlamydia trachomatis* a cause of prostatitis? *Journal of Urology*, **134**, 711.

Schaeffer, A. J. (1987). Multiclinic study of norfloxacin for treatment of urinary tract infections. *American Journal of Medicine*, **82**(Suppl. B), 53–8.

Schaeffer, A. J. and Darras, F. S. (1990). The efficacy of norfloxacin in the treatment of chronic bacterial prostatitis refractory to trimethoprim-sulfamethoxazole and/or carbenicillin. *Journal of Urology*, **144**, 690–3.

Schaeffer, A. J., Wendel, E. F., Dunn, J. K., and Grayhack, J. T. (1981). Prevalence and significance of prostatic inflammation. *Journal of Urology*, **125**, 215–19.

Scully, B. E. (1990). Pharmacology of the fluoroquinolones. *Urology*, **35**(Suppl.), 8–11.

Sergura, J. W., Opitz, J. L., and Greene, L. F. (1979). Prostatosis, prostatitis or pelvic floor tension myalgia? *Journal of Urology*, **122**, 168–72.

Shafik, A. (1991). Anal submucosal injection: A new route for drug administration. *Urology*, **37**, 61–4.

Shortliffe, L. M. D. and Wehner, N. (1986). The characterization of bacterial and non-bacterial prostatitis by prostatic immunoglobulins. *Medicine*, **65**, 399–414.

Shortliffe, L. M. D., Wehner, N., and Stamey, T. A. (1981). The detection of a local prostatic immunologic response to bacterial prostatitis. *Journal of Urology*, **125**, 509–15.

Shortliffe, L. M. D., *et al.* (1985). Measurement of chlamydial and ureaplasma antibodies in serum and prostatic fluid of men with nonbacterial prostatitis (abstract). *Journal of Urology*, **133**(4), part 2, 276A.

Silver, T. M., *et al.* (1976). The radiological spectrum of acute pyelonephritis in adults and adolescents. *Radiology*, **118**, 65–9.

Sinaki, M., Merritt, J. L., and Stillwell, G. K. (1977). Tension myalgia of the pelvic floor. *Mayo Clinic Proceedings*, **52**, 717–21.

Sutor, D. J. and Wooley, S. E. (1974). The crystalline composition of prostatic calculi. *British Journal of Urology*, **46**, 533–5.

Stamey, T. A. (1973). The role of introital enterobacteria in recurrent urinary tract infections. *Journal of Urology*, **109**, 467–72.

Stamey, T. A. (ed.) (1980). *Pathogenesis and treatment of urinary tract infections*, p. 344. Williams and Wilkins, Baltimore, MD.

Teillac, P. (1991). Management of urinary tract infection in elderly men. *European Urology*, **1**, 19–23.

Tolkoff-Rubin, N. E. and Rubin, R. H. (1987). New approaches to the treatment of urinary tract infection. *American Journal of Medicine*, **82**(Suppl.), 270–7.

Weidner, W., Schiefer, H. G., and Dalhoff, A. (1987). Treatment of chronic bacterial prostatitis with ciprofloxacin results of a one year follow-up study. *American Journal of Medicine*, **82**(Suppl.), 280–3.

Weidner, W., Schiefer, H. G., and Krauss, H. (1988). Role of *Chlamydia trachomatis* and Mycoplasmas in chronic prostatitis. A review. *Urology International*, **43**, 167–73.

Weidner, W., Schiefer, H. G., and Brahler, E. (1991). Refractory chronic bacterial prostatitis. A re-evaluation of ciprofloxacin treatment after a median follow-up of 30 months. *Journal of Urology*, **146**, 350–2.

Winberg, J. (1989). The prepuce: A mistake of nature? *Lancet*, **3**, 598–9.

Winningham, D. G., Nemoy, N. J., and Stamey, T. A. (1968). Diffusion of antibiotics from plasma into prostatic fluid. *Nature*, **219**, 139–43.

Wiswell, T. E. and Smith, F. R. (1985). Decreased incidence of urinary tract infections in circumcised male infants. *Pediatrics*, **75**, 901–3.

Wolfson, J. S. and Hooper, D. C. (1985). The fluoroquinolones: Structures, mechanism of action and resistance, and spectra of activity in vitro. *Antimicrobial Agents and Chemotherapeutics*, **28**, 581–6.

Wolfson, S. A., Kalmanson, G. M., Rubin, M. E. and Guzed, L. B. (1965). Epidemiology of bacteriuria in a predominantly geriatric male population. *American Journal of Medical Science*, **250**, 163–73.

14

Tuberculosis, leprosy, and other mycobacterial diseases

John B. Eastwood, Susan. A. Dilly, and John M. Grange

Classification and characteristics of mycobacteria

In 1898, the generic name *Mycobacterium* was given to a group of bacteria which included the tubercle and leprosy bacilli and a few environmental isolates. These shared a peculiar staining property—the ability to retain the colour imparted by arylmethane dyes after treatment with dilute mineral acids. For this reason, members of this genus are often termed 'acid-fast bacilli'.

One of the most notable characteristics of the mycobacteria is their possession of thick, lipid-rich cell walls which are the most complex yet found in nature. Being rich in lipids, mycobacteria are hydrophobic and often grow as a mould-like pellicle on liquid media: this is the origin of the name *Mycobacterium* (fungus-bacterium).

The genus *Mycobacterium* contains over 50 species; 41 were included in the *Approved lists of bacterial names* (Skerman *et al.* 1980) and some have been described subsequently (Grange 1990). The species are divisible into two main groups, the rapid- and slow-growers. There are also a few species, notably the leprosy bacillus (*M. leprae*), that have never been convincingly cultivated *in vitro*.

From a clinical standpoint, the most important species are those causing serious and widespread human disease. These include *M. leprae* and a group of closely related species termed the tuberculosis complex or the mammalian tubercle bacilli—*M. tuberculosis* (the human tubercle bacillus), *M. bovis* (the bovine tubercle bacillus, but also an important cause of human disease), and *M. africanum* (a group of strains with rather variable properties mostly isolated from human beings in Equatorial Africa).

The tuberculosis complex also contains *M. microti*, a very rare cause of tuberculosis in voles and other small mammals but not in man, and bacille Calmette–Guérin (BCG), a living vaccine strain which was derived from a tubercle bacillus of bovine origin and attenuated by multiple subculture. Most other species in this genus are free-living environmental saprophytes and are particularly associated with water. Thus, they are found in wet soil, marshland (particularly sphagnum marshes), lakes, streams, rivers, and estuaries (Collins *et al.* 1984). Some species, notably *M. kansasii*, *M. xenopi*, and *M. gordonae* colonize piped water supplies. Mycobacteria may also occur as saprophytes in animal and human intestines and may be isolated from faeces and soil contaminated by animal faeces.

Some of the environmental mycobacteria cause opportunist disease in human beings and animals (Table 14.1). Most are slow-growing, although two fast-growing species, *M. chelonae* and *M. fortuitum*, may be pathogenic. These rapid growers were originally isolated from the turtle and frog respectively and, in the older literature, were referred to as the 'cold-blooded tubercle bacilli'.

Among the slow-growing opportunist pathogens, the most widespread and frequently encountered are *M. avium*, the avian tubercle bacillus, and *M. intracellulare*. These species are very closely related and are often grouped together as *M. avium-intracellulare* (MAI) or the *M. avium* complex (MAC). In recent years, this complex has emerged as a common cause of opportunist infection in patients with AIDS (Pitchenik and Fertel 1992).

Mycobacterium avium-intracellulare and *M. kansasii* are found world-wide. Other species are more geographically restricted. Thus *M. xenopi* is frequently isolated from clinical and environmental specimens in London, southern coastal region of England, and northern France but it is relatively uncommon elsewhere.

Although rarely causing disease, environmental mycobacteria readily gain access to the human body by drinking, washing, and bathing, and by inhalation of aerosols. Therefore, they are frequently isolated from the pharynx, intestinal tract, and the external genitalia. For this reason, great care is required in the in-

Table 14.1 Mycobacteria associated with human disease

Obligate pathogens		
M. tuberculosis	Human tubercle bacillus	
M. bovis	Bovine tubercle bacillus	
M. africanum		
M. leprae	Leprosy bacillus	
Causes of named mycobacterial disease		
M. marinum	Swimming pool (or fish tank) granuloma	
M. ulcerans	Buruli ulcer (an uncommon tropical disease)	
Slow-growing mycobacteria causing non-specific tuberculosis-like disease		
M. avium[a]	*M. scrofulaceum*	*M. malmoense*
M. xenopi	*M. simiae*	*M. szulgai*
M. asiaticum	*M. haemophilum*	
M. gordonae	*M. kansasii*	
M. intracellulare[a]		
Fast-growing pathogens		
M. chelonae[b]		
M. fortuitum		

Note: The mycobacteria in this table other than 'obligate pathogens' are often referred to as 'environmental saprophytes'.

[a]Often grouped together as *M. avium-intracellulare* (MAI).

[b]*M. abscessus* in the older literature

terpretation of positive microscopic examinations for acid-fast bacilli and of cultures from urine of mycobacteria other than members of the tuberculosis complex. Care is required in the collection of urine samples as there have been a number of clusters of positive cultures of environmental mycobacteria due to collection of urine into non-sterile containers (Collins *et al.* 1984).

From 1980 to 1989, a total of 572 environmental mycobacteria cultured from urine in south-eastern England were submitted to the regional tuberculosis laboratory but, with five possible exceptions, all were casual isolates of species known to be present in the environment (Grange and Yates 1992). The older literature states that *M. smegmatis* is a common contaminant of the external genitalia. In fact, this is a rarely encountered species, accounting for less than 1 per cent of isolates from urine in south-eastern England. It is possible that this name was applied to many rapidly growing species that are now identified by their own names.

Tuberculosis

Epidemiology

About one-third of the world's population has been infected by *M. tuberculosis* and about 8 million new cases of post-primary tuberculosis develop from this infected pool annually (Kochi 1991). The incidence of tuberculosis is increasing world-wide, partly due to the HIV pandemic. By 1992 there were an estimated 4 million persons dually infected by *M. tuberculosis* and HIV and about 400 000 new cases of HIV-related tuberculosis, 5 per cent of the global total of tuberculosis annually (Narain *et al.* 1992).

Human tuberculosis is usually the result of the inhalation of small numbers of tubercle bacilli in moist droplets expectorated by patients with infectious or 'open' pulmonary tuberculosis. More rarely, it is caused by drinking milk contaminated by *M. bovis.*

Analysis of 13 634 cases of non-pulmonary tuberculosis in five studies revealed that genitourinary disease was the second most common form, exceeded only be lymphadenopathy, and that it accounted for 27 per cent of the cases (Kennedy 1989). The proportion of cases of tuberculosis involving the genitourinary system in a population depends on the ethnic origin and age of the patients. Reports from several developed countries show that ethnic minority populations, notably those of Indian subcontinent (ISC) origin, often have a relatively higher incidence of extra-pulmonary lesions than the indigenous population. The incidence of genitourinary tuberculosis in the ISC group is, however, less than expected for reasons that are unclear (Ormerod 1993). Studies in south-eastern England (Table 14.2) show that the percentage of patients with extra-pulmonary manifestations of tuberculosis is higher in those of ISC ethnic origin (46 per cent) than in those of European ethnic origin (19 per cent), but genitourinary disease is relatively less common in the ISC group (8 per cent) than in the European

Table 14.2 Distribution of extra-pulmonary manifestations of tuberculosis according to site (1984–91)

Site	European			ISC		
	Males	Females	Total	Males	Females	Total
Extra-pulmonary (EP)[*]						
Genitourinary	136 (35)	61 (16)	197 (25)	72 (9)	54 (7)	126 (8)
Lymph node	104 (27)	171 (44)	275 (36)	406 (53)	588 (60)	894 (56)
Bone/joint	68 (18)	76 (20)	144 (19)	155 (20)	141 (17)	296 (19)
Abdomen	21 (6)	34 (9)	55 (7)	55 (7)	64 (8)	119 (7)
Neurological	13 (3)	19 (5)	32 (4)	28 (4)	27 (3)	55 (3)
Disseminated	24 (6)	1 (<1)	25 (3)	7 (1)	3 (<1)	10 (1)
Other/unknown	19 (5)	25 (6)	44 (6)	50 (6)	43 (5)	93 (5)
Total	385	387	772	773	820	1593
Pulmonary only	2299	1014	3313	1062	796	1858
Grand total	2684	1401	4085	1835	1616	3451
Patients with EP lesions	14%	28%	19%	42%	51%	46%

The patients are of European and Indian subcontinent (ISC) origin in south-eastern England. Numbers of individuals in other ethnic groups were too small for meaningful comparisons to be made (percentages in brackets).

[*]Some patients also had pulmonary lesions.

group (25 per cent). Table 14.2 also shows that genitourinary disease, unlike most other forms of non-pulmonary tuberculosis, is relatively more frequent in males than in females in both ethnic groups.

In countries where tuberculosis is common among younger members of the population, genitourinary tuberculosis tends to involve an older age group than other forms of the disease. This age difference is less obvious where, as a result of disease control, tuberculosis is predominantly of the post-primary type in older persons. In the United States and Canada, the peak age of patients with genitourinary tuberculosis has been found to be higher than that of those with lymphadenitis but lower than that of those with bone and joint disease (Kennedy 1989). Similar trends are evident in the ethnic European population of south-eastern England where lymphatic, genitourinary, and bone and joint tuberculosis are most prevalent in the 20–30, 50–60, and 70–80 age groups, respectively.

As a result of control measures, tuberculosis due to *M. bovis* is uncommon in industrially developed nations and most cases are due to re-activation of dormant infection acquired many years previously. Renal disease is a rare manifestation of primary tuberculosis due to *M. bovis* but is a relatively common form of post-primary disease. Since the commencement of a survey in 1977, almost all cases of tuberculosis due to *M. bovis* in south-eastern England have been post-primary and about 25 per cent have involved the genitourinary system (Yates and Grange 1988). A bizarre epidemiological feature of this form of tuberculosis is transmission of the disease back to cattle by infected farm workers urinating in cowsheds. Several such cases have been reported in Europe and one farm worker infected 48 cows in four different herds (Schliesser 1974).

Pathogenesis

In developed countries, infection by tubercle bacilli almost always occurs via the respiratory tract. Since the eradication of bovine tuberculosis, infection via the oropharynx and intestine is rare. Little is known of the early events in man following inhalation of tubercle bacilli but studies in the rabbit show that bacilli are taken up by alveolar macrophages. The bacilli once established replicate, kill the macrophage, and are taken up by other macrophages and by polymorphonuclear neutrophils, resulting in a localized and non-specific inflammatory lesion. Bacilli are transported to the local lymph nodes where secondary lesions develop. From these lymph nodes there can be generalized haematogenous spread.

Specific cell-mediated immunity, not to be confused with delayed type hypersensitivity manifested as a positive tuberculin test, develops within a week or two of infection. This immunity is due to presentation of mycobacterial antigen to T-helper cells, resulting in their activation, proliferation, and secretion of macrophage-activating cytokines, notably interferon-gamma (IFNγ). The IFNγ activates a hydroxylase in the macrophage, enabling it to convert vitamin D into the active metabolite calcitriol. This, in turn, primes the macrophage for release of tumour necrosis factor (TNF) which appears to play an important role in the formation of the granuloma (Kindler *et al.* 1989).

In most infected people, provided the immune response is normal, primary tuberculosis does not become clinically apparent. The exact mechanism of protective cell-mediated immunity in tuberculosis in man is poorly understood. Bacillary killing by macrophages is probably involved, although attempts to demonstrate such killing *in vitro* have usually proved unsuccessful. Cytotoxic T cells and natural killer cells play a key role in protective immunity in tuberculosis by lysing effete macrophages harbouring tubercle bacilli, probably in the cytoplasm rather than in phagosomes, thereby enabling the bacilli to be engulfed and destroyed by immunologically competent phagocytes. It appears likely that an entire granuloma is required for protection as this is able to create an anoxic and acidic micro-environment that inhibits bacterial growth (Lowrie 1990). On the other hand, such conditions appear to favour the development of bacterial persistence, whereby *M. tuberculosis* may lie dormant, or almost dormant, in tissues for years or decades.

Overt primary tuberculosis occurs in about 5 per cent of infected people. This may be manifested by progression of the primary complex or by development of disease in a distant organ (e.g. meninges, bone, and kidney), as a result of the initial haematogenous spread. Primary renal tuberculosis tends to present later than other primary extra-pulmonary forms (Wallgren 1948). Dissemination also occurs when a tuberculous lesion erodes the wall of a major blood vessel and large numbers of bacilli are released into the bloodstream. This leads to miliary tuberculosis so named on account of the numerous millet seed-like granulomas throughout the body. The kidney is often involved in miliary tuberculosis but local manifestations are overshadowed by the severe systemic effects. Most infected individuals who do not manifest overt primary disease remain healthy but about 5 per cent subsequently develop post-primary disease which is characterized by extensive tissue necrosis. In HIV-positive persons overt tuberculosis develops much more commonly, estimated at about 10 per cent annually.

In addition to the development of protective immunity, infected individuals develop a characteristic tissue-necrotizing reaction, originally described by Koch in the guinea-pig, and termed the 'Koch phenomenon'. Like protective immunity, the mechanism of this reaction is poorly understood. As mentioned above, there is evidence that tumour necrosis factor (TNF), probably cell membrane-bound, is required for the maturation of macrophages to epithelioid cells and for their aggregation in the granuloma. In Koch-type reactivity there is an uncontrolled release of TNF, triggered by cell wall components of the tubercle bacillus, together with sensitization of surrounding cells to the toxic effect of this cytokine, resulting in excessive tissue necrosis (Rook and Al Attiyah 1991). TNF causes damage to the endothelium of blood vessels and the resulting haemostasis and infarction may lead to further tissue necrosis. Tuberculin reactivity develops 3–10 weeks after infection. It is a complex phenomenon, bearing no direct relation to either protective or tissue necrotizing immune responses.

There has been considerable debate as to whether protective immunity and necrotizing hypersensitivity are quantitatively different manifestations of the same immune process or of different, and perhaps mutually exclusive, processes (Bothamley and Grange 1991). The latter concept has received strong support from the description of two different T-helper cell activities, TH1 and TH2, the cytokine patterns of which could well be responsible for the two different types of immune reactivity in tuberculosis (Mosmann 1991).

As a result of the phenomenon of persistence, endogenous re-activation leading to post-primary tuberculosis may occur years or even decades after the initial infection, although similar disease may be due to exogenous re-infection. Post-primary tuberculosis is usually characterized by excessive tissue destruction as a result of the necrotizing Koch-type reactivity. In the lung, this necrosis generates cavities communicating with the bronchi, thereby enabling bacilli to be transmitted to other individuals. It has, however, the beneficial effect of limiting dissemination by the haematogenous and lymphatic routes and the disease is thus usually localized. Cavities also occur in the kidney as a result of lesions eroding into the renal pelvis and discharging their softened, necrotic contents. Both cavity formation and localization of disease are compromised in immunosuppressed persons.

Re-activation tuberculosis may occur in the genitourinary tract. This has, for example, been evident in the case of post-primary tuberculosis due to *M. bovis*; as mentioned above, about 25 per cent of such cases in south-eastern England involve this site.

In the kidney, granulomas resulting from the implantation of small numbers of tubercle bacilli during early haematogenous spread usually appear first in association with glomeruli, probably because of the high blood flow and favourable oxygen tension. Typically, at this stage, the cortical granulomas are bilateral but they remain dormant until factors, often unknown, permit the bacilli to proliferate. The enlarging granulomas may rupture into the proximal tubule enabling bacilli to reach the loop of Henle where it is thought they survive well because of impaired phagocytosis in the hypertonic environment. Their continued proliferation and the host's immune response leads to granuloma formation in the medulla. The disease process may be sufficiently destructive to cause papillary necrosis and there may be rupture through the calyceal wall. By this means, bacilli can reach the renal pelvis, ureter, bladder, prostate, and epididymis. Apart from this direct spread there can be dissemination of bacilli via the local lymphatics to reach these parts of the genitourinary tract. Furthermore, there may be direct haematogenous spread from the lung or other site of primary infection which explains why there can sometimes be genital involvement without the urinary tract being affected.

Clinical manifestations

'Classical' urogenital tuberculosis

Tuberculosis of the urinary tract is easily overlooked. Lattimer (1965) described 25 physicians with renal tuberculosis, 18 of whom presented only after advanced cavitating disease had developed. It is not uncommon for the diagnosis to be made either at operation or on post-mortem examination.

In practice, most patients present with lower urinary tract symptoms typical of 'conventional' bacterial cystitis. It is only when the patient fails to respond to the usual antibacterial agents or when urine examination reveals pyuria in the absence of a positive culture on routine media that further investigation is instigated. Other symptoms of urinary tract tuberculosis that might suggest conventional bacterial urinary infection include dysuria, back, flank or suprapubic pain, haematuria, frequency, and nocturia. Renal colic is unusual but can occur in up to 10 per cent of patients (Pasternack and Rubin 1993). Constitutional symptoms, such as fever, weight loss, and night sweats, are unusual and indicate the need to search for other foci of tuberculosis. Interestingly, Simon *et al.* (1977), reported that only a third of patients with urinary tract tuberculosis had an abnormal chest X-ray.

When renal tuberculosis is advanced and bilateral there may be reduction of glomerular filtration rate (GFR) due to generalized destruction of the parenchyma and in some patients this progresses to end-stage renal failure. A more common cause for loss of GFR is ureteric and bladder involvement due to seeding of *M. tuberculosis* into the urine. Such seeding can lead to ureteric scarring with distortion and urinary tract obstruction. Similarly, there can be considerable fibrosis and contraction of the bladder.

In the male, genital tuberculosis usually results from seeding from infected urine and the most common manifestation is epididymo-orchitis. Tuberculous prostatitis also occurs. It is important that the urinary tract of patients with genital tuberculosis is investigated since 75 per cent of patients with epididymo-orchitis already have evidence of urinary tract involvement. tuberculosis of the urethra and penis is uncommon but can present with papulo-necrotic skin lesions, fistulae, and genital ulceration. Although infection usually results from direct seeding of infected urine, penile tuberculosis can be acquired by direct inoculation from contaminated surgical instruments or clothing, and from ritual circumcision (Annobil *et al.* 1990). In the female, tuberculosis of the genital tract is accompanied by urinary tract tuberculosis in less than 5 per cent of cases (i.e. far less commonly than in the male). Pasternack and Rubin (1993) suggest that this difference is due to the fact that tuberculosis of the female genital tract is almost always the result of haematogenous spread alone.

Tuberculous interstitial nephritis (Figs 14.1 and 14.2)

It is now clear that a more insidious form of renal tuberculosis occurs. Mallinson *et al.* (1981) described three patients (two from the Indian subcontinent and one from West Africa) with advanced renal failure in whom imaging had revealed equal-sized smooth kidneys without evidence of calcification or gross anatomical distortion. In none were tubercle bacilli found in the urine. Renal histology revealed interstitial infiltrates with chronic inflammatory cells and granulomas in all three patients and there was caseation in two. In two, acid-fast bacilli were identified with appropriate stains. In two patients there was evidence of tuberculosis on chest X-ray and one patient had tuberculous peritonitis. The important point in this report is that there can be tuberculous

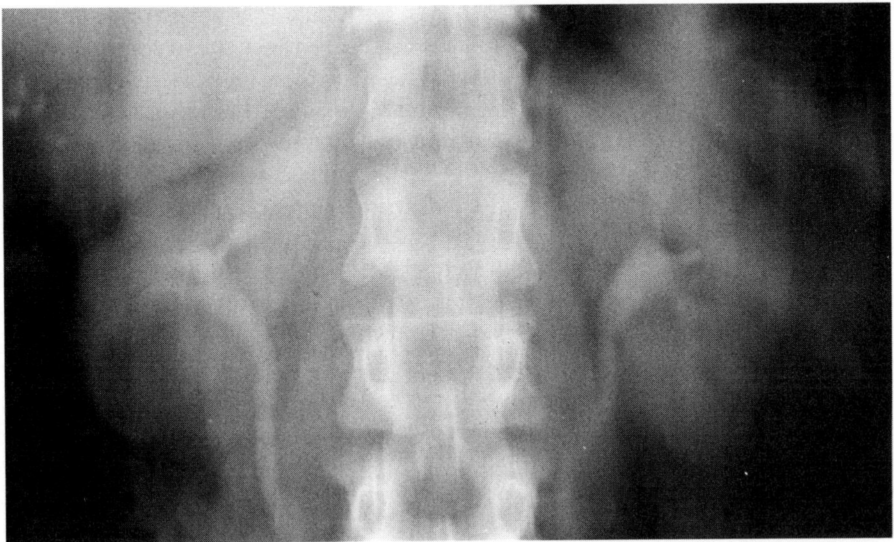

Fig. 14.1 Tuberculous interstitial nephritis. An IVU film (9 cm tomographic cut). Kidneys are of reduced volume but without specific diagnostic features. (Patient is a Ugandan-Asian woman described by Benn *et al.* (1988); GFR, 17 ml/min; plasma creatinine, 238 μmol/l.)

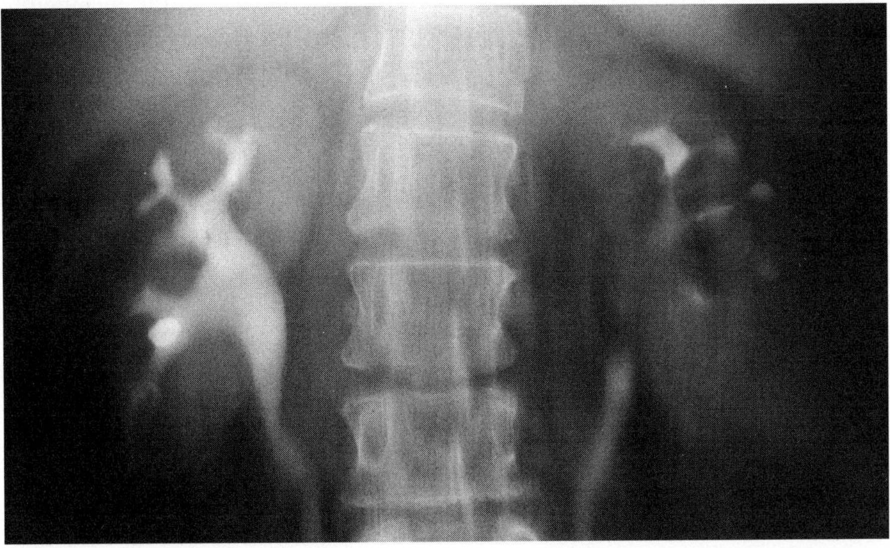

Fig. 14.2 Tuberculous interstitial nephritis. An IVU film (8 cm tomographic cut). There is evidence of widespread loss of papillae. (Burmese woman aged 70; GFR, 11 ml/min; plasma creatinine, 274 μmol/l.)

involvement of the kidneys, sufficient to cause renal failure, in the absence of either the typical renal destruction with calcification and fibrosis or urinary tract obstruction. In a review of 3500 renal biopsies carried out over 14 years, Mignon *et al.* (1984) reported that they had found interstitial granulomas in 24. Three of these patients had tuberculosis and in one acid-fast bacilli were found in the kidney.

Benn and colleagues (1988) reported a Ugandan-Asian woman (urea, 13.3 mmol/1; creatinine, 260 μmol/1; creatinine clearance, 17 ml/min) with equal-sized smooth kidneys on intravenous urography (IVU) (Fig. 14.1), in whom renal biopsy showed interstitial fibrosis with epithelioid and giant cell granulomas (see Fig. 14.4), one of which showed caseation. Acid-fast bacilli were not seen in the biopsy and *M. tuberculosis* was not grown from biopsy material or urine. She had a strongly positive Mantoux test and treatment with anti-tuberculosis drugs for 12 months was associated with improvement in GFR (creatinine, 223 μmol/1; creatinine clearance, 39 ml/min) over the next three years. In this patient, tuberculosis had not been considered before the biopsy because, unlike the cases of Mallinson *et al.* (1981), there was no other evidence of tuberculosis and five of the six midstream samples of urine (MSSUs) were free of leucocytes.

Tuberculosis and glomerular disease

Chronic tuberculosis commonly gives rise to amyloidosis and in India is a common cause of renal amyloid (Chugh *et al.* 1981). Glomerulonephritis as a complication of tuberculosis is uncommon. In 1979, Hariprasad *et al.* reported a patient with dense deposit disease and tuberculosis. In 1983, Shribman *et al.* reported a patient with miliary tuberculosis who had focal proliferative glomerulonephritis. There was granular staining for IgA, IgM, and C3 in the mesangium and around capillary loops but granulomas were not seen. Interestingly, similar renal histology has been documented in lepromatous leprosy (Iveson *et al.* 1975).

End-stage renal disease

Tuberculosis is an important cause of progressive renal failure as, unlike most other causes, it is theoretically preventable and easily treatable (Benn *et al.* 1988). In 1991, the European Dialysis and Transplant Association (EDTA) registry reported that 195 (0.65 per cent) of 30 064 new patients assigned a renal diagnosis among the 35 countries reporting to EDTA had renal failure on the basis of renal tuberculosis, an incidence similar to that of earlier years (Table 14.3). The country with the largest incidence was Greece at 4.51 per cent (Mallick 1993). Other important contributors were Portugal, Belgium, Spain, Italy, and Yugoslavia (Fig. 14.3). In a recent report from Portugal, Neves *et al.* (1993) show that there can be local areas of high incidence. Over a 10-year period in the Algarve tuberculosis was the cause of renal failure in as many as 12 of 345 patients starting haemodialysis In some instances, the patients presented terminally without having had any symptoms of tuberculosis.

It is possible that the number of patients with urinary tract tuberculosis as a cause of end-stage renal disease is being generally underestimated as, although it

Table 14.3 Tuberculosis as a cause of end-stage renal disease in 35 countries (EDTA)

Year	Males			Females			All		
	n	(%)	Total	n	(%)	Total	n	(%)	Total
1984	114	(0.93)	12 283	86	(0.97)	8 853	200	(0.95)	21 136
1985	96	(0.72)	13 339	82	(0.86)	9 557	178	(0.78)	22 896
1989	96	(0.62)	15 476	77	(0.70)	10 925	174	(0.66)	26 401
1990	62	(0.46)	13 512	54	(0.59)	9 458	116	(0.51)	22 970
1991	114	(0.64)	17 696	81	(0.65)	12 368	195	(0.65)	30 064

EDTA: European Dialysis and Transplant Association Registry, Tuberculosis = code 91.
n = number of new patients with renal tuberculosis; T = total number of new patients assigned a renal diagnosis.

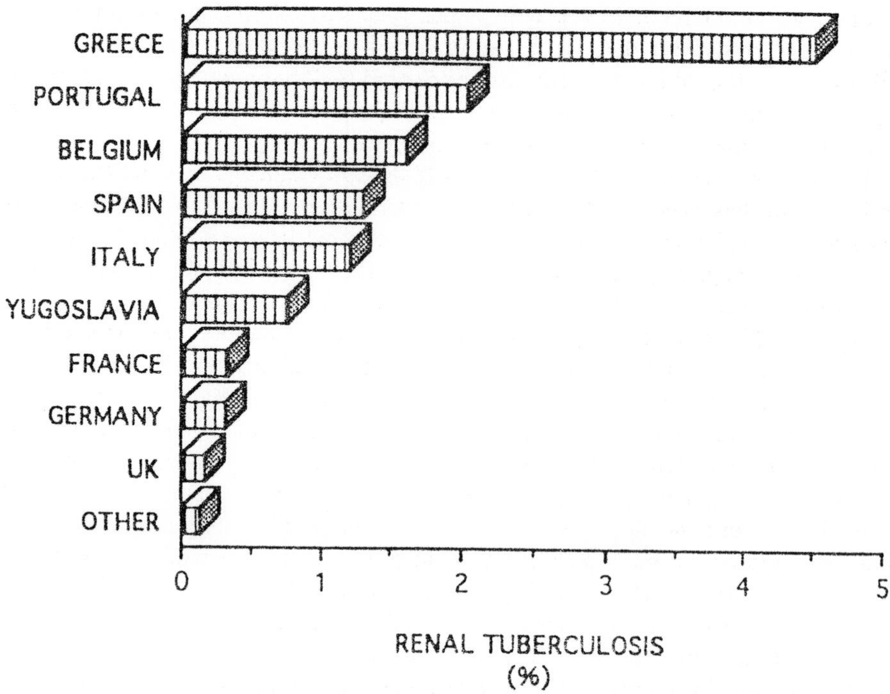

Fig. 14.3 Reported frequency of tuberculosis as a cause of end-stage renal disease in 35 countries in 1991. Percentages are numbers of new cases as a proportion of total new patients assigned a primary renal diagnosis. (EDTA Registry data for 1991, Mallick 1993.)

is possible that most individuals with classical urinary tract tuberculosis will be identified, the interstitial form can easily be overlooked. Hence it is important that the diagnosis is considered in all patients with equal-sized smooth kidneys without a clear-cut renal diagnosis, especially in high-risk groups (Mallinson *et al.* 1981; Morgan *et al.* 1990).

Dialysis and transplant patients

Tuberculosis is a problem in dialysis and transplant patients. In haemodialysis patients it often presents in an insidious manner with anorexia, low-grade fever, and weight loss. In some reports the majority of cases have been extra-pulmonary or, occasionally, miliary (Sasaki *et al.* 1979; Hussein *et al.* 1990). Tuberculosis appears to be much more common among haemodialysis patients than in the general population (Smith 1982) and the type of presentation suggests that dialysis is associated with re-activation of quiescent disease. In this context it is important to realize that among predominantly Caucasian populations there may be a significant excess of individuals from ethnic minorities who have renal failure (Pazianas *et al.* 1991; Roderick *et al.* 1994), and that some of these also have a higher incidence of tuberculosis (Kwan *et al.* 1991).

There are fewer reports in patients undergoing CAPD (continuous ambulatory peritoneal dialysis) but there is no reason to suspect that re-activation of tuberculosis is any less likely to occur in these patients. There are now a number of reports of tuberculous peritonitis in CAPD patients (Cheng *et al.* 1989; Tan *et al.* 1991; Ahijado *et al.* 1991; Ong *et al.* 1992).

Tuberculosis has always been a worrying clinical challenge in renal transplant patients but has received less attention than opportunist infections such as *Pneumocystis carinii* and cytomegalovirus. When renal transplantation had been a part of nephrological practice for 30 years, Lichtenstein and MacGregor (1983) on reviewing the literature, found only 42 cases of tuberculosis in patients with transplants. More recently, Qunibi *et al.* (1990) have described 14 cases among their 403 renal transplant patients. They found the annual incidence of tuberculosis in these patients in Saudi Arabia to be about 50 times greater than in their general population. A particular finding among their patients and in published reports comprising 130 patients in all was a high proportion of miliary infections (64.3 per cent in their series of 14, and 38.5 per cent of the total of 130). They found no difference in the risk of developing tuberculosis between those who did or did not have a positive tuberculin test. In one of the patients of Qunibi *et al.* (1990), *M. tuberculosis* was acquired with the transplant kidney as had been described in an earlier report (Peters *et al.* 1984). In a series of 633 renal transplant patients, Higgins et al. (1991) found that there were no cases of tuberculosis among patients receiving chemoprophylaxis but six cases among 27 high-risk patients who did not receive chemoprophylaxis.

It is widely believed that treatment with corticosteroids predisposes to the re-activation of tuberculosis, but the evidence for this is weak. Nevertheless, the American Thoracic Society recommends that patients with healed pulmonary tuberculosis who are given long-term corticosteroids should be given isoniazid chemoprophylaxis for one year (American Thoracic Society 1974). This subject has been further explored by Bateman (1993). Qunibi *et al.* (1990) suggest that isoniazid 300 mg daily with pyridoxine 25–50 mg daily should be given for one year to all patients on steroids with one of the following: a history of inadequately treated tuberculosis; an abnormal chest X-ray; a positive tuberculin test > 10 mm in diameter; and contact with a case of active tuberculosis. Preventive therapy should also be given to tuberculin-negative patients who receive a kidney from a tuberculin-positive donor.

Laboratory diagnosis

The best containers for urine samples are sterile 28 ml glass or plastic screw-capped bottles (Universal Containers). Early morning midstream specimens should be collected on three successive days. If the patient experiences difficulty in voiding urine directly into such containers, any alternative collecting vessel must be sterile. Specimens should be delivered to the laboratory with a minimum of delay otherwise contaminating bacteria will replicate. If delays are unavoidable, specimens should be refrigerated but not frozen.

As discussed above, laboratory tests on urine for the diagnosis of mycobacterial disease may be compromised by contamination by environmental mycobacteria. In particular, detection of acid-fast bacilli by direct microscopic examination of centrifuged urine deposits should be viewed with great suspicion. Urine contains contaminating non-acid-fast organisms which, unless destroyed or inhibited, will overgrow the culture medium. Urine must therefore be 'decontaminated' before inoculation on to appropriate media. This is usually achieved by treating centrifuged urine deposits with an acid (e.g. 4 per cent sulphuric acid), standing for 15–40 minutes, adding 15 ml of sterile water, re-centrifuging, and inoculating media with the deposit. An alternative to decontamination is the use of a medium containing a 'cocktail' of antibiotics that kill virtually all fungi and bacteria other than mycobacteria. Tissue biopsies are homogenized in a Griffith tube or similar grinding device and inoculated on to suitable media. The need for decontamination is determined by the site of origin of the tissue. Better culture results are obtained from biopsy of tissue surrounding necrotic lesions than from the necrotic material itself as free fatty acids in the latter may kill any mycobacteria that are present.

The definitive histological diagnosis of mycobacterial infection at any site is made by detecting acid-fast bacteria. This requires staining by the Ziehl–Neelsen technique which involves de-colorizing with acid or a mixture of acid and alcohol. The mycobacteria will appear as red rods with this method but the degree of acid and alcohol fastness varies with species and environmental conditions. Between 10^4 and 10^5 bacteria per millilitre of tissue need to be present to allow reliable visual detection.

Traditionally, mycobacteria are cultured on egg-based media, such as Löwenstein–Jensen medium, but there is a delay of 2 to 8 weeks before growth of tubercle bacilli is visible. More rapid results are obtainable by radiometric techniques, whereas molecular methods, such as the polymerase chain reaction (PCR), offer the prospect of even more rapid diagnosis.

Identification of mycobacteria and tests for susceptibility to antimicrobial agents are usually undertaken in reference centres. The traditional methods are rather slow but DNA probes for identification and radiometric methods for drug susceptibility tests, where available, enable results to be issued more rapidly.

Laboratory procedures for isolation, identification, and sensitivity testing of mycobacteria are described in detail by Collins *et al.* (1985).

Histopathology

Tuberculosis in the kidney may be miliary or cavitary (Heptinstall 1992). In miliary tuberculosis, the kidney is speckled with hard, white, 1–3 mm nodules, whereas in cavitary or 'caseous and ulcerative' tuberculosis, there is destruction of the parenchyma. The classical finding in both forms is the granuloma which may caseate, the centre becoming necrotic and having a macroscopic resemblance to cheese.

Initially, the granulomas are small, situated in the cortex, and bilateral. They are centred on capillaries, especially those within the glomerular tuft but some-

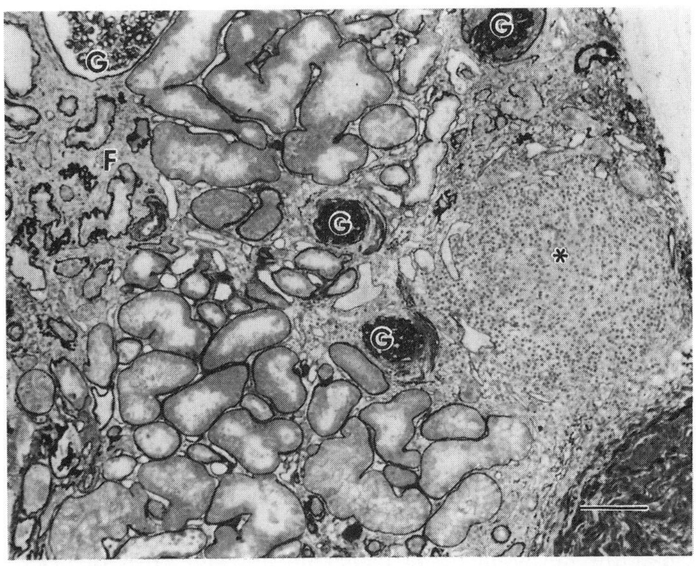

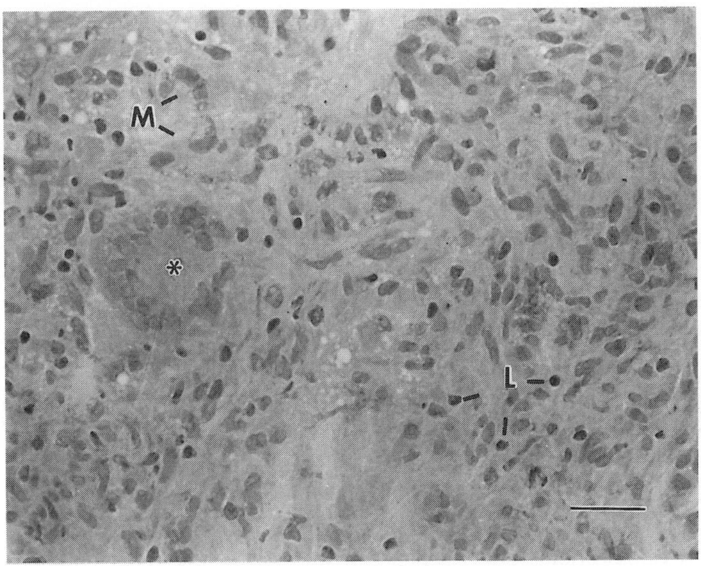

Fig. 14.4 Tubulo-interstitial disease with granulomata. Photomicrographs of the renal biopsy from the patient whose X-ray is shown in Fig. 14.1. *Upper*. The low power view shows one normal and three sclerosed glomeruli (G), focal tubular atrophy and interstitial fibrosis (F), and a large granuloma (*). (Scale bar, 100 μm, Jones methenamine silver stain.) *Lower*. The higher power view is of a granuloma with lymphocytes (L), epithelioid macrophages, (M) and a Langhans-type giant cell (*) with its peripheral palisade of nuclei. (Scale bar, 50 μm, haematoxylin and eosin stain.)

times those related to the collecting ducts and convoluted tubules. These lesions are usually asymptomatic. Symptoms occur when the lesions are more extensive and involve the medulla. Individual papillae may be damaged or several may be involved. These areas may coalesce with destruction of a large amount of renal parenchyma. The first radiologically detectable lesion is often that due to an infected focus ulcerating through the tip of a calyx. This allows spread of bacteria throughout the renal pelvis and down the ureter to the bladder. Tissue destruction and granuloma formation are associated with fibrosis which can lead to strictures and, hence, to obstructive damage to any area of the renal tract.

Ureteric stricture can lead to a tuberculous pyonephrosis while obstruction of the neck of a calyx may lead to replacement of the involved renal lobule by an encapsulated caseous mass. The most common sites for obstruction are the neck of a calyx, the pelviureteric junction, the mid-ureter, the ureterovesical junction, and, in females, the point where the ureter passes under the broad ligament. The bladder may be affected with ulceration of the mucosa and fibrosis of the wall, leading to persistent symptoms of cystitis and eventual reduction in bladder capacity (Laidlaw 1976). Effective chemotherapy can promote healing of active lesions without the development of damaging fibrosis. Areas of inactive chronic disease already containing fibrous tissue and caseous material do not improve on treatment.

Involvement of the urethra is uncommon despite the fact that it must convey infected urine. Ross (1953) reported nine cases of urethral involvement in 469 men with genitourinary tuberculosis and O'Flynn (1970) described 10 cases of urethral stricture in 762 cases. In general, urethral tuberculosis is difficult to diagnose and may present with unusual fistulae involving the perineum, anus, and rectum, or as long strictures that are difficult to treat (Symes and Blandy 1973).

Tuberculous epididymo-orchitis generally presents with swelling of the testis or epididymis and there may be associated abscesses or sinuses. Patients may have no previous history of tuberculosis so epididymo-orchitis may be the presenting feature; histological examination providing the diagnosis. IVU examination may, however, reveal upper renal tract changes consistent with tuberculosis in up to 75 per cent of cases (Ferrie and Rundle 1983).

Calcification is common in renal tuberculosis and appears to have increased in incidence with the advent of effective chemotherapy. In the 1930s, fewer than 10 per cent of cases of renal tuberculosis showed calcification but this has more than doubled in series reported since the introduction of anti-tuberculosis drugs. It is possible that some of the increase is explained by patients surviving long enough to develop calcification. The calcification may be in the renal parenchyma or the wall of the urinary tract. There may be calculi. In 740 cases of genitourinary tuberculosis, Ross (1970) found calcification in 24 per cent of the kidneys. This included five stag-horn calculi, 14 ureteric stones, and seven bladder stones. Finally, the end-stage kidney may have focal or diffuse dystrophic calcification resulting in a so-called 'cement' kidney. Radiologically, this can give a 'cumulus cloud' appearance.

One feature of renal tuberculosis is the tendency for leukoplakia to develop in the renal pelvis. This is probably simply a result of chronic inflammation leading to conversion of normal transitional epithelium to squamous epithelium with associated hyperplasia and keratinization. Large amounts of keratin may flake off into the pelvis to form a mass which may cause local obstruction. The passage of keratinous debris may give rise to repeated episodes of renal colic. These problems with keratin were more common before the chemotherapeutic era but there have been occasional recent cases (Byrd *et al.* 1976).

The microscopic features of tuberculosis are not site-specific but vary depending on the stage of the disease and the immunity of the patient. Histological material may show typical granulomas or may show only lymphocytes and plasma cells in the interstitium without any epithelioid or giant cells. A classical granuloma is a collection of macrophages, many of which have the appearance of epithelioid cells, surrounded by a variable number of lymphocytes and plasma cells. In addition, there may be Langhans giant cells which are multinucleate epithelioid cells with the nuclei arranged as a peripheral horseshoe (Fig. 14.4). A feature of tuberculous granulomas is central caseation and peripheral fibrosis, probably partly due to the immune response and partly due to the healing process. Attempts at healing can result in small fibrous nodules and calcific foci.

The tissues responses are affected by the immune status of the patient. Attempts have been made to delineate a spectrum analogous to that of leprosy for patients with tuberculosis but there has been limited success owing to great intrinsic differences between the two diseases. Nevertheless, in some forms of tuberculosis, notably chronic skin disease (lupus vulgaris), there are non-necrotic granulomas and no detectable acid-fast bacilli, whereas immunosuppressed patients, including those with AIDS, may have disseminated lesions teeming with tubercle bacilli but little or no macrophage activation and granuloma formation (Ridley and Ridley 1987). The most common pattern of tissue response lies in between these forms, with caseous granulomas and small numbers of tubercle bacilli. In this intermediate group, there are no histological features that provide useful indicators of prognosis (Lucas 1988).

Tuberculosis is not the only cause of granulomas, although the presence of caseation is rare in granulomas occurring in other disease. Other potentially granulomatous conditions include sarcoidosis, Wegener's granulomatosis, reaction to foreign/abnormal material (e.g. myeloma protein, ruptured tubules, crystals), leprosy, brucellosis, and certain fungal infections.

*Imaging**

Intravenous urography is very useful in the detection of urinary tract tuberculosis because of its ability to detect calcification, to provide a detailed image of anatomy, and to show the multiple lesions that commonly occur (Chapter 4, Figs 4.26, 4.29, 4.31).

Renal tuberculosis may be unilateral or bilateral. Calcification is seen in about 30 per cent or cases (Roylance *et al.* 1970). It may have a variety of patterns—

*The figures referred to in this section can be found in Chapter 4.

punctate, speckled, or hazy. In advanced tuberculosis the whole pelvicalyceal system and ureter may be outlined by calcification—the so-called tuberculosis autonephrectomy (Fig. 4.27).

Early tuberculosis is seen as irregularity of the papillary margins with reduced contrast medium density in the affected areas. Cavities, either smooth or irregular, then develop and communicate with the pelvicalyceal system (Fig. 4.28). As destruction progresses there is associated parenchymal loss. Fibrosis leads to strictures. When these affect the calyceal infundibula there is no calyceal filling at urography and the infundibulum shows a typical 'pinched-off' appearance (Fig. 4.30). Fibrosis at the pelviureteric junction causes obstruction at this level. Local granuloma formation or dilated obstructed calyces that do not fill with contrast medium may produce a mass effect (Fig. 4.30). Extension of infection into the perinephric space with abscess formation may occur. Fistulae may develop, particularly to the skin and gut. To show them fully, retrograde ureterography or sinography may be required.

Ureteric and bladder tuberculosis are usually secondary to renal tuberculosis and signs of renal abnormality are therefore present. The earliest ureteric change is ulceration but this is rarely demonstrated radiologically. Stricturing then occurs and there may be associated filling defects if there is florid granuloma formation. As fibrosis progresses the ureter shortens and becomes thick-walled. Vesicoureteric junction incompetence may occur and lead to vesicoureteric reflux. The bladder wall thickens and granulomas may cause filling defects. With generalized involvement, bladder capacity is reduced. Calcification in the ureter and bladder only occurs with fairly advanced disease. Calcification may also occurs in the seminal vesicles, vas, and prostate if these are involved.

Ultrasonography shows many of the changes of advanced disease such as pelvicalyceal dilatation, local collections, and calcification (Schaffer *et al.* 1983). However, it is a less sensitive detector than urography, even of advanced disease (Premkumar *et al.* 1987).

Computed tomography is a good method for demonstrating the many changes in advanced disease: calcification, pelvicalyceal dilatation, scars, strictures, and extra-renal spread (Fig. 4.31) (Goldman et al. 1985; Premkumar et al. 1987). Its sensitivity in early disease has not been assessed but is likely to be less than urography because it shows less detailed pelvicalyceal anatomy.

Follow-up studies of patients on chemotherapy reveal that ureteric strictures may develop during treatment. They may occur at sites apparently normal on the urogram obtained at presentation, presumably because mucosal ulceration at the affected site was not visualized. A limited urogram is the best method of looking for ureteric strictures and their effects on the upper tracts (Fig. 4.32).

Treatment (Table 14.4)

Although most clinical trials of anti-tuberculosis drug regimens have involved pulmonary disease, modern short-course chemotherapy appears effective in all forms of tuberculosis, including those involving the genitourinary system. A

Table 14.4 Daily doses of first- and second- line anti-tuberculosis drugs

Drug	Adults	Children
Rifampicin	450 mg, bodyweight <50 kg 600 mg, bodyweight ≥50 kg	Up to 20 mg/kg (maximum 60 mg)
Isoniazid	200–300 mg	10 mg/kg
Pyrazinamide	1.5 g, bodyweight <50 kg 2.0 g, bodyweight ≥50 kg	35 mg/kg
Ethambutol*	15–25 mg/kg	15–25 mg/kg
Streptomycin	750 mg if bodyweight <50 kg 1.0 g if bodyweight ≥50 kg 750 mg if age >40 yrs	20–30 mg/kg (maximum 1.0 g)
Thiacetazone	150 mg	4 mg/kg
PAS	8–12 g (divided doses)	200 mg/kg
Ethionamide	750 mg (divided doses)	15 mg/kg
Cycloserine	500 mg (divided doses)	Not recommended

*The 25 mg/kg dose should not be given for more than 2 months; additional therapy should be at 15 mg/kg. Ethambutol may cause ocular toxicity. Visual acuity should be checked regularly and ethambutol should not be given to children not old enough to be tested for visual acuity.
From Grange (1988), with permission.

number of regimens have been described but most are based on an intensive phase of treatment lasting two months, during which almost all tubercle bacilli are killed, and a continuation phase lasting four months, during which the few remaining 'persisters' are killed (Girling 1989). The usual first-line drugs used in the intensive phase are rifampicin, isoniazid, pyrazinamide, and ethambutol. Streptomycin is sometimes used in the intensive phase, especially in regions where resistance to one or more of the first-line drugs is common, but it has the disadvantage that it must be injected. The usual drugs used in the continuation phase are rifampicin and isoniazid.

The drugs are usually given daily but if supervision of therapy is not easily arranged they may be given twice or thrice weekly, either throughout or for the continuation phase only.

Other anti-tuberculosis drugs include thiacetazone, para-aminosalicylic acid (PAS), ethionamide, prothionamide, cycloserine, kanamycin, viomycin, capreomycin, quinolones (e.g. ofloxacin), and the newer macrolides, but these are less effective and often more toxic and/or costly than the first-line drugs. Their use is usually restricted to treatment of tuberculosis caused by multi-drug-resistant bacilli.

Rifampicin, isoniazid, pyrazinamide, ethionamide, and prothionamide are either eliminated in the bile or metabolized so they may be given in normal doses to patients with impaired renal function. Ethambutol is eliminated predominantly by the kidney and reduced doses should be given according to GFR: 25 mg should be given three times weekly if the GFR is between 50 and

100 ml/min and twice weekly if it is between 30 and 50 ml/min (Mitchison and Ellard 1980; Girling 1989). Streptomycin and other aminoglycosides are excreted entirely by the kidney and are nephrotoxic in some patients; their use should be avoided if possible if there is impairment of renal function. It should be remembered that, although it is relatively easy to achieve urine sterility with modern therapeutic regimes, it takes much longer to eradicate organisms from the tissues of the renal tract (Osterhage *et al.* 1980).

Encephalopathy is a rare complication of isoniazid therapy and its incidence is reduced by the prophylactic use of pyridoxine, 25–50 mg/day. A few cases have been described in dialysis patients despite pyridoxine prophylaxis but resolution has occurred on cessation of isoniazid therapy (Cheung *et al.* 1993).

In renal transplant patients, care should be taken with rifampicin as it increases catabolism of steroids and cyclosporin. Streptomycin is contraindicated in patients on cyclosporin as there is a significant risk of nephrotoxicity. The role of preventive anti-tuberculosis therapy in renal transplant patients is controversial.

Leprosy

Leprosy and renal disease

Renal damage is an important cause of morbidity and mortality in patients with leprosy although direct involvement of the kidney by *Mycobacterium leprae* appears to be an unusual occurrence. It has been postulated that renal tissue is more resistant than other organs to invasion by this bacillus (Gupta *et al.* 1977). Although epithelioid granulomas compatible with lepromas have been observed in this organ, a review of the literature by Al-Mohaya *et al.* (1988) revealed no reports of acid-fast bacilli being detected. On the other hand, many different renal diseases, including interstitial nephritis, secondary amyloidosis, and most histological forms of glomerulonephritis, have been reported in leprosy patients (Mittal *et al.* 1972; Iveson *et al.* 1975; Ng *et al.* 1981; Date *et al.* 1985, Chopra *et al.* 1991). Autopsy studies have revealed that between 11 and 38 per cent of patients with leprosy die of renal failure due to glomerulonephritis or amyloidosis (Ridley 1988), but the incidence of milder or resolving renal disease detectable by percutaneous renal biopsy is higher (Date and Johny 1975).

Glomerulonephritis occurs most frequently in patients with multi-bacillary (lepromatous and borderline lepromatous) leprosy and is due to deposition of immune complexes in the glomeruli (Date and Johny 1975; Ng *et al.* 1981). Although abnormalities in renal function occur during acute episodes of the immune complex disease erythema nodosum leprosum (ENL), opinions differ as to whether glomerulonephritis is more common in patients with ENL (Drutz and Gutman 1973; Ng *et al.* 1981; Al-Mohaya *et al.* 1988). It has also been observed that repeated episodes of ENL are a strong predisposing factor for amyloidosis (McAdam *et al.* 1975).

Amyloidosis is also associated with multi-bacillary leprosy and its geographical incidence varies considerably. There have been a few reports of renal failure in leprosy patients as a complication of rifampicin therapy (Gupta *et al.* 1992).

Roselino *et al.* (1993) report four renal transplant patients with leprosy. Two had the disease before transplantation and did not relapse; the other two presented with new disease (one lepromatous, one borderline) and in one the disease responded well to dapsone.

Environmental mycobacterial disease

Urinary tract involvement

Disease of the genitourinary system due to environmental mycobacteria is exceedingly rare. Diagnosis poses serious problems in view of the frequency with which such bacteria are harmless contaminants of urine. Brooker and Aufderheide (1980) proposed six criteria for the diagnosis of such disease:

(1) symptoms of chronic or recurrent genitourinary infection;
(2) radiological or endoscopic evidence of genitourinary disease;
(3) abnormalities on urine analysis;
(4) failure to isolate other urinary tract pathogens;
(5) repeated isolations of the same mycobacterial species; and
(6) histological demonstration of granulomas and, preferably, acid-fast bacilli.

The first four criteria should alert the clinician to the possibility of a mycobacterial aetiology, the fifth strongly suggests the diagnosis, but only the sixth is confirmatory. A retrospective application of these criteria failed to confirm the diagnosis in 19 supposed cases (Brooker and Aufderheide 1980).

The few confirmed cases of renal disease were caused by *M. intracellulare*, termed the 'Battey bacillus' in the older literature. Two such patients were treated successfully by nephrectomy (Faber *et al.* 1965, Pergament *et al.* 1974) and one by nephroureterectomy (Newman 1970). A further patient with pulmonary disease due to a slow-growing, non-chromogenic mycobacterium (a description compatible with *M. intracellulare*) developed a renal abscess due to an identical strain (Tsai *et al.* 1968). Three cases of epididymitis have been reported, one due to *M. xenopi* (Engbaek *et al.* 1967) and two to *M. kansasii* (Wood *et al.* 1956; Hepper *et al.* 1971). Both *M. xenopi* and *M. fortuitum* were isolated from a case of prostatitis with a granulomatous appearance compatible with mycobacterial disease (Lee *et al.* 1977).

Complicating end-stage renal disease and its treatment

Renal transplantation and the accompanying iatrogenic immunosuppression predispose the patient to mycobacterial disease (Sinnott and Emmanuel 1990). The incidence of such disease in these patients is much higher than in the general population and in 25–40 per cent of cases the cause is an environmental mycobacterium. The appearance of tuberculosis is usually the result of reactivation of dormant foci and the disease may be confined to the lung or involve many organs. Disease due to environmental mycobacteria may also be localized to the lung or disseminated, but is usually mainly a cutaneous problem. When it is cutaneous the organism is usually *M. haemophilum*, *M. marinum*, *M. chelonae*, or *M. fortuitum*. Indeed, the great majority of reported cases of *M. haemophilum* infection have been cases of cutaneous involvement in renal transplant recipients.

Two different mycobacterial diseases may occur in the same patient. Koizumi and Sommers (1980) describe a patient who developed tuberculosis culture-positive for *M. tuberculosis*, four years after renal transplantation. The following year, after an episode of transplant rejection treated with methylprednisolone, the patient developed a radiological opacity in the left lower lobe of the lung which, on excision and culture, yielded a heavy growth of *M. xenopi*.

Symptoms of mycobacterial disease are often masked by the immunosuppression so diagnosis is not easy and thus often delayed. Mortality is around 30 per cent. Therapy of diseases caused by environmental mycobacteria is by agents appropriate to the species.

Small clusters and isolated cases of disseminated disease due to *M. chelonae* have occurred in patients on haemodialysis (Lowrie *et al.* 1990). In some cases, the cause was contamination of the dialysis machine by *M. chelonae*, probably from the local water supply. In one such case (Azadian *et al.* 1981), the identity of isolates from the patient and from the water-softener resin used to purify the water in a hospital haemodialysis unit was established by isoelectric focusing patterns of mycobacterial enzymes (Sparks and Ross 1981).

Environmental mycobacterial disease is a complication of intermittent chronic peritoneal dialysis. Band *et al.* (1981) reviewed 17 cases, all due to *M. chelonae*. As in the case of haemodialysis, the cause appeared to be use of contaminated equipment. This complication is less frequently encountered with CAPD (chronic ambulatory peritoneal dialysis). Dunmire and Breyer (1991) reviewed nine cases: four due to *M. fortuitum*; three to *M. chelonae*; and one each to *M. gastri* and *M. avium-intracellulare*. *Mycobacterium gastri* is not a known mycobacterial pathogen and, under this circumstance, it may be acting more as a saprophyte. A case due to *M. kansasii* has also been reported (Giladi *et al.* 1991). Treatment, which is usually successful, involves drainage of residual fluid, removal of the catheter (essential for success), and appropriate chemotherapy. Complications include abdominal abscesses, fistulae, and adhesions. In practice, most patients with mycobacterial peritonitis need to be transferred to haemodialysis (White *et al.* 1993).

Special problems of immunocompromised patients

Until the advent of the HIV pandemic, disseminated disease due to environmental mycobacteria was an uncommon complication of congenital or acquired immunosuppression. The genitourinary tract may be involved as a manifestation of the disseminated disease.

In a study of the isolation of mycobacteria from HIV positive patients in south-eastern England, environmental mycobacteria were isolated relatively infrequently from the urine or genitourinary tract, relative to other sites (Yates *et al.* 1993). Strains of *M. avium-intracellulare* (MAI) were isolated from 407 patients but from the urine of only 12 of them (2.9 per cent). In all of these cases MAI was isolated from multiple sites. A total of 229 other environmental mycobacteria were isolated from 209 patients, in nine cases (4.3 per cent) from urine. Six of these were single isolates (two *M. chelonae*, two *M. fortuitum*, one *M. gordonae*, and one *M. xenopi*) and were probably casual contaminants. In the other three cases, all *M. kansasii*, there were isolations from other sites, suggesting disseminated infection. It is possible that the low isolation rate of mycobacteria from urine in HIV/AIDS patients is artefactual. Owing to the high incidence of contaminating mycobacteria, many centres may not examine urine when there is evidence of mycobacterial disease involving other sites.

Conclusion

The association of disease of the kidneys and urinary tract with mycobacterial infection is of two kinds. First, mycobacteria (especially *M. tuberculosis*) may cause renal and urinary tract disease which, occasionally, leads to renal failure. Secondly, patients with renal failure, especially when treated by dialysis or transplantation, are more susceptible both to reactivation of latent mycobacterial disease (usually tuberculosis) or to disease due to recent infection (especially by environmental mycobacteria). A further association is that some patients with renal disease, notably vasculitides and certain forms of glomerulonephritis, require treatment with immunosuppressive drugs that render them more susceptible to mycobacterial disease. The development of unexplained fever, malaise, and weight loss in these patients and in renal transplant recipients should lead to a suspicion of mycobacterial disease.

Patients with chronic renal failure, including those treated by haemodialysis or CAPD need careful attention to drug dosages when treatment for mycobacterial disease is indicated. A further complication in renal transplant patients is the interaction between cyclosporin, tacrolimus (FK506) and other immunosuppressive drugs with some of the antibacterial agents used in the treatment of mycobacterial disease.

Acknowledgements

We are grateful to Professor Netar Mallick for facilitating access to the EDTA Registry data. We also thank Miss Marion Amos for secretarial assistance.

References

Ahijado, F., *et al.* (1991). Tuberculous peritonitis on CAPD. *Contributions to Nephrology*, **89**, 79–86.

Al-Mohaya, S. A., Coode, P. E., AlKhder, A. A., and Suhaibani, M. O. (1988). Renal granuloma and mesangial proliferative glomerulo-nephritis in leprosy. *International Journal of Leprosy*, **56**, 599–602.

American Thoracic Society (1974). Preventative therapy of tuberculosis infection. *American Review of Respiratory Disease*, **110**, 371–4.

Annobil, S. H., Al Hilfi, A., and Kazi, T. (1990). Primary tuberculosis of the penis in an infant. *Tubercle*, **71**, 229–30.

Azadian, B. S., *et al.* (1981). Disseminated infection with *Mycobacterium chelonei* in a haemodialysis patient. *Tubercle*, **62**, 281–4.

Band, J. D., Ward, J. I., and Fraser, D. W. (1981). Peritonitis due to a *Mycobacterium chelonei*-like organism associated with intermittent chronic peritoneal dialysis. *Journal of Infectious Diseases*, **145**, 9–17.

Bateman, E. D. (1993). Is tuberculosis prophylaxis necessary for patients receiving corticosteroids for respiratory disease? *Respiratory Medicine*, **87**, 485–7.

Benn, J. J., Scoble, J. E., Thomas, A. C., Eastwood, J. B. (1988). Cryptogenic tuberculosis as a preventable cause of end-stage renal failure. *American Journal of Nephrology*, **8**, 306–8.

Bothamley, G. H. and Grange, J. M. (1991). The Koch phenomenon and delayed hypersensitivity 1891–1991. *Tubercle*, **72**, 7–11.

Brooker, W. J. and Aufderheide, A. C. (1980). Genitourinary tract infections due to atypical mycobacteria. *Journal of Urology*, **124**, 242–4.

Byrd, R. B., Viner, N. A., Omell, G. H., and Trunk, G. (1976). Leukoplakia associated with renal tuberculosis in the chemotherapeutic era. *British Journal of Urology*, **48**, 377–81.

Cheng, I. K., Chan, P. C., and Chan, M. K. (1989). Tuberculous peritonitis complicating long-term peritoneal dialysis. *American Journal of Nephrology*, **9**, 155–61.

Cheung, W. C., Lo, C. Y., Lo, W. K., Ip, M., and Cheng, I. K. (1993). Isoniazid induced encephalopathy in dialysis patients. *Tubercle and Lung Disease*, **74**, 136–9.

Chugh, K. S., Singhal, P. C., Sakhuja, V., Datta, B. N., Jain, S. K., and Dash, S. C. (1981). Pattern of renal amyloidosis in Indian patients. *Postgraduate Medical Journal*, **57**, 31–5.

Chopra, N. K., Lakhani, J. D., Pande, R. S., Modi, K. B., and Pasle, R. K. (1991). Renal involvement in leprosy. *Journal of the Association of Physicians of India*, **39**, 165–7.

Collins, C. H., Grange, J. M., and Yates, M. D. (1984) Mycobacteria in water. *Journal of Applied Bacteriology*, **57**, 193–211.

Collins, C. H., Grange, J. M., and Yates, M. D. (1985). *Organisation and practice in tuberculosis bacteriology*. Butterworths, London.

Date, A. and Johny, K. V. (1975). Glomerular subepithelial deposits in lepromatous leprosy. *American Journal of Tropical Medicine and Hygiene*, **24**; 853–5.

Date, A., Harihar, S., and Jeyavarthini, S. E. (1985). Renal lesions and other major findings in necropsies of 133 patients with leprosy. *International Journal of Leprosy*, **53**, 455–60.

Drutz, D. J. and Gutman, R. A. (1973). Renal manifestations of leprosy: glomerulonephritis—a complication of erythema nodosum leprosum. *American Journal of Tropical Medicine and Hygiene*, **22**, 496–502.

Dunmire, R. B. and Breyer, J. A. (1991). Non-tuberculous mycobacterial peritonitis during chronic ambulatory peritoneal dialysis: case report and review of diagnostic and therapeutic strategies. *American Journal of Kidney Disease*, **18**, 126–30.

Engbaek, H. C., Vergmann, B., and Baess, I. (1967). *Mycobacterium xenopi*: a bacteriological study of *M. xenopi*, including case reports of Danish patients. *Acta Pathologica et Microbiologica Scandinavica*, **69**, 576–94.

Faber, D. R., *et al.* (1965). Idiopathic unilateral renal hematuria associated with atypical acid-fast bacillus, Battey type: cure by partial nephrectomy. *Journal of Urology*, **93**, 435–9.

Ferrie, B. G. and Rundle, J. S. H. (1983). Tuberculous epididymo-orchitis. A review of 20 cases. *British Journal of Urology*, **55**, 437–9.

Giladi, M., Lee, B. E., Berlin, O. G., and Panosian, C. B. (1992). Peritonitis caused by *Mycobacterium kansasii* in a patient undergoing continuous ambulatory peritoneal dialysis. *American Journal of Kidney Diseases*, **19**, 597–9.

Girling, D. J. (1989). The chemotherapy of tuberculosis. In *The biology of the mycobacteria*, (ed. C. Ratledge, J. L. Stanford, and J. M. Grange), Vol. 3, pp. 285–323. Academic Press, New York.

Goldman, S. M., Fishman, E. K., Hartman, D. S., Kim, Y. C. and Siegelman, S. S. (1985). Computed tomography of renal tuberculosis and its pathological correlates. *Journal of Computer Assisted Tomography*, **9**, 771–6.

Grange, J. M. (1988). *Mycobacteria and human disease*, p. 157, Edward Arnold, London.

Grange, J. M. (1990) The mycobacteria. In *Topley and Wilson's principles of bacteriology, virology and immunity*, (ed. M. T. Parker and B. I. Duerden), (8th edn), Vol. 2, pp. 73–101. Edward Arnold, London.

Grange, J. M. and Yates, M. D. (1992). Survey of mycobacteria isolated from urine and the genito-urinary tract in South-East England from 1980 to 1989. *British Journal of Urology*, **69**, 640–6.

Gupta, A., Sakhuja, V., Gupta, K. L., and Chugh, K. S. (1992). Intravascular hemolysis and acute renal failure following intermittent rifampin therapy. *International Journal of Leprosy and Other Mycobacterial Diseases*, **60**, 185–8.

Gupta, J. C., Diwakar, R., Singh, S., Gupta, D. K., and Panda, P. K. (1977). A histopathological study of renal biopsies in 50 cases of leprosy. *International Journal of Leprosy*, **45**, 167–70.

Hariprasad, M. K., Dodelson, R., Eisinger, R. P., and Gary, N. E. (1979). Dense deposit disease in tuberculosis. *New York State Journal of Medicine*, **79**, 2084–5.

Hepper, N. G., Karlson, A. G., and Leary, F. J. (1971). Genito-urinary infection due to *Mycobacterium kansasii*. *Mayo Clinic Proceedings*, **446**, 387–90.

Heptinstall, R. H. (1992). Renal manifestations of various infective conditions. In *Pathology of the kidney* (4th edn), (ed. R. H. Heptinstall), pp. 1936–9. Little Brown, Boston.

Higgins, R. M., *et al.* (1991). Mycobacterial infections after renal transplantation. *Quarterly Journal of Medicine*, **78**, 145–53.

Hussein, M. M., Bakir, N., and Roujouleh, H. (1990). Tuberculosis in patients undergoing maintenance dialysis. *Nephrology Dialysis Transplantation*, **5**, 584–7.

Iveson, J. M., McDougall, A. C., Leathem, A. J., and Harris, H. J. (1975). Lepromatous leprosy presenting with polyarthritis, myositis and immune-complex glomerulonephritis. *British Medical Journal*, **3**, 619–21.

Kennedy, D. H. (1989). Extrapulmonary tuberculosis. In *The biology of the mycobacteria*, (ed. C. Ratledge, J. L. Stanford, and J. M. Grange), Vol. 3, pp. 245–84. New York, Academic Press.

Kindler, V., *et al.* (1989). The inducing role of tumour necrosis factor in the development of bactericidal granulomas during BCG infection. *Cell*, **56**, 731.

Kochi, A. (1991). The global tuberculosis situation and the new control strategy of the World Organisation. *Tubercle*, **72**, 1–6.

Koizumi, J. H. and Sommers, H. M. (1980). *Mycobacterium xenopi* and pulmonary disease. *American Journal of Clinical Pathology*, **73**, 826–30.

Kwan, J. T., Hart, P. D., Raftery, M. J., Cunningham, J., and Marsh, F. P. (1991). Mycobacterial infection is an important infective complication in British Asian dialysis patients. *Journal of Hospital Infection*, **19**, 249–55.

Laidlaw, M. (1976). Renal tuberculosis. In *Scientific foundations of urology*, (ed. D. Innes Williams and G. D. Chisholm), Vol. 1. Heinemann, London.

Lattimer, J. K. (1965). Renal tuberculosis. *New England Journal of Medicine*, **273**, 208–11.

Lee, L. W., *et al.* (1977). Granulomatous prostatitis: association with isolation of *Mycobacterium fortuitum*. *Journal of the American Medical Association*, **237**, 2408–9.

Lichtenstein, I. H. and MacGregor, R. R. (1983). Mycobacterial infections in renal transplant recipients: report of five cases and review of the literature. *Reviews of Infectious Diseases*, **5**, 216–26.

Lowrie, D. B. (1990). Is macrophage death on the field of battle essential to victory, or a tactical weakness in immunity against tuberculosis? *Clinical and Experimental Immunology* 80; 301–3.

Lowrie, P. W., *et al.* (1990). *Mycobacterium chelonei* infections among patients receiving high-flow dialysis in a haemodialysis clinic in California. *Journal of Infectious Diseases*, **1161**, 85–90.

Lucas S. B. (1988). Histopathology of leprosy and tuberculosis—an overview. *British Medical Bulletin* 44; 584–99.

Mallick, N. P. (1993). *European Dialysis and Transplant Association Registry*. St. Thomas' Hospital, London. [Personal communication.]

Mallinson, W. J. W., Fuller, R. W., Levison, D. A., Baker, L. R. I., and Cattell, W. R. (1981). Diffuse interstitial renal tuberculosis—an unusual cause of renal failure. *Quarterly Journal of Medicine*, **50**, 137–48.

McAdam, K. P. W. J., Anders, R. F., Smith, S. R., Russell, D. A., Price, M. A. (1975). Association of amyloidosis with erythema nodosum leprosum reactions and recurrent neutrophil leucocytosis in leprosy. *Lancet*, **3**, 572–6.

Mignon, F., Mery, J. P., Mougenot, B., Ronco, P., Roland, J., and Morel-Maroger, L. (1984). Granulomatous interstitial nephritis. In *Advances in nephrology*, Vol. 13 (ed. J F. Bach, J. Grosnier, J. L. Funch-Brentano, J. P. Grönfeld, W. H. Maxwell, pp. 218–45). Year Book Publishers, Chicago.

Mitchison, D. A. and Ellard, G. A. (1980). Tuberculosis in patients having dialysis. *British Medical Journal*, **1**, 1186; 1533.

Mittal, M. M., Agarwal, S. C., Maheshwari, H. B., and Kumar, S. (1972). Renal lesions in leprosy. *Archives of Pathology*, **93**, 8–12.

Morgan, S. H., Eastwood, J. B., and Baker, L. R. I. (1990). Tuberculous interstitial nephritis—the tip of an iceberg. *Tubercle*, **71**, 5–6.

Mosmann, T. R. (1991). Regulation of immune responses by T cells with different cytokine secretor phenotypes. Role of a new cytokine: cytokine synthesis inhibitory factor (IL 10). *International Archives of Allergy and Applied Immunology*, **94**, 110–5.

Narain, J. P., Raviglione, M. C., and Kochi, A. (1992). *HIV-associated tuberculosis in developing countries: epidemiology and strategies for prevention*, Pub. WHO/TB/92.164. World Health Organization, Geneva.

Neves, P. L., *et al.* (1993). Unusual presentation of renal tuberculosis: End-stage renal disease. *Nephrology, Dialysis, Transplantation*, **8**, 288–9.

Newman, H. (1970). Renal disease associated with atypical mycobacteria, Battey type: case report. *Journal of Urology*, **103**, 403–5.

Ng, W. L., Scollard, D. M., and Hua, A. (1981). Glomerulonephritis in leprosy. *American Journal of Clinical Pathology*, **76**, 321–9.

O'Flynn, D. (1970). Treatment of genito-urinary tuberculosis. *British Journal of Urology*, **42**, 667–71.

Ong, A. C., Scoble, J. E., Baillod, R. A., Fernando, O. N., Sweny, P., and Moorhead, J. F. (1992). Tuberculous peritonitis complicating peritoneal dialysis: a case for early diagnostic laparotomy. *Nephrology Dialysis Transplantation*, **7**, 443–6.

Ormerod, L. P. (1993). Why does genito-urinary tuberculosis occur less often than expected in the ethnic Indian subcontinent population living in the United Kingdom? *Journal of Infection*, **27**, 27–32.

Osterhage, H. R., Fischer, V., and Haubensak, K. (1980). Positive histological tuberculous findings despite stable sterility of the urine on culture. Results of 111 nephrectomies and partial nephrectomies. *European Urology*, **6**, 116–8.

Pasternack, M. S. and Rubin, R. H. (1993). Urinary tract tuberculosis. In *Diseases of the kidney*, (ed. R. W. Schrier and C. W. Gottschalk), (5th edn), p. 915. Churchill Livingstone, London.

Pazianas, M., Eastwood, J. B., MacRae, K. D., and Phillips, M. E. (1991). Racial origin and primary renal diagnosis in 771 patients with end-stage renal disease. *Nephrology Dialysis Transplantation*, **6**, 931–5.

Pergament, M., Gonzalez, R., and Fraley, E. E. (1974). Atypical mycobacterioses of the urinary tract: a case report of extensive disease caused by the Battey bacillus. *Journal of the American Medical Association*, **229**, 816–17.

Peters, F. T., Reiter, C. G., and Boswell, R. L. (1984). Transmission of tuberculosis by kidney transplantation. *Transplantation*, **38**. 514–16.

Pitchenik, A. E. and Fertel, D. (1992). Medical management of AIDS patients: tuberculosis and non-tuberculous mycobacterial disease. *Medical Clinics of North America*, **76**, 121–71.

Premkumar, A., Latimer, M., and Newhouse, J. H. (1987). CT and sonography of advanced urinary tract tuberculosis. *American Journal of Roentgenology*, **148**, 65–9.

Qunibi, W. Y., *et al.* (1990). Mycobacterial infection after renal transplantation—a report of 14 cases and review of the literature. *Quarterly Journal of Medicine*, **77**, 1039–60.

Ridley, D. S. and Ridley, M. J. (1987). Rationale for the histological spectrum of tuberculosis. A basis for classification. *Pathology*, **19**, 186–92.

Ridley, D. S. (1988). *Pathogenesis of leprosy and related diseases*, pp. 89–90. John Wright, London.

Roderick, P. J., Jones, I., Raleigh, V. S., McGeown, M., and Mallick, N. (1994). Population need for renal replacement therapy in Thames regions: ethnic dimension. *British Medical Journal*, **309**, 1111–4.

Rook, G. A. W. and Al Attiyah, R. (1991). Cytokines and the Koch phenomenon. *Tubercle*, **72**, 13–20.

Roselino, A. M., de Almeida, A. M., Foss, N. T., Raspanti, E. O., and Ferraz, A. S. (1993). Renal transplantation in leprosy patients. *International Journal of Leprosy and Other Mycobacterial Diseases*, **61**, 102–5.

Ross, J. C. (1953). Renal tuberculosis. *British Journal of Urology*, **25**, 277–92.

Ross, J. C. (1970). Calcification in genito-urinary tuberculosis. *British Journal of Urology*, **42**, 656–60.

Roylance, J., Penry, J. B., Davies, E. R., and Roberts, M. (1970). The radiology of tuberculosis of the urinary tract. *Clinical Radiology*, **21**, 163–70.

Sasaki, S., *et al.* (1979). Ten years' survey of dialysis-associated tuberculosis. *Nephron*, **24**, 141–5.

Schaffer, R., Becker, J. A., and Goodman, J. (1983). Sonography of tuberculous kidney. *Urology*, **22**, 209–11.

Schliesser, T. (1974). Die Bekampfung der Rindertuberkulose—Tierversuch der Vergangenheit. *Praxis der Pneumonologie vereinigt mit der Tuberkulosearzt*, **28** (Suppl.), 870–4.

Shribman, J. H., Eastwood, J. B., and Uff, J. S. (1983). Immune-complex nephritis complicating miliary tuberculosis. *British Medical Journal*, **287**, 1593–4.

Simon, H. B., Weinstein, A. J., Pasternack, M. S., Swartz, M. N., and Kunz, L. J. (1977). Genito-urinary tuberculosis: Clinical features in a general hospital population. *American Journal of Medicine*, **63**, 410–20.

Sinnott, J. T. and Emmanuel, P. J. (1990). Mycobacterial infections in the transplant patient. *Seminars in Respiratory Infections*, **5**, 65–71.

Skerman, V. D. B., McGowan, V., and Sneath, P. H. A. (1980). Approved list of bacterial names. *International Journal of Systematic Bacteriology*, **30**, 225–420.

Smith, E. C. (1982). Tuberculosis in dialysis patients. *International Journal of Artificial Organs*, **5**, 11–12.

Sparks, J. and Ross, G. W. (1981). Isoelectric focusing studies on *Mycobacterium chelonei*. *Tubercle*, **62**, 289–93.

Symes, J. M. and Blandy, J. P. (1973). Tuberculosis of the male urethra. *British Journal of Urology*, **45**, 432–6.

Tan, D., Fein, P. A., Jorden, A., and Avram, M. M. (1991). Successful treatment of tuberculous peritonitis while maintaining patient on CAPD. *Advances in Peritoneal Dialysis*, **7**, 102–4.

Tsai, S. H., Yue, W. Y., and Duthoy, E. J. (1968). Roentgen aspects of chronic pulmonary mycobacteriosis. An analysis of 18 cases including one with renal involvement. *Radiology*, **90**, 306–10.

Wallgren, A. (1948). The 'timetable' of tuberculosis. *Tubercle*, **29**, 245–51.

White, R., *et al.* (1993). Non-tuberculous mycobacterial infections in continuous ambulatory peritoneal dialysis patients. *American Journal of Kidney Diseases*, **22**, 581–7.

Wood, L. E., Buhler, V. B., and Pollak, A. (1956). Human infection with the 'yellow' acid fast bacillus: a report of fifteen additional cases. *American Review of Tuberculosis and Pulmonary Diseases*, **73**, 917–29.

Yates, M. D. and Grange, J. M. (1988). Incidence and nature of human tuberculosis due to bovine tubercle bacilli in South East England: 1977–1987. *Epidemiology and Infection*, **101**, 225–9.

Yates, M. D., Pozniak, A., and Grange, J. M. (1993). Isolation of mycobacteria from patients seropositive for the human immunodeficiency virus (HIV) in South East England: 1984–1992. *Thorax*, **48**, 990–5.

15

Fungal infections of the urinary tract

R. J. Hay

Introduction

Fungal infections or mycoses are some of the most common diseases of man. These include thrush (candidosis) and ringworm (dermatophytosis) as well as systemic infections which are important complications of the management of the seriously ill and immunocompromised patient (Warnock and Richardson 1991). Involvement of the kidney or upper urinary tract may occur during the course of bloodstream dissemination of systemic infection or by direct contamination during the course of surgery. Lower urinary tract infection occurs spontaneously or as a result of bladder catheterization.

Classification of fungal infection

The main fungal infections seen in man are caused by either unicellular fungi, yeasts, or mould fungi which grow to form chains of joined cells. These infections are usually divided into superficial, subcutaneous, and deep mycoses. A classification is given in Table 15.1.

Superficial mycoses include common infections, such as ringworm (tinea pedis, tinea capitis), superficial candidosis, or thrush and *Malassezia* infections. The subcutaneous mycoses are rare and are mainly confined to the tropics and subtropics. They usually develop after percutaneous inoculation of organisms. Systemic mycoses are divided into those infections which only occur in the compromised patient, the opportunistic infections, and those which are mainly found in defined endemic areas and can develop in otherwise healthy individuals (Warnock and Richardson 1991).

Endemic mycoses, which include histoplasmosis and coccidioidomycosis, develop after inhalation and the primary site of infection is the lung. A significant proportion of these infections are subclinical. In endemic areas, an estimate of exposure can be obtained by determining the percentage of positive skin tests in the community. Changes in host immune status will affect the clinical manifestations of these endemic diseases. Histoplasmosis in AIDS patients, for instance, has distinct clinical features such as *Histoplasma* septicaemia and usually presents as a widely disseminated infection. In contrast, opportunistic infections only occur where there is some form of host abnormality predisposing to infection (Weber and Rutala 1989). In many cases this is

Table 15.1 The mycoses

Superficial mycoses
Dermatophytosis (ringworm)
Superficial candidosis (oral, cutaneous, vaginal)
Malassezia infections
Miscellaneous (tinea nigra, white piedra)
Subcutaneous mycoses
Mycetoma
Sporotrichosis
Chromoblastomycosis
Systemic mycoses
(1) Opportunists
systemic candidosis
aspergillosis
cryptococcosis
mucormycosis
(2) Endemic mycoses
histoplasmosis
coccidioidomycosis
paracoccidioidomycosis
blastomycosis
penicilliosis

immunologically related, but other factors such as diabetes, the presence of prosthetic material, or an exposed epithelial surface may determine invasion.

Superficial invasion of the lower genital or urinary tracts is seen in superficial candidosis. Infection of the kidney may follow haematogenous dissemination of any systemic fungal infection but it is most common with systemic candidosis. Infection of the renal pelvis or ureter may also follow dissemination of infection or may arise following surgery to the area. Less commonly it occurs without any obvious predisposition.

Factors predisposing to fungal infection

Immunological defence against fungi is either T lymphocyte- or phagocyte-mediated. Patients who are particularly prone to fungal infection include those with defective numbers of functioning T lymphocytes (e.g. HIV infection) or neutrophil defects (e.g. leukaemic patients). Particular fungal infections are more likely to occur in patients in each of these groups. Cryptococcosis is more common in those with T cell abnormalities and aspergillosis is mainly, but not exclusively, seen in neutropenic patients. Superficial candidosis may occur in patients with either T cell or neutrophil abnormalities but systemic *Candida* infections are mainly found in those with neutropenia.

In addition to these specific immunological abnormalities the presence of synthetic materials, such as intravenous or intraperitoneal catheters, predispose to infection. This is mainly seen with candidosis where organisms can adhere through fungal glycopeptide surface receptors to epithelium or a plastic prosthesis. This process of adherence is enhanced if the surface of the prosthesis is coated with certain proteins such as fibrin.

Therapeutic considerations

Therapy of fungal infections involves the use of a distinct group of antimicrobials (Warnock and Richardson 1991; Medoff *et al.* 1983). There are three main families of antifungal drugs: the polyenes, the azoles, and the allylamines. There is also a miscellaneous group of compounds such as flucytosine and griseofulvin which do not belong to a single family of drugs (Table 15.2). This is

Table 15.2 Antifungal drugs

Polyenes
Amphotericin B (AMB)*
Nystatin
Natamycin
Lipid-complexed AMB*
Azoles
Imidazoles
miconazole*
clotrimazole
econazole
ketoconazole*
sulconazole
tioconazole
Triazoles
fluconazole*
itraconazole*
Allylamines
Terbinafine
Naftifine
Morpholines
Amorolfine
Miscellaneous
Griseofulvin
Ciclopiroxolamine
Tolnaftate
Flucytosine (5FC)*

*Antifungal drugs available for systemic mycoses.

not a static picture as there are new groups of antifungals continually under development. These include new azole or polyene derivatives, the morpholine antifungals such as amorolfine, a new fungal sterol biosynthesis inhibitor, and cell wall antagonists such as the echinocandins (e.g. cilofungin), or the nikkomycins.

The polyene, amphotericin B, has long been the mainstay of antifungal chemotherapy (Medoff and Kobayashi 1980). It is given intravenously in does of 0.5–1.0 mg/kg daily. As it is mainly metabolized in the liver, adjustment of dosage is unnecessary in renal failure unless there is evidence that the drug itself is contributing to renal impairment. Although it is effective against a wide range of organisms it can cause a number of major adverse events, such as renal tubular damage and reduced renal plasma flow, as well as hypokalaemia and anaemia (Butler *et al.* 1964). Hyperpyrexia, prostration, and hypotension can follow infusions. Different methods have been devised to reduce the frequency and severity of these reactions, such as slow infusions, a gradual increase in daily dosage, and the use of anthistamines, hydrocortisone, pethidine, and amiloride, to control symptoms. In severely ill patients rapid escalation of dosage is advisable starting with half the maximum dose, which is given very slowly for the first hour to monitor for adverse reactions. The full dose is given 24 hours later. The frequency of side-effects can also be reduced by using a liposome-encapsulated formulation of the drug that allows physicians to give doses up to 6 mg/kg daily without significant adverse reactions (Chopra *et al.* 1991; Meunier *et al.* 1991). Other lipid complexes of amphotericin B are being developed. The use of a mixed intra-lipid and amphotericin B preparation has also been suggested as a means of treating systemic fungal infections (Moreau *et al.* 1992). At present, there is insufficient data on both efficacy and safety to encourage its use.

With the conventional preparation, amphotericin B is present in low concentrations in the urine and it will commonly be necessary to use a combination of drugs for urinary tract infection. Lipsome-encapsulated amphotericin B accumulates in low concentrations in the renal parenchyma and urine. Toxicity is less but concentrations are also low so there is no particular advantage to using it in renal infections.

The azole drugs include two imidazoles which can be used for systemic therapy, ketoconazole and miconazole, as well as the triazoles, fluconazole and itraconazole (Warnock and Richardson 1991). High urine concentrations can be obtained with fluconazole but it is less active against mould fungi such as aspergilli. Some non-*albicans Candida* species such as *C. krusei* and *C. glabrata* are often insensitive to fluconazole. The usual doses of fluconazole in systemic mycoses are between 200–600 mg daily and the drug can be given orally or intravenously. As fluconazole is largely excreted via the kidney some adjustment of dose is advised in patients with renal impairment even though no adverse reactions have been ascribed to high serum levels of the drug. Generally, after two daily doses the dosage interval should be lengthened to 48 hours in those with creatinine clearances of 20–40 ml/min or 72 hours in those with creatinine clearances of 10–20 ml/min. With patients on regular dialysis one dose is given post-dialysis. Itraconazole has a wider spectrum of activity than fluconazole but does not produce high urine levels. It is an oral drug employed in doses of 100–400 mg daily. Neither ketoconazole nor miconazole are commonly used for systemic fungal infections, although the latter is effective in infections caused by the fungus, *Pseudallescheria boydii*. None of the azoles are known to cause serious adverse reactions affecting renal function.

Flucytosine is another systemic antifungal drug which can be used in urinary infections due to *Candida* but can cause significant bone marrow toxicity with neutropenia and thrombocytopenia at blood levels above 100 mg/l. Its principal route of elimination is renal and the dose must be reduced in patients with renal impairment. The dose in those with normal renal function is about 120 mg/kg/day divided into four equal doses. In neonates, a smaller dose of 60–80 mg/kg/day is used as the half life of the drug is slightly longer than in adults (Drouhet *et al.* 1974). Regular monitoring of blood flucytosine levels is important. Generally, these should be maintained between 40 and 60 mg/l 1–2 hours post-dose. Instructions for modifying the dose in the presence of renal impairment are given in Table 15.3. Primary or secondary resistance to this drug is also well described. The secondary resistance generally follows continuous long-term use of the drug over several weeks.

Table 15.3 Dose reduction of flucytosine (5FC) for patients with impaired renal function

Creatinine clearance	Total daily dose	Interval between doses
<40 ml/min	120–150 mg/kg	6 h
20–40 ml/min	50–100 mg/kg	12 h
10–20 ml/min	25–50 mg/kg	24 h
Patients on:		
(a) Haemodialysis	25–50 mg/kg	Post-dialysis
(b) CAPD	25–50 mg/kg	Daily

After Scholer (1980).

A summary of the antifungals used in the management of disease of the urinary tract is given in Table 15.4.

The urinary tract and mycoses

Infections of the upper urinary tract are seen in a number of systemic mycoses but are most common with candidosis (Weber and Rutala 1989). Lower urinary tract infection with candidosis is also well described. Disseminated fungal infections caused by *Aspergillus*, *Fusarium*, and *Trichosporon* may lead specifically to renal invasion. Kidney infections may also occur with dissemination of other infections, notably histoplasmosis, coccidioidomycosis, paracoccidioidomycosis,

Table 15.4 Drugs used for fungal infections of the renal tract

Disease	Drug	Potential problems	Dose/day
Disseminated candidosis	Amphotericin B (AMB)	Low urinary levels Drug-related toxicity	0.6–1.0 mg/kg
	Fluconazole	Resistance (non-*albicans Candida* spp.) Reduce dose in renal impairment	200–600 mg; 4–6 mg/kg in infants
	Flucytosine (5FC) and AMB	Reduce dose of 5FC in renal impairment Drug-related toxicity	AMB 0.6–0.8 mg/kg 5FC 120 mg/kg*
Candiduria not associated with dissemination	Fluconazole	Resistance (non-*albicans Candida* spp.) Reduce dose in renal impairment	As above
	Flucytosine (5FC)	Resistance Drug-related toxicity Reduce dose of 5FC in renal impairment	As above minus AMB
Other infections (e.g. *Aspergillus*)	Fluconazole	Resistance (non-*albicans Candida* spp.) Reduce dose in renal impairment Sensitivity of organism	200–600 mg
	Itraconazole	Low urine levels	100–400 mg

*Flucytosine doses for patients with renal impairment are given in Table 15.3.

and blastomycosis. Symptoms or signs of kidney involvement are usually masked by other manifestations of a severe disseminated infection such as weight loss, lymphadenopathy, meningitis, or cough. It is often difficult to be certain that isolation of fungi in urine is a sign of disseminated infection, focal disease affecting the collecting systems or lower tract infection. The various possibilities are discussed below.

Candidosis

Yeasts of the genus *Candida* are common causes of human disease. While usually *C. albicans* is the main culprit, other non-*albicans* species of *Candida* may also be involved. Disease due to these fungi may be superficial or deep; deep focal infections such as bladder infections may also occur. The main clinical forms of deep *Candida* infection are:

- Candidemia
- Focal deep candidosis, e.g.,
  - *Candida* cystitis
  - *Candida* infection of the renal pelvis without evidence of septicaemia
- Disseminated candidosis

Candidemia refers to the isolation of *Candida* from blood culture without evidence of local infection including lack of renal invasion.

Disseminated candidosis

In disseminated candidosis haematogenous spread of organisms is followed by invasion of different organs. Culture of *Candida* from urine in a patient with signs of septicaemia indicates renal involvement. Renal impairment may occur but other factors, such as shock or the use of amphotericin B, may be involved. Symptoms include pyrexia and loin pain, but weakness and muscle tenderness as well as evidence of invasion of other sites, such as visual impairment, tend to dominate. Frequency and painful micturition are less common. There may be microscopic haematuria.

In neonates, a group predisposed to *Candida* septicaemia, there are variations in this mode of presentation. The main differences between adult and neonatal disseminated candidosis are due to the high incidence in the latter of ventriculitis or meningitis and renal involvement. The high frequency of meningitis in neonates with *Candida* septicaemia is often associated with a prior intraventricular haemorrhage. Pyrexia is present but signs of meningitis and irritability may develop. Significant and irreversible renal impairment may occur (Noe and Tonkin 1982). This may be accompanied by renal enlargement seen on ultrasound or computed tomography (CT) scans or even noted clinically (Kinjanar *et al.* 1986). Enlargement of the renal pelvis and partial obstruction due to masses of fungal filaments or hyphae in the tubules and collecting ducts may occur. Microscopy of suprapubic urine aspirates may show similar tangled masses of *Candida*.

Neonatal *Candida* septicaemia most commonly occurs in those born at under 30-weeks' gestational age. Entry of *Candida* is thought to be related to umbilical or peripheral vein cannulation.

In all cases, diagnosis is based on the isolation and identification of *Candida* from a normally sterile site such as blood or a suprapubic aspirate of urine. At present, other measures, such as serology or antigen detection, have proved disappointing in the diagnosis of these infections. Antibodies to *Candida* are often present in low titre both in normal individuals and in the immunocompromised patient with candidosis. Antigen detection systems using latex agglutination or enzyme-linked immunosorbant assay (ELISA) frequently fail to pick up early infections. Histopathological confirmation of *Candida* infection is diagnostic but often impracticable.

Treatment of *Candida* septicaemia with renal involvement is no different to other forms of disseminated candidosis, amphotericin B or fluconazole being the main treatments used. The duration of treatment will depend on the resolution of lesions and the results of cultures. Three weeks' therapy is probably a minimum. The presence of *Candida* in the urine is often taken to be an indication that flucytosine should be added to amphotericin B although objective evidence of the value of the combination is not available (Wong-Beringer *et al.* 1992). Renal invasion in neonates can proceed rapidly and in some cases a kidney can be virtually destroyed by infection before treatment can be initiated. For this reason treatment should commence quickly in neonatal candidosis (Noe and Tonkin 1982). The same drugs are used as for *Candida* septicaemia in adults. Management of renal candidosis where there is no sign of septicaemia is discussed below.

Candida infections not associated with septicaemia

Upper urinary tract infections

Yeast infections of the upper urinary tract without evidence of blood stream spread may be caused by a number of different *Candida* species. Moulds including *Aspergillus, Paecilomyces*, and dematiaceous (pigmented) fungal species may also cause this type of infection (Turck and Stamm 1981).

Infection of the renal pelvis caused by *Candida* generally follows surgical manipulation of the ureters or surgery to the pelviureteric junction. Intra-operative contamination or post-operative contamination via a ureterostomy are causes of infection. The presence of a synthetic surface, such as a ureteric catheter, suture or ureterostomy tube, predisposes to infection. It may arise *de novo* and rarely without any identifiable predisposition. In those cases where there have been no surgical procedures it is likely that the organisms have disseminated to the kidney through the bloodstream. Many fungi then proliferate in the renal tubules, and pelvic invasion may merely represent an extension of renal infection. It may also follow renal papillary necrosis, where tissue debris is thought to provide a focus for infection (Tomashefski and Abramowsky 1981). Although there have been no large published series this complication appears to be more common in diabetic patients (Klimek *et al.* 1979). Other predisposing factors include pre-existing urinary tract pathology and renal transplantation where structural anomalies or foreign material, such as sutures, provide a nidus of infection (Hamory and Wenzel 1978). It is, however, an uncommon infection.

The main organisms involved are *Candida* spp., *C. albicans* being the most common cause. Other species, such as *C. tropicalis*, may also be implicated. Non-*albicans Candida* species are more commonly found in this localized form of renal candidosis than in disseminated *Candida* infections.

Infection may be symptom-free or present with fever and malaise. Dull loin pain, frequency, and painful micturition may also develop. Renal colic may be associated with the passage of mycelial masses or fungus balls down the ureter. Renal colic does not indicate a particular infection as both yeast and mycelial fungi may form fungal balls. Occasionally, long-standing infection may result in obstruction at the pelviureteric junction with the appearance of hydro- or pyonephrosis (Alkalay *et al.* 1991; Corbella *et al.* 1992). A perinephric abscess may develop and renal papillary necrosis (Tomashefski and Abramowsky 1981) has been recorded in such patients. In premature infants renal pelvic obstruction is a complication of disseminated candidosis.

Diagnosis involves the identification of the causative fungus by microscopy and culture of urine or ureterostomy cannulae. Attempts to correlate specific levels of yeasts in urine or other features, such as haematuria or hyphal formation with renal parenchymal invasion, have not been successful (Kozinn *et al.* 1978.) There are, however, other clues to pelvic invasion by fungi. The presence of fungal balls may show up as filling defects in the renal pelvis on CT scans, US, or IVU (intravenous urography) (Goodman *et al.* 1992). The organisms can also be identified as mycelial tangles on microscopy of spun urine samples and, indeed, can often be seen with the naked eye. Serology may occasionally help in following the course of therapy with candidosis, although the frequency of the isolation of unusual organisms in this form of infection reduces the value of serology since there are no diagnostic serological tests for the whole range of potential pathogens.

Treatment is difficult because it depends on the identification of the organism. There are two elements to therapy: (1) the removal, where possible, of any prosthetic material; and (2) chemotherapy. The choice of drug is largely determined by three factors: the drug sensitivity of the fungus, the penetration of the drug into the area, and the likely need for long-term therapy (Wong-Beringer *et al.* 1992; Alkalay *et al.* 1991). The drugs which give the highest urine concentrations are fluconazole and flucytosine. Fluconazole is mainly active against *C. albicans* and some other yeasts. It is not effective against *C. krusei*, *C. glabrata*, and certain other yeasts. The development of drug resistance to flucytosine is a potential problem. Amphotericin B given by intravenous route does not enter the urine in sufficient quantities, although a combination of amphotericin B and flucytosine has been recommended. Retrograde irrigation has not been shown to be effective and care needs to be exercised in using amphotericin B in this context given its known toxicity for the renal tubules.

There are no studies on which to base an accurate estimate of the most appropriate duration of treatment. If using an oral drug, at least two months will be necessary and longer if the urine is not sterile. Patients may relapse and close follow-up is advisable. If cultures remain positive while the patient is still receiving therapy, the organisms should be tested for drug resistance.

Infections of the lower urinary tract

Fungal infection of the bladder is generally caused by *Candida* species. Affected patients commonly have either an indwelling catheter or have received courses of antibiotics. Symptoms are often minimal, although frequency as well as pain and discomfort on micturition are common. The urine is often cloudy, sometimes completely opaque, and may have a yeasty smell. The diagnosis is confirmed by microscopy and culture. Often, the isolation of *Candida* from urine, candiduria, is an unexpected finding. The presence of candiduria should be re-checked ensuring there is no contamination from vaginal or subprepucal colonization. If candiduria is confirmed in the asymptomatic patient it is important to exclude this as the result of disseminated infection or renal parenchymal invasion.

There has been uncertainty in the past over the most appropriate therapy. It is certainly important to eliminate predisposing factors such as the removal of catheters (Wong-Beringer *et al.* 1992). Chemotherapy with fluconazole (100 mg/day for 7–10 days) is appropriate in most cases, although for certain non-*albicans Candida* species flucytosine is often effective.

The management of candiduria

Management of the patient who presents with candiduria is a common and difficult problem. As can be see from the foregoing there are three main explanations for positive urine cultures: (1) disseminated candidosis affecting the kidney; (2) infection of the collecting system often localized to the renal pelvis, (3) and bladder infection. The differential diagnosis is based on a combination of clinical judgement and laboratory investigation. Important points which may assist establish the diagnosis and site of infection in the patient with candiduria are as follows:

1. It is necessary to establish whether there is any evidence of systemic spread which would support a diagnosis of *Candida* septicaemia. This includes examining specific sites such as the eyes, liver, or spleen for evidence of infection. The presence of predisposing factors, such as neutropenia, favour the development of disseminated candidosis as does the presence of *Candida* endocarditis. Blood cultures should be taken to exclude *Candida* septicaemia. If any are positive it is advisable to treat the patient for a disseminated infection.

2. Renal pelvic infection occurs in less severely ill patients although, as has been stated before, it may develop in patients with septicaemia. It is important to recognize this complication, particularly in neonates, in view of the risk of renal obstruction. The development of renal colic, the presence of underlying diabetes, or previous upper renal tract surgery, and the isolation of mould fungi or non-*albicans Candida* species in culture should alert the clinician to the possibility of infection of the upper urinary tract. Imaging of the upper urinary tract by IVU, US, or CT is then indicated (Kinjanar *et al.* 1986). The presence of mycelial balls in urine is suggestive of upper urinary tract infection although occasionally these may form in bladder infections.

3. Typically, *Candida* cystitis presents with suprapubic pain, pyrexia, and frequency, as well as painful micturition. These symptoms alone may suggest the diagnosis. The isolation of *Candida* from urine in these circumstances is not necessarily an indication for specific treatment as stopping antibiotics and removing catheters may bring about a recovery. This is especially true of asymptomatic candiduria found by chance. Urine samples should be re-examined for candiduria 7–10 days following discontinuation of antibiotics or removal of the catheter to ensure spontaneous clearance. Persistant candiduria merits careful review for evidence of upper tract infection and for the need for treatment with fluconazole.

Unfortunately, it is not always possible to localize the extent of urinary *Candida* infection with precision. Laboratory tests, including serology and quantitative urine cultures, are unhelpful (Kozinn *et al.* 1978). It is usually preferable to treat the worst scenario.

Aspergillosis and other fungal infections

Renal *Aspergillus* infections may occur during bloodstream dissemination or arise as an infection of the renal pelvis (Weber and Rutala 1989). The same factors described for candidosis predispose to pelvic infection. The usual organism is *Aspergillus fumigatus* but other species, such as *A. flavus*, *A. niger* and *A. terreus*, may cause disease. These latter species are particularly common in patients presenting with infections of the renal pelvis. Renal pelvis infection presents in an identical fashion to *Candida* infection at this site. The diagnosis is only established by urine culture. Microscopy of urinary sediments is usually insufficient for identification of the fungi concerned.

Treatment of renal or pelvic infections is difficult as the drugs that are most active against mould fungi do not enter the urine in sufficient concentrations. Amphotericin B or itraconazole are usually used in disseminated infections. Itraconazole, either on its own, or in combination with flucytosine, is a reasonable choice for localized infections affecting the renal pelvis and collecting ducts. An alternative is amphotericin B and flucytosine. Where possible, cultures should be tested for *in vitro* sensitivity to antifungals as this may widen the choice of treatment.

Other mould fungi, such as *Pseudallescheria* or *Paecilomyces*, occasionally cause infection affecting the collecting system. Their management is identical to that for aspergillosis.

More rarely, other pathogenic fungi, such as the zygomycetes which include *Rhizomucor* and *Rhizopus* spp., can cause infections of the kidneys during the course of dissemination. This pattern of mucormycosis is mainly seen in severely neutropenic patients. Renal lesions rarely occur during dissemination of *Cryptococcus neoformans*. In AIDS patients chronic infection of the prostate by *Cryptococcus* commonly occurs. Apart from low pelvic pain this produces few symptoms but may be a cause of positive urine cultures.

Dissemination to the kidneys from a pulmonary focus can occur with most of the endemic systemic mycoses such as histoplasmosis, coccidioidomycosis, blastomycosis, and paracoccidioidomycosis. Chronic epididymitis may follow dissemination in blastomycosis.

Fungal infections in the immunocompromised patient

Patients who have received solid organ transplants, including renal transplants are more susceptible to fungal infection as a result of the use of steroids, azathioprine, and cyclosporin (Dummer *et al.* 1983). Because cyclosporin A has some antifungal activity it is possible that the frequency of fungal infection may be lower in patients receiving this drug although there are no human studies to confirm this. Oral candidosis, dermatophytosis, and pityriasis versicolor are all seen in transplanted patients. Among systemic infections candidosis, invasive aspergillosis, cryptococcosis, and mucormycosis may all be involved. Infections due to aspergilli may be sporadic with cases presenting in clusters. This results from exposure of groups of patient to peaks of environmental exposure related to building work carried out in the vicinity of the ward area or other causes such as contaminated ventilation systems. Clustering of cases of aspergillosis should alert clinicians to the possibility of a point source of infection.

AIDS patients are also susceptible to disseminated fungal infections such as cryptococcosis, histoplasmosis, and penicilliosis. Disseminated candidosis and aspergillosis have been recorded but are less common.

Neutropenic patients, including those under treatment for leukaemia, and bone marrow transplant (BMT) recipients are susceptible to aspergillosis and disseminated candidosis. Renal involvement may occur in these patients as a result of disseminated infection.

Treatment of these infections has been described previously. In addition, antifungals have been used as prophylactic agents to prevent infection in these severely immunocompromised patients. Until recently there has been little evidence that this approach will prevent systemic fungal infections, although most antifungals including topical amphotericin B (lozenges) and nystatin (suspension, tablets), or systematically active compounds, such as ketoconazole and itraconazole, will reduce the risk of oropharyngeal candidosis. A recent study in BMT patients showed a small but significant reduction in systemic mycoses in those receiving fluconazole prophylaxis (Goodman *et al.* 1992). There are some potential problems with this approach, such as the risk of infection or colonization with other pathogens like *C. krusei* and aspergilli that are resistant to fluconazole. For this reason many units still prefer to use topical prophylaxis rather than fluconazole.200–600 mg

References

Alkalay, A. L., Srugo, I., Blifield, C., Komaiko, M. S., and Pomerance, J. J. (1991). Noninvasive medical management of fungus ball uropathy in a premature infant. *American Journal of Perinatology*, **8**, 330.

Butler, W. T., Bennett. J. E., Alling, D., and Wertlake, P. T. (1964). Nephrotoxicity of amphotericin B: early and late effects in 81 patients. *Annals of Internal Medicine*, **61**, 175.

Chopra, R., Blair, S., Strang, J., Cervi, P., Patterson, K. G., and Goldstone, A. H. (1991). Liposomal amphotericin B (AmBisome) in the treatment of fungal infections in neutropenic patients. *Journal of Antimicrobial Chemotherapy*, **28**(Suppl. A), 45.

Corbella, X., Carratala, J., Castells, M., and Berlanga B. (1992). Fluconazole treatment in Torulopsis glabrata upper urinary tract infection causing obstruction. *Journal of Urology*, **147**, 1116.

Drouhet, E., Borderon, J. C., Borderon, E., and Boulard, P. (1974). Evolution des concentrations seriques de 5-fluorocytosine chez les premature. *Bulletin de la Société Française de Mycologie Medicale*, **3**, 37.

Dummer, J. S., Hardy, A., Poorsatter, A., and Ho, M. (1983). Early infections in kidney, heart and liver transplant recipients on cyclosporin. *Transplantation*, **36**, 259.

Goodman, J. L., *et al.* (1992). A controlled trial of fluconazole to prevent fungal infections in patients undergoing bone marrow transplantation. *New England Journal of Medicine*, **326**, 845.

Harmony, B. H. and Wenzel, R. P. (1978). Hospital-associated candiduria: predisposing factors and review of the literature. *Journal of Urology*, **120**, 444.

Kinjanar, C., Cramer, B. C., Reid, W. D., and Andrews, W. L. (1986). Neonatal renal candidiasis: sonographic diagnosis. *American Journal of Roentgenology*, **147**, 801.

Klimek J. J., Sayers, R., Kelmas, B. W., and Quintiliani, R. (1979). Statistical analysis of factors predisposing to candiduria. *Connecticut Medicine*, **43**, 364.

Kozinn, P. J., Taschdjian, C. L., Goldberg, P. K., Wise, G. J., Toni, E. F., and Seelig, M. S. (1978). Advances in the diagnosis of renal candidiasis. *Journal of Urology*, **119**, 184.

Medoff, G. and Kobayashi, G. A. (1980). The polyenes. In *Antifungal chemotherapy*, (ed. D. C. E. Speller), p. 3. Wiley, Chichester.

Medoff, G., Brajtburg, J., and Kobayashi, G. S. (1983). Antifungal agents useful in therapy of systemic fungal infections. *Annual Reviews of Pharmacology and Toxicology*, **2**, 303.

Meunier, F., Prentice, H. G., and Ringden, O. (1991). Liposomal amphotericin B (AmBisome): safety data from a phase II/III clinical trial. *Journal of Antimicrobial Chemotherapy*, **28**(Suppl. A), 83.

Moreau, P., Milpied, N., Fayette, N., Ramee, J.-F., and Harousseau, J.-L. (1992). Reduced renal toxicity and improved clinical tolerance of amphotericin B mixed with intralipid compared with conventional amphotericin B in neutropenic patients. *Journal of Antimicrobial Chemotherapy*, **30**, 535.

Noe, H. N. and Tonkin, I. L. D. (1982). Renal candidiasis in the neonate. *Journal of Urology*, **127**, 517.

Scholer, H. (1980). Flucytosine. In *Antifungal chemotherapy*, (ed. D. C. E. Speller), p. 84. Wiley, Chichester.

Tomashefski, J. F. and Abramowsky, C. R. (1981). Candida associated renal papillary necrosis. *American Journal of Clinical Pathology*, **75**, 190.

Turck, M. and Stamm, W. E. (1981). Nosocomial infection of the urinary tract. *American Journal of Medicine*, **70**, 581.

Warnock, D. W. and Richardson, M. D. (ed.) (1991). *Fungal infection in the immunocompromised patient*. Wiley, Chichester.

Weber, D. J. and Rutala, W. A. (1989). Epidemiology of hospital acquired fungal infections. In *Diagnosis and therapy of systemic fungal infections*, (ed. K. Holmberg and R. Meyer). Raven Press, New York.

Wong-Beringer, A., Jacobs, R. A., and Guglielmo, B. J. (1992). Treatment of funguria. *Journal of the American Medical Association*, **267**, 2780.

Index